Guidelines for Nurse Practitioners in Gynecologic Settings

10th Edition

Joellen W. Hawkins, RN, PhD, WHNP-BC, FAAN, FAANP, has been a women's health nurse practitioner since 1969 and is professor emerita of William F. Connell School of Nursing at Boston College where, from 1983 to 2007, she was the coordinator of the women's health nurse practitioner program, teaching clinical and theory courses for that program, as well as the advanced practice role course. Currently, she is writer in residence at Simmons College, Department of Nursing, Boston. For 30 years, she practiced as a WHNP in Rhode Island, Connecticut, and Massachusetts. Her research includes abuse during pregnancy; screening for abuse; coalition building to address violence in a community; and historical work on individual nurses, advanced practice nursing, and women's health nurse practitioners. She is the chief nursing consultant for *Taber's Cyclopedic Medical Dictionary* T-22. She is the author or editor of 36 books and more than 100 articles in professional journals.

Diane M. Roberto-Nichols, BS, APRN-C, has practiced as an OB/GYN nurse practitioner for more than 30 years. She practices at Ellington OB/GYN Associates in Ellington, Connecticut and at the University of Connecticut Student Health Services (Storrs). Her practice focus has been on women's health, starting as coordinator of the Women's Health Clinic at the University of Connecticut–Storrs where she was instrumental in making contraception and confidential health care available to female students. She also codeveloped a protocol and implemented an assault crisis center for sexually and physically abused students at the university, as well as coauthored the protocols that served as the prototype for this book. She continues to provide education and health care to women throughout their life span.

J. Lynn Stanley-Haney, MA, APRN-C, is an adult medicine nurse practitioner with special practice areas in gynecology and psychiatry. Her current practice includes Ellington OB/GYN Associates in Ellington, Connecticut, Eastern Connecticut State University Counseling and Psychological Services (Willimantic, Connecticut), and private practice in psychotherapy and psychotherapeutic medication management. Since certification in 1980, she has pursued advocacy in women's health and access to care. As the director of nursing for the University of Connecticut Student Health Services (1978–1993), she worked with their Women's Health Clinic in assuring quality of care and also provided direct care to students. Along with her long-time colleague and coauthor Diane M. Roberto-Nichols, she codeveloped and implemented a 24-hour sexual assault crisis service for physically abused and sexually assaulted women students, as well as coauthored the protocols that served as the prototype for this book. Since leaving the university, she has worked to implement and manage, as well as practice clinically in, state-funded school-based health services.

Guidelines for Nurse Practitioners in Gynecologic Settings

10th Edition

Joellen W. Hawkins, RN, PhD, WHNP-BC,
FAAN, FAANP
Diane M. Roberto-Nichols, BS, APRN-C
J. Lynn Stanley-Haney, MA, APRN-C

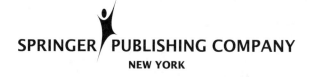

SPRINGER PUBLISHING COMPANY
NEW YORK

Springer Publishing Company, LLC
11 West 42nd Street
New York, NY 10036
www.springerpub.com

Acquisitions Editor: Margaret Zuccarini
Production Editor: Lindsay Claire
Composition: Absolute Service, Inc.

ISBN: 978-0-8261-2962-8
E-book ISBN: 978-0-8261-2963-5
Printable Patient Education Handouts ISBN: 978-0-8261-9351-3

14/5

The author and the publisher of this Work have made every effort to use sources believed to be reliable to provide information that is accurate and compatible with the standards generally accepted at the time of publication. Because medical science is continually advancing, our knowledge base continues to expand. Therefore, as new information becomes available, changes in procedures become necessary. We recommend that the reader always consult current research and specific institutional policies before performing any clinical procedure. The author and publisher shall not be liable for any special, consequential, or exemplary damages resulting, in whole or in part, from the readers' use of, or reliance on, the information contained in this book. The publisher has no responsibility for the persistence or accuracy of URLs for external or third-party Internet websites referred to in this publication and does not guarantee that any content on such websites is, or will remain, accurate or appropriate.

PDF versions of the Patient Information and Consent Forms (Appendix A) and the Patient Education Handouts (Appendix I) are available at www.springerpub.com/hawkins10

Library of Congress Cataloging-in-Publication Data

Hawkins, Joellen Watson.
  Guidelines for nurse practitioners in gynecologic settings / Joellen W. Hawkins, Diane M. Roberto-Nichols, J. Lynn Stanley-Haney. — 10th ed.
    p. ; cm.
  Includes bibliographical references and index.
  ISBN 978-0-8261-2962-8 — ISBN 978-0-8261-2963-5 (e-book)
  1. Gynecologic nursing. 2. Nursing care plans. I. Roberto-Nichols, Diane M. II. Stanley-Haney, J. Lynn. III. Title.
  [DNLM: 1. Genital Diseases, Female—nursing. 2. Nurse Practitioners. 3. Nursing Care—methods. 4. Patient Care Planning. WY 156.7]
  RG105.H368 2012
  618.1'0231—dc23
                        2011029340

Special discounts on bulk quantities of our books are available to corporations, professional associations, pharmaceutical companies, health care organizations, and other qualifying groups.

If you are interested in a custom book, including chapters from more than one of our titles, we can provide that service as well.

For details, please contact:
Special Sales Department, Springer Publishing Company, LLC
11 West 42nd Street, 15th Floor, New York, NY 10036-8002
Phone: 877-687-7476 or 212-431-4370; Fax: 212-941-7842
Email: sales@springerpub.com

Printed in the United States of America by McNaughton & Gunn.

Contents

PART III: GUIDELINES FOR MANAGING WOMEN'S HEALTH CONDITIONS

PART IV: APPENDICES

Contributors

Rosanna DeMarco, PhD, PHCNS-BC, ACRN, FAAN
Associate Professor in Community Health
William F. Connell School of Nursing
Boston College
Chestnut Hill, MA

Christine S. Edgerton, RN, WHNP-BC, MS
Nurse Practitioner, Breast Care Center
Beth Israel Deaconess Medical Center
Boston, MA

Mary Finnigan, BA, MA
Coordinator, Natural Family Planning
Archdiocese of Boston
Boston, MA

Linda Hansen-Rodier, MS, RN, WHNP-BC
Dermatology Nurse Practitioner
Northeast Dermatology Associates
North Andover, MA

Amy J. Kassirer, MSW, RNP, WHNP-BC
Family Nurse Practitioner with a specialization in addiction
Preventive Medicine Associates, Inc. (Norton Family Practice)
Norton, MA

Foreword

There is empiric support that patient outcomes are improved when clinical care is based on rigorously designed studies.[1] However, it often takes years for research findings to be incorporated into practice. Until the *research-practice gap* closes, clinical guidelines are one of the best ways for clinicians to stay up to date in practice and to apply the best available evidence to their care of patients.

The landmark 10th edition of this classic clinical reference provides the busy clinician with a "one-stop" comprehensive guide to women's health for all nurse practitioners who care for women across the life span. The book is consistently organized and includes essential components of the history, diagnostic workup, treatment and management guidelines for most common health issues and problems specific to providing gynecologic care to women. For the first time, this edition reorganizes content for easier access by presenting general guidelines for women's health care in a separate section, discrete from the disorders guidelines. A second, short section presents guidelines for contraception and preconception care, separating these guidelines from those relating to disorders or conditions of concern. The editors present more than 50 additional guidelines that provide sound clinical guidance for managing the most common clinical conditions seen in women's health care. This new organization presents the clinician with a sparkling new resource that is an easily accessible, comprehensive collection of clinically reliable women's health care guidelines.

I expect that clinicians will join me in welcoming the land-mark 10th edition of this classic reference, containing updated clinical content, additional resources, new organization, and patient education recommendations.

NOTE

1. B. M. Melnyk, E. Fineout-Overholt, S. B. Stillwell, & K. M. Williamson (2010). Evidence-based practice: The seven steps of evidence-based practice. *American Journal of Nursing, 110*(1), 51–53.

R. *Mimi Secor, MS, MEd, FNP-BC, FAANP*
Family Nurse Practitioner/Consultant,
Specializing in Women's Health
National NP Radio Host–ReachMD
"Partners in Practice"

Preface

The 10th edition of *Guidelines for Nurse Practitioners in Gynecologic Settings* is designed to assist nurse practitioners, nurse midwives, clinical nurse specialists, physician assistants, students preparing for these roles, and other health professionals who care for women across the life span and in community health care settings. The issues about which women may seek care range from common gynecologic concerns, including infections and sexually transmitted diseases, and navigating life transitions such as fertility control and preparing for pregnancy, to menopause and incontinence. Women also seek care and assistance when they encounter abuse or struggle with weight management, osteoporosis, smoking cessation, stress management, mental health issues, and risks for heart disease and breast cancer. The clinical guidelines, appendices, and bibliographies for this edition have been extensively revised and rewritten to address these concerns, using best-evidence data from the literature when those data are available.

The three principal authors of the guidelines are nurse practitioners who have practiced for decades in women's health care settings. All were actively involved in the publication of the first edition and have continued to be responsible for updating these guidelines for each edition of the book. Several guidelines were developed by nurse practitioner colleagues with expertise in particular specialty areas within women's health care.

This 10th edition has several special features to assist you in your practice, including the following:

- A new chapter on well women annual examination.
- An enhanced mental health chapter that details an approach to discontinuation of SSRI/SNRIs.
- A bibliography for each guideline, plus one or more websites at the end of each chapter.

- Guidelines for sexually transmitted diseases, vaginitis, and vaginosis reflect the CDC *Sexually Transmitted Diseases Treatment Guidelines 2010.*
- Guidelines for the management of cytological abnormalities and cervical intraepithelial neoplasia reflect the recommendations of the American Society for Colposcopy and Cervical Pathology (ASCCP) Consensus Conference 2006 (www.asccp.org).
- The information on hormone therapy, menopause, and osteoporosis reflects evidence-based practice generated through analysis of the emerging data from the *Women's Health Initiative* and other studies.
- Information on contraception is based on research articles and on the 2010 adaptation of the World Health Organization's 2009 4th edition of *Medical Eligibility Criteria for Contraceptive Use.*
- Information on natural family planning has changed significantly, and the revised guidelines, prepared by an expert NFP educator, reflect those changes.

Three special new features are designed to facilitate clinical use in primary care:

- New, spiral binding to ensure these clinical guidelines will lay flat for easy reference
- Availability of the Patient Education Handouts in PDF format
- New organization of the book

New four-part organization includes the following:

I. General Guidelines for Women's Health Care—presents six chapters that cover the well woman exam, safe practices for clinicians, complementary and alternative therapies (CAMs), smoking cessation, weight management, and guidelines for assessing victims of abuse and violence.
II. Guidelines for Contraception and Preconception Care—presents two chapters, the cover methods of contraception and family planning and the preconception care.
III. Guidelines for Managing Women's Health Conditions—presents guidelines on 50 discrete disorders that are grouped into 13 chapters. Within each chapter, the disorders are organized alphabetically for ultimate ease of use.
IV. Appendices—presents nine invaluable clinical resources such as screening tools, consent forms, and patient education handouts. The patient information and consent forms (Appendix A) and the patient education handouts (Appendix I) are available in PDF format at www.springerpub.com/hawkins10.

Our extensive revisions reflect new information for all the guidelines, including contraceptive methods, CAMs, medical abortion, and breast conditions. Each patient information handout has been revised and updated, as have the consent forms. All the bibliographies are new and reflect the latest literature and evidence-based practice. We hope that you— our colleagues, students preparing for a career as nurse practitioners and nurse–midwives, as well as for other health care professions—will find this 10th edition to be an invaluable resource as you strive, as we have, to provide the best possible care for your patients.

Joellen W. Hawkins
Diane M. Roberto-Nichols
J. Lynn Stanley-Haney

Acknowledgments

The authors would like to thank our publishers, colleagues, and all those who have helped make this 10th edition a reality. The section on Dysesthetic Vulvodynia was developed by Linda Hansen Rodier, MS, RN, WHCNP, Dermatology Nurse Practitioner, Dartmouth-Hitchcock Dermatology Clinic, Manchester, New Hampshire. Summary of mucus descriptions is by the late Eleanor S. Tabeek, RN, CNM, PhD; updated by Mary Finnigan, BA, MA.

General Guidelines for Women's Health Care

Well Woman Initial/Annual Gynecologic Exam

1

I. DEFINITION

The initial visit to a gynecologic clinician for the purpose of a comprehensive health history and a physical exam including, but not limited to, a breast exam, pelvic exam, Pap smear, and other laboratory work as indicated by age and history

II. HISTORY

A. Medical history
   1. General health status
   2. Recent changes in health status
   3. Allergies
   4. Surgeries
   5. Significant injuries
   6. Current medications, including herbs and supplements
   7. Last colonoscopy if age appropriate
   8. Vaccination status. Is the woman up to date on age-appropriate vaccines? Refer to the Centers for Disease Control and Prevention (CDC) vaccination guidelines for current recommendations. Federal law requires that each patient receive a Vaccination Information Statement (VIS) prior to being given any immunization. A copy of the VIS can be found on the CDC site (www.cdc.gov/vaccines).
   9. Birth control history, past and present
B. Recent changes in immediate family history
C. Gynecologic history
   1. Menstrual history
      a. Last menstrual period (LMP)
      b. Menarche
      c. Interval
      d. Duration
      e. Flow
      f. Dysmenorrhea
      g. Recent changes in pattern/flow, others
D. Urinary tract history
   1. History of past infections: how often, treatment, approximate date of last infection
   2. Current problems (discomfort, pressure, incontinence)
   3. History of genitourinary (GU) surgery
E. Pap smear history
   1. Date of last Pap smear
   2. Abnormal Pap smear history (approximate dates, clinical intervention)
F. Sexual history
   1. Sexual orientation
   2. Age at first sexual experience/intercourse
   3. Number of sexual partners
   4. Length of time with present partner

    5. Issues related to sexual function
      a. Libido
      b. Dyspareunia
      c. Postcoital bleeding
G. Social history
    1. Date of birth
    2. Smoking history
      a. Age at first cigarette
      b. Number of cigarettes/packs smoked each day
      c. Desire for smoking cessation
        i. Prior attempts
        ii. Method(s) used
        iii. Was it successful; if not, would the patient like to try again
    3. Alcohol use
      a. Age at first drink
      b. Current use; how many drinks per day/week
      c. What type of alcohol
      d. Has the patient, or any family member/friends, felt or expressed concern? Does alcohol use cause issues/problems in the home or workplace? If so, a referral to a therapist might be considered and discussed.
    4. Recreational drug use
      a. Past use
      b. Present use
      c. Has the use of substances caused difficulties with relationships or in the workplace? If so, a referral might be considered and discussed.
    5. Exercise history
      a. Does the woman exercise; what kind of exercise, for how long, and how often?
      b. Has this pattern changed from a previous pattern? In what way?
    6. Abuse history
      a. Was the woman abused as a child (physical abuse, mental abuse, sexual abuse)?
      b. Is there a history of domestic violence? Does the woman feel safe at home? Does she fear harm for herself or her children?
      c. If abuse is current and the woman agrees, efforts to reach local social services that deal with abuse should be noted and a plan of action developed. If the woman is not ready to act, it would be appropriate to give her the names and numbers of local resources and strategize how she can safely keep these numbers where she can find them.
      d. Women at risk should be encouraged to develop a plan for a quick departure from their residence. This plan should include, but not be limited to, bringing cash, birth certificates/passports for self and children, a spare set of car keys, copies

of prescriptions for self and children, and a pre-thought-out safe haven (*see abuse and violence guidelines in Chapter 6*).

7. Nutritional/dietary history
    a. Is the woman happy with her current weight?
    b. Does she consider her diet well balanced?
    c. Has she actively attempted to lose weight?
    d. If so, what plans or methods has she used? Has she taken any weight loss medication (prescription or over the counter [OTC])? Has this been successful?
    e. Nutritional counseling may be appropriate
8. Safe sex practices
    a. Use of condom (past and present)
    b. Avoiding unsafe situations involving use of alcohol, drugs, and casual, unprotected sex

III. PHYSICAL EXAM
A. Vital signs
B. Weight/height/body mass index (BMI)
C. General exam
    1. Skin
    2. Head/eyes, ears, nose, throat (EENT)
    3. Thyroid
    4. Lymph nodes
    5. Heart
    6. Lungs
    7. Abdomen
    8. Extremities
    9. Breasts
D. Gynecologic exam
    1. External genitalia
    2. Vagina
    3. Cervix
    4. Uterus
    5. Adnexa
    6. Rectum

IV. LABORATORY
A. Urine dipstick/culture as indicated
B. Pap smear as indicated (*refer to Pap smear guidelines in Chapter 10*)
C. Sexually transmitted disease (STD) testing as indicated by age and history
D. Vaginal cultures if indicated
E. General hematologic screening as indicated by age, health history, and access to other routine health care. Example: If the woman has no primary care provider and has not had a baseline lipid level, fasting blood sugar, and any other laboratory tests that seem to be indicated, then it would seem appropriate to do the laboratory tests and refer the patient out as indicated.

V. TREATMENT/INTERVENTION
  A. Order mammogram/bone density testing as indicated by age and history
  B. Teach and/or reinforce self breast examination (SBE)
  C. Order laboratory tests as indicated
  D. Administer/refer for vaccines as appropriate to setting
  E. Teach as appropriate to history and physical findings, including, but not limited to, changes in Pap smear guidelines, diet, exercise, vaccines, smoking cessation, alcohol use, safe sex, STD testing, and general safety
  F. Prescribe for birth control method chosen, or any other treatment indicated by findings
  G. Allow time for questions and concerns. Make future appointment(s) for discussion or evaluation of specific problems or concerns raised during the visit.
  H. Refer to other care providers as appropriate

Note: This chapter is an ideal and comprehensive guideline obviously created to encourage the most thorough and ideal initial annual exam. Clearly, this guideline is meant to be adapted to your setting and time constraints. Follow-up annual exam should include review and update of initial information.

Safe Practices for Clinicians

2

I. SAFE PRACTICES FOR CLINICIANS[1]

A. Dispose of all needles, scalpels, capillary tubes, glass slides, lancets, and other sharp items in puncture-resistant containers. Handle as little as possible (i.e., do not recap needles); use safety needles when available.

B. Wear gloves *when anticipating* exposure to body fluids, including for phlebotomy and for handling specimens (urine, blood, stool, sputum, vaginal secretions), and for contact with any mucous membranes (vaginal, oral, nasal, rectal) and open wounds. Do not substitute gloves for handwashing, however.

C. Wear gloves, gowns, masks, and goggles as appropriate when there is to be extensive contact with body fluids as during surgery or delivery; wear double gloves for surgical procedures when possible. Change any blood-stained clothing as soon as possible.

D. Wash thoroughly (with copious amounts of soap and water) following any skin contact with patient's body fluids.

E. Wear gloves on both hands for vaginal and rectal exams; use careful technique to keep one hand clean when handling clean materials such as containers for Pap smears or examination lights; wash after examination is completed. Goggles are now recommended for vaginal examinations and phlebotomy in ambulatory as well as inpatient settings.

F. Change gloves for rectal examination after vaginal examination or for fitting a diaphragm after pelvic examination.

G. Avoid contamination of surfaces in the examining room or laboratory with body fluids from patients.

H. Use chlorine bleach solution 1:10 in a spray bottle to clean examining table and other surfaces and items contaminated with body fluids. Several other commercial products with longer shelf life are available for this use. Wear gloves for clean-up.

I. Keep hands from becoming dry and cracked.

J. Follow Centers for Disease Control and Prevention (CDC) and Occupational Safety and Health Administration (OSHA) recommendations and updates for protection of self and patients (http://www.cdc.gov; http://www.osha.gov).

K. Assume every patient has the potential to be infected with hepatitis, AIDS, or to be HIV positive and protect him or her and yourself with good technique.

L. Educate staff and patients about modes of infection, protection, and address myths to dispel unwarranted fears.

See Bibliographies.
Website:http://www.osha.gov/pls/oshaweb/owadisp.show_document?p_table=STANDARDS&p_id=10051

NOTE

1. Adapted from material developed by R. M. C. Secor (1997). Vaginal microscopy: Refining the nurse practitioner's technique. *Clinical Excellence for Nurse Practitioners, 1*(1), 29–34; and H. A. Carcio, & M. C. Secor (2010). Vaginal microscopy. In *Advanced health assessment of women: Clinical skills and procedures* (2nd ed.). New York, NY: Springer Publishing.

Complementary and Alternative Therapies[1]

3

Increasingly, women are using complementary and alternative medicine (CAM) therapies for preventative and palliative care as alternative or adjunct therapies to their traditional medical care. In the following, we will present an overview of the most commonly used therapies for perimenopause, premenstrual syndrome (PMS), and depression. Pregnant and lactating women should not use any CAM therapies without consulting with their care provider.

I. DEFINITION

Alternative therapies refer to treatment approaches that, although used for many years, have not been evaluated and tested by conventional methods. The term *complementary therapies* is used to convey the concept that these therapies are often used in conjunction with conventional medically accepted treatments. When looked at in this manner, the term assumes a more holistic view of women's health care needs.

II. TYPES

A. The following are therapies commonly used by women:
1. Vitamins
2. Minerals
3. Herbals and other naturally occurring substances
4. Phytoestrogens (dietary)
5. Natural estrogen
6. Natural progesterones
7. Acupuncture
8. Biofeedback/hypnosis
9. Homeopathy
10. Naturopathy
11. Therapeutic touch, massage, Reiki
12. Traditional medicines
    a. Ayurveda
    b. Traditional Chinese medicines
    c. Tibetan
    d. Wise woman traditional
    e. Herbalism
    f. These traditional methods may have
        i. Complex theoretic structure
        ii. Literature-based traditions
        iii. Classic gynecologic texts
        iv. Materia medica with specific herbs for reproductive and gynecologic problems
13. Therapies based on oral tradition

III. REASONS FOR SELECTION/USE OF CAM

A. Preference for more "natural" treatment
B. Belief in unconventional (non-Western) medicine

C. Concern about potential side effects of conventional medicines and treatments
D. Dissatisfaction with or lack of confidence in conventional methods
E. Desire to have control over one's own health and health care
F. Being raised in a culture that believes in and uses CAM therapies
G. Belief in the body's ability to heal itself

IV. PROBLEMS AND CONCERNS
A. Lack of systemized research and sufficiently well-designed studies to measure safety and efficacy
B. Self-medication based on insufficient information
C. Lack of standardization of therapeutics
D. Failure to inform health care practitioner of CAM use; supplements can interact with prescription or over-the-counter (OTC) medications

V. CAUTIONS
A. Remember, "natural" is not synonymous with safe.
B. CAM should be used only for minor problems, not for conditions that have potential to be life altering or life threatening.
C. CAM should not be used in pregnancy or breastfeeding without discussion with an allopathic or osteopathic health care practitioner.
D. Use should be limited to recommended dosages for recommended time frames.
E. Users need to be knowledgeable about CAM methods. Do not use CAM therapy that you have not personally researched and understand its use. The Internet should not be the only source of research and information.
F. Use should begin with a smaller than recommended dose to observe for adverse reaction.
G. Buy or seek therapies only from reputable manufacturers and practitioners. Remember that in the United States, herbal and other natural preparations are regulated only as dietary supplements. They are not standardized or regulated by the U.S. Food and Drug Administration (FDA).

VI. FREQUENTLY USED/RECOMMENDED CAM THERAPIES
A. Menopause
  1. B Complex vitamins
    a. Usual dose 50 to 300 mg daily
    b. Conditions
      i. Stress/depression
      ii. Water retention
    c. Toxicity/adverse effects
      i. None known

2. Vitamin C
   a. Usual dose 500 mg daily
   b. Conditions
      i. Free radical scavenger/antioxidant
      ii. Linked with raising levels high-density lipoprotein (HDL) and lowering levels low-density lipoprotein (LDL)
      iii. Maintaining bone structures
      iv. Maintaining healthy connective tissues
   c. Toxicity/adverse effects
      i. Use with caution and medical supervision if history of compromised kidney function
      ii. Increased doses (5,000 mg/day) associated with intestinal gas and loose stool; if history of reflux, take buffered vitamin C
3. Vitamin D
   a. Usual daily dose 600 to 800 IU (this recommendation is changing as researchers and clinicians study the role of vitamin D)[2]
   b. Conditions
      i. Vitamin D at 400 IU per day under age 70
      ii. Vitamin D at 600 IU daily for women over age 70; for women with darker skin, 1,000 IU daily as well as for elders without sun exposure
      iii. Serum levels of 25–hydroxyvitamin D in the range of 20 to 30 mg are sufficient for bone health
      iv. Vitamin D intake should not be more that 4,000 IU daily without consultation with a health care practitioner
   c. Currently, the role of vitamin D in providing protection from falls, hypotension, hypertension, cancer and possibly auto-immune diseases continues to unfold
   d. Conditions
      i. Osteoporosis—increase mineral absorption, bone mineralization
4. Vitamin E
   a. Usual daily dose 400 to 800 IU may be used up to 1,200 IU safely
   b. Conditions
      i. Hot flashes
      ii. Cardiovascular prevention (remains controversial), poor circulation
      iii. Atrophic vaginitis
   c. Toxicity/adverse effects
      i. Use with caution if patient is on high blood pressure medication (may decrease blood pressure)
      ii. Use with caution or not at all if patient is on anticoagulant therapy
      iii. Using more than recommended dose can result in nausea, flatulence, diarrhea, heart palpitations, fainting (all reversible with dose decrease)

5. Calcium
   a. Usual daily dose in divided doses 1,000 to 2,500 mg—should be used in conjunction with vitamin D to aid in bone remineralization
      i. Adolescents should be taking 1,000 to 2,500 mg daily
      ii. Pregnant women 19 to 50 should be taking 1,000 to 2,500 mg daily
      iii. Breast-feeding women 19 to 50 should be taking 1,000 to 2,500 mg daily
      iv. Women up to age 50 should be taking 1,200 to 2,000 mg daily
      v. After age 50, women should be taking 1,200 to 2,000 mg daily
      vi. Remember, calcium should be taken in divided doses
      vii. Women should be advised not to take more than 2,500 mg per day from diet and supplements, unless advised by a provider
   b. Conditions
      i. Osteoporosis (prevention and treatment) provides reintegration of calcium into bones
      ii. Hypertension—aids in contraction and expansion of heart muscle
   c. Toxicity/adverse effects
      i. Calcium has no known toxic effects in doses 2,000 mg or less (caution in use of antacids as calcium supplements; in addition to calcium many of these products contain aluminum that interferes with calcium absorption)
      ii. Too much calcium from supplements may increase the risk of kidney stones and possibly heart attacks
6. Essential fatty acids (EFAs)
   a. Usual daily dose omega-3/omega-6 (3,000–4,000 mg/day)
   b. Conditions
      i. Hot flashes, vaginal atrophy, mood swings and irritability, bloating and fluid retention, decreased libido
      ii. Cardiovascular disease osteoporosis: A correct balance of EFAs is essential for the rebuilding and production of new cells and to decrease inflammation and modulate hormone imbalance
      iii. EFAs consist of eicosapentaenoic acid omega-3 (EPA), docosahexaenoic acid omega-3 (DHA), and gamma-linolenic acid omega-6 (GLA)
   c. Toxicity/adverse effects
      i. No known adverse effects
7. Coenzyme Q10 (ubiquinone)
   a. Usual daily dose 30 to 100 mg
   b. Conditions
      i. The name ubiquinone is appropriate because coenzyme Q10 is found everywhere in the body; a powerful

antioxidant, it stimulates the immune system, increases tissue oxygenation, and has vital antiaging effects. Extensive research has been done regarding its impact on heart disease. It is mentioned here because of its preventative effects.
   c. Toxicity/adverse effects
      i. No known adverse effects
8. Dong quai (*Angelica sinensis*)
   a. Usual daily dosage—consult preparation instructions
   b. Conditions
      i. Hot flashes, irritability, insomnia, restlessness, night sweats, headaches, toxicity, menstrual migraine
   c. Toxicity/adverse effects
      i. No known toxicity; may cause minor gastrointestinal (GI) upset (do not use dong quai during menses if hypermenorrhea is a problem). Interacts with and increases the activity of the anticoagulant drug warfarin. This can lead to increased bleeding.
      ii. Avoid use in pregnancy and lactation
9. Chasteberry (*Vitex agnus-castus*)
   a. Usual daily dosage—consult individual preparation
   b. Conditions
      i. Mood swings, irritability, depression, balances estrogen–progesterone levels in the body
      ii. Hot flashes—balances estrogen, progesterone
   c. Toxicity/adverse effects
      i. Usually without adverse effects—rarely causes nausea, diarrhea, weight gain, fatigue, headaches, allergic rash, alopecia, acne—spontaneously disappear when discontinued
10. Black cohosh (*Cimicifuga racemosa*) does not act like estrogen as previously thought. It has good safety record.
   a. Usual daily dosage—consult individual preparation
      i. Counsel women that therapeutic effects generally begin after 2 weeks and that maximum effects are usually seen within 8 weeks
   b. Conditions
      i. Hot flashes
      ii. Fatigue
      iii. Irritability
      iv. Night sweats
      v. Headaches
      vi. Insomnia
      vii. Heart palpitations
   c. Toxicity/adverse effects
      i. Low incidence of adverse effects with moderate dose
         a) Avoid during pregnancy and lactation

        b) Avoid the use in women with aspirin sensitivity because it contains salicylates

    ii. Overdose of black cohosh may cause nausea, vomiting, dizziness, and nervous system and visual disturbances

11. Ginkgo biloba
    a. Usual daily dosage—consult preparation directions
    b. Conditions
        i. Circulation
        ii. Cognitive impairment, forgetfulness
        iii. Cold hands and feet
        iv. Antitoxin/anti-inflammatory
    c. Toxicity/adverse effects
        i. Headaches
        ii. Nausea
        iii. Heart palpitations
        iv. Dizziness
        v. Allergic skin reactions
        vi. Do not use if taking aspirin, anticoagulants, or prior to surgery
        vii. Do not use if patient has a history of seizure disorder

12. St. John's wort (*hypericum perforatum*)
    a. Usual daily dose—300 mg (range in clinical trials has indicated a dosage of 900 mg daily in three divided doses)
    b. Conditions
        i. Depression, anxiety, sleep disorders, smoking cessation
    c. Toxicity/adverse effects
        i. May alter liver enzyme function in processing some drugs, including HIV medications, digoxin, warfarin, oral contraceptives, antidepressants
        ii. Because of numerous interactions, women should check with all care providers prior to using
        iii. Adverse reactions include:
            a) Dry mouth
            b) Nausea
            c) Change in bowel habits
            d) Photo sensitivity
            e) Fatigue
            f) Dizziness
            g) Insomnia
            h) Headache

13. Ginseng
    a. There are three kinds of ginseng: Asian (Chinese or Korean), American, and Siberian. The first two are authentic ginseng. Siberian ginseng is not; however, it looks similar and has similar effects on the body.
        i. Usual daily dose 100 to 400 mg/day—varies with origin and preparation

      b. Conditions (It is advised to limit use to 3 consecutive months then take a 3-month break before resuming.)
- i. Stress
- ii. Fatigue
- iii. Loss of libido
- iv. Depression
- v. Vaginal dryness—ginseng has a direct estrogenic effect

      c. Toxicity/adverse effects
- i. CNS symptoms, headache, confusion, drowsiness
- ii. GI problems; vomiting, abdominal pain
- iii. Lowered blood pressure
- iv. Should not be used by women with:
  - a) Inflammatory bowel disease
  - b) Multiple sclerosis
  - c) Rheumatoid arthritis and systemic lupus
  - d) Allergic rhinitis, asthma or eczema

14. Dietary phytoestrogens are naturally found in foods. These compounds may produce effects similar to estrogen; found in cereal, legumes, and grasses.
    - a. There are three main groups of phytoestrogens: isoflavones, lignans, and coumestans
      - i. Isoflavones are found in soy, garbanzo beans, and other legumes. They may be consumed in the form of soy, miso, and tofu.
      - ii. Lignans are found in seed oils such as flaxseed
      - iii. Coumestans are found in red clover, sunflower seeds, and bean sprouts
    - b. Phytoestrogens are thought to be helpful in minimizing hot flashes, maintaining bone density, and lowering cholesterol, LDLs, and triglycerides
    - c. Natural progesterones manufactured from wild yams—patients should be discouraged from using OTC preparations of topical progestins for their progesterone imbalance since there is no standardized compounding. Replacement hormones are usually synthesized.

15. Melatonin is helpful with sleep disturbances: difficulty falling asleep and waking in the middle of the night, unable to go back to sleep, and for short-term regulation of sleep patterns such as jetlag or transient insomnia
    - a. Sleep disorders
      - i. Difficulty falling asleep—melatonin 5 mg, 3 to 4 hours before bedtime for at least 4 weeks
      - ii. Difficulty staying asleep—a controlled release dose 2 hours before bedtime
    - b. Contraindicated in pregnancy, lactation, and in women with autoimmune illnesses

    c. Adverse reactions include:
       i. Depression
      ii. Dizziness
     iii. Excessive daytime somnolence
     iv. Headache
      v. Nausea
    d. Avoid driving after ingestion of melatonin

16. Other
    a. Relaxation techniques
    b. Biofeedback
    c. Meditation
    d. Tai Chi and Qigong
    e. Yoga
    These techniques can be helpful in helping the body regain homeostasis, thus making it more possible to adapt to change without increasing stress
    f. Ayurvedic and Chinese herbals may also be used. There are several preparations on the market. These include:
      i. Meno-care used to alleviate palpitations, insomnia, mood swings, and hot flashes. Usual dose—one tablet twice a day.
     ii. Geriforte used to address the overall stress of aging. Usual dose—two tablets twice a day. Source: health food store or through the manufacturer, Himalaya, in the United States (1-800-869-4640)
     iii. Nukeba Zhen Wan (women's precious teapills)—an herbal blend, generally used to address low estrogen levels, hot flashes, forgetfulness, confusion, insomnia, and tearfulness. Usual dose—on an empty stomach:
        a) Take 4 to 6 tablets daily divided into three doses or may take in two divided doses or one dose in the morning and one dose in the afternoon
        b) May take up to 9 to 12 tablets to alleviate severe symptoms
        If no relief, see licensed clinician.
     iv) Er Xian Tang Wan (two immortals teapills) helpful in fatigue, hot flashes, night sweats, low libido. Usual daily dose is 8 pills 3 times a day.
    These herbals may be found in health food stores or ordered from Ethical Nutrients (1-800-638-2848). Although these preparations are easily available, consultation with an Ayurvedic or Chinese medicine clinician is recommended.
    g. Homeopathic remedies are based on the premise that the body has the capacity to heal itself. Formulas are compounded that use very minute quantities of an agent to trigger the body's innate capacity to heal. Preparations specific to a symptom can be found in health food stores for

self-treatment. Homeopathic practitioners are also available to work with a patient to customize preparations to fit the person's symptoms.

VII. PREMENSTRUAL SYNDROME
  A. B complex
    1. Usual dose 50 to 300 mg/day
    2. Symptoms
      a. Stress/depression
      b. Water retention (especially B_6)
    3. Toxicity/adverse effects
      a. none known
  B. Vitamin B_6, usual dose 100 to 200 mg/day
  C. Magnesium, usual dose 400 mg/day
  D. Vitamin E, usual dose 400 to 600mg/day
  E. Chromium, usual dose 250 μg daily or twice a day to reduce sugar cravings
  F. EFAs—also helpful with dysmenorrhea
    1. Usual daily dose—as indicated on individual preparation/no daily optimum dose
    2. Conditions
      a. Help to reduce depression, irritability, cramps, nausea, bloating, and headaches. Correct balance of EFAs is essential for the rebuilding and production of new cells—decrease inflammation, moderate hormone imbalance.
  G. Licorice (*Glycyrrhiza glabra*)
    1. Usual daily dose varies with preparation
    2. Conditions addressed—estrogen-like activity helps in irritability, mood swings, stimulates adrenal glands
    3. Toxicities—should not be used by women with kidney problems, high blood pressure, patients taking potassium. Not advisable for use in persons who are on low salt diets or persons taking diuretics, corticoid treatments, cardiac glycosides, or medications for hypertension.
  H. Black cohosh (*Cimicifuga racemosa*)
    1. Usual daily dosage—as indicated on individual preparation
    2. Conditions
      a. Nervousness
      b. Irritability
      c. Sleep disturbances
      d. Depressive moods
      e. Headache
  I. Evening primrose oil
    1. Usual daily dosage—as indicated on individual preparation
    2. Conditions addressed
      a. Vasomotor symptoms
      b. Cyclical breast tenderness

3. Toxicities
   a. Should not be used by women with seizure disorders
J. St. John's wort
   1. Usual daily dosage—as indicated on individual preparations
   2. Conditions addressed
      a. May be helpful in alleviating the CNS anxiety and irritability of PMS
   3. Toxicities
      a. Should not be used by women on oral contraceptives because there may be a decrease in contraceptive effect
      b. Should not be used concurrently with psychotropic medication
      c. Side effects may include
         i. Dry mouth
         ii. GI—nausea, diarrhea
         iii. Fatigue
         iv. Insomnia
         v. Headache
         vi. Jitteriness

VIII. DEPRESSION
   A. SAMe (S-adenosylmthionine)
      1. Usual daily dosage 200 to 1,600 mg/day with onset of effect usually seen in 1 to 2 weeks
      2. Conditions addressed
         a. Depression
         b. Dysthemia
         c. Seasonal affective disorder
      3. Toxicities/interactions
         a. No safety concerns identified
         b. No interactions documented
         c. SAMe should not be used in women suspected of being bipolar. Use may cause increased anxiety and mania
   B. St. John's wort
      1. Usual dosage—as indicated on individual preparations
      2. Conditions addressed
         a. Mild, moderate depression
            i. The use of St. John's wort has not been demonstrated to be effective for severe depression
         b. Dysthemia
      3. Toxicities/interactions
         a. *See Frequently Used/Recommended CAM Therapies, **VI.J***

See Appendix F and Bibliographies.
Websites: http://www.ncbi.nlm.nih.gov/pubmed?term=complementary%20 alternative%20medicine; http://nccam.nih.gov/; http://www.therapeutic-touch .org; American Botanical Council: http://www.herbalgram.org/herbalgram

NOTES

1. Consult guideline on emotional/mental health issues found in Chapter 11.
2. A. C. Ross, J. E. Manson, S. A. Abrams, J. F. Aloia, P. M. Brannon, S. K. Clinton, et al. (2011). The 2011 report on dietary reference intakes for calcium and vitamin D from the Institute on Mendicine: What clinicians need to know. *Journal of Clinical Endocrinology & Metabolism, 96*(1), 53–58. doi:10.1210/jc.2010-2704.

Smoking Cessation

4

I. DEFINITION

Smoking is the leading cause of preventable illness and premature death in the United States, causing approximately 440,000 deaths annually. An estimated 40 million Americans smoke, and it has been estimated that of this number, 70% want to quit. Quitting involves the process of fighting both the physical and psychological dependence of smoking. It is believed that nicotine is as addictive as cocaine, opiates, amphetamines, and alcohol. Nicotine dependence is not limited to smoking cigarettes, but also associated with smokeless tobacco such as loose leaf pouches, plugs, twists or snuff, and chewing tobacco. Nicotine dependence is classified as a substance-use disorder in *DSM-IV*.

II. ETIOLOGY

A. The nicotine contained in inhaled cigarette smoke reaches the brain in approximately 10 seconds. Once received in the brain, nicotine causes the brain to release dopamine and norepinephrine. When nicotine is inhaled in a regular fashion, the brain accepts the chemicals by increasing the number of nicotine receptor sites. This mechanism is believed to underlie nicotine dependence. When inhaled nicotine binds to these receptor sites, it causes arousal, stimulation, increased heart rate, and increased blood pressure. These physical reactions cause the smoker to experience mood elevation, reduced anxiety, and stimulation within seconds of inhalation. Signs and symptoms of withdrawal may begin within a few hours of the last cigarette, peak at 48 to 72 hours, and return to baseline 3 to 4 weeks after quitting.

B. Problems associated with smoking
   1. Pregnancy complications: low birth weight, miscarriage, preterm delivery, placenta previa, placenta abruption, premature rupture of membranes
   2. Increased asthma and other respiratory problems in children exposed to secondhand smoke
   3. Increased risk for developing cataracts and macular degeneration
   4. Increased risk for cancer (esophageal, bladder, kidney, pancreatic, leukemia, breast, gynecologic)
   5. Gastric and duodenal ulcers
   6. Premature wrinkling of the skin
   7. Decreased bone density, osteoporosis, fractures
   8. Impotence and fertility problems
   9. Pneumonia, chronic obstructive pulmonary disease, poor asthma control, coughing, wheezing, dyspnea
   10. Decreased high-density lipoprotein (HDL)
   11. Peripheral vascular disease
   12. Periodontal and dental diseases; oral cancers
   13. Depression
   14. Contributes to early onset of menopause

III. BARRIERS TO SMOKING CESSATION
A. Physical dependence/addiction
1. Withdrawal symptoms
a. Depressed mood/anxiety
b. Insomnia
c. Irritability
d. Difficulty concentrating
e. Increased appetite—weight gain
f. Anger
g. Restlessness
h. Frustration
i. Increased heart rate
B. Psychological dependence
1. Behaviors associated with smoking become integrated into a person's routine
2. Smoking once integrated into routine becomes associated with pleasure and enjoyment
3. Smoking may also be used to cope with stress or lessen negative emotions

IV. HISTORY
A. Risk assessment
1. Ask all patients at annual visit, Do you smoke?
2. How many cigarettes a day? For how long?
3. How soon after awakening do you smoke your first cigarette?
4. Do you wake at night to smoke?
5. Is it difficult for you to observe "no smoking" rules?
6. Which cigarette would be hardest to give up?
7. Do you smoke more cigarettes in the first hours of your days than at other times?
8. Have you ever attempted to stop smoking?
9. If yes, what got in your way?
10. Smoking assessment questionnaire may be used, for example, the Fagerstrom[1] test for nicotine dependence
B. What the patient may present with
1. Nagging, chronic cough
2. Sinus congestion
3. Shortness of breath
4. Fatigue
5. Elevated blood pressure
6. Inability to meet physical challenges (run for a bus, play with young children)
7. Decreased fertility
8. Osteoporosis, decreased bone density
9. Premature wrinkling
10. Gum disease

C. Additional questions to be asked
   1. Pregnancy complications
   2. History of abnormal Pap smears
   3. History of, or presently existing, cancer
   4. Fractures
   5. Cataracts/glaucoma
   6. Problems with cold hands or feet or leg pain
   7. Diabetes
   8. Gastric or duodenal ulcer
   9. Current medicines including herbals, homeopathics, vitamins
   10. Use of smokeless preparations

V. PHYSICAL EXAMINATION
A. Vital signs
   1. Temperature
   2. Pulse, respirations
   3. Blood pressure
B. Skin
   1. Observe for color, tone, and premature wrinkling
C. Eyes, ears, nose, throat
   1. Thorough examination of oral cavity; observe dental cavities, stained teeth, tongue or buccal lesions, gum disease, foul breath
D. Lungs
   1. Listen for adventitious sounds (wheezes, rales, crackles)
E. Breast examination
F. Abdominal examination
G. Gynecologic examination (Pap smears, cultures, bimanual)
H. Extremities
   1. Observe extremities for signs of circulatory, peripheral vessel involvement, pulses, and pedal edema

VI. LABORATORY EXAMINATION
A. Complete blood count (elevated hematocrit, white blood cells, platelets, decreased leukocytes)
B. Lipid level (decreased HDL)
C. Consider
   1. Vitamin C level (decreased)
   2. Serum uric acid (decreased)
   3. Serum albumin (decreased)
   4. Pulmonary function tests

VII. DIFFERENTIAL DIAGNOSIS
A. Per physical findings
B. Depression
C. Anxiety

VIII. TREATMENT
A. Intervention needs to be multifaceted and tailored to each patient's needs—multiple nicotine medication interventions may be used simultaneously without adverse effect
B. Any approach needs to include information regarding the following:
1. A clear, strong stop smoking message
2. Risks associated with smoking
3. Benefits of cessation, advise all users to stop
4. Addictive components of smoking
5. What to expect during withdrawal period
6. Potential risk of relapse
C. Personalize the risks to each individual. Relate the individual's current health problems or findings on physical examination to the effects of smoking.
D. Emphasize how smoking cessation can reward the individual
E. If the patient indicates a willingness to quit, form a contract for a quit date. This date should be within a short time frame (1–2 weeks). A notation of this date should be made and the clinician should reinforce the contract with a phone call.
F. Factors involved in successful cessation efforts include:
1. Timely intervention and motivation by clinician
2. Individual's desire and motivation
3. Multifaceted program
4. Individualization of method and program to patient's situation
G. Methods (may be used individually or in conjunction with each other)
1. Behavioral
a. Draft a list of reasons to quit smoking and the rewards of quitting. This list should be kept with the person and reviewed when the urge to smoke "hits" and he or she is in need of reinforcement.
b. Inform family and friends and ask for their support and encouragement
c. Smoker should keep a journal. In precessation stage, the smoker can use the journal to record each cigarette smoked, the social cues experienced, the setting, the intensity of the craving, and the time of day. This can help identify the individual's triggers and assist smoker to adapt strategies and coping skills to get past the triggers. Keeping a journal during cessation is helpful for expressing feelings and recording the steps of the journey.
d. Patient should avoid alcohol, which weakens resolve
e. Patient should throw out all cigarettes, ashtrays, and so forth
f. Patient should avoid being around smokers
g. If possible, patient should establish a "no smoking" living space

    h. Patient should increase exercise level (walking, weight lifting, yoga). Exercise assists in weight management, stress reduction, and sense of well-being.

    i. Consider use of meditation or relaxation tapes

    j. Patient should learn cognitive and behavioral strategies to reduce negative mood

2. Nicotine replacement: The theory behind nicotine replacement therapy is that by replacing the nicotine, the smoker can deal with the emotional factors and use behavioral changes without having to deal with the full impact of physical withdrawal at the same time

    a. Gum—offers episodic satisfaction for nicotine craving as it arises

       i. Nicotine polacrilex (Nicorette) 2 mg per piece (maximum 30 pieces per day)

       ii. Nicotine polacrilex (Nicorette DS) 4 mg per piece (maximum 20 pieces per day)

      iii. Adverse effects

         a) Mouth sores

         b) Dyspepsia

         c) Hiccup

         d) Jaw ache

         e) 10% of those who use gum may become dependent requiring long-term use (1–2 years) to remain abstinent

    b. Transdermal patches. If a patient chooses to use the patch, there should be a contract not to smoke during its use.

       i. Nicotine transdermal therapeutic system (Habitrol) 21 mg/day (24 hours) for 4 to 6 weeks, then 14 mg/day for 2 to 4 weeks, then 7 mg/day for 2 to 4 weeks

       ii. Nicotine transdermal system (NicoDerm CQ) 21 mg/day (24 hours) for 4 to 6 weeks, then 14 mg/day for 2 to 4 weeks, then 7 mg/day for 4 to 6 weeks

      iii. Nicotine transdermal system (Nicotrol) 15 mg/day (16 hours) for 4 to 6 weeks

      iv. Nicotine transdermal system (ProStep) 22 mg/day (24 hours) for 4 to 8 weeks, then 11 mg/day for 2 to 4 weeks

       v. Adverse effects

         a) Skin reactions

         b) Insomnia

         c) Vivid dreams

         d) Myalgia

      vi. If vivid dreams and/or insomnia are a problem, the patient may remove the patch prior to retiring and apply new patch on arising. *Note:* If waking during the night is a problem, the 24-hour patches may provide more relief.

c. Nasal spray—has the advantage of being an accelerated delivery system, delivering nicotine on demand (within 10 seconds) as a cigarette does

   i. Nicotine nasal spray (Nicotrol NS) one spray (0.5 mg) in each nostril (8–40 mg/day) to a maximum of 5 times per hour or 40 times per 24 hours. Maximum: 3 months treatment

   ii. Adverse effects

     a) Higher incidence of dependence

     b) Nasal irritation

     c) Throat irritation

     d) Rhinitis

     e) Sneezing

     f) Watering eyes

     g) Coughing

   iii. Contraindicated in women with nasal polyps or other chronic nasal disorders

d. Nicotrol inhaler 10 mg/cartridge (4 mg delivered) 6 to 16 cartridges/day for up to 12 weeks, reduce gradually over 12 more weeks then discontinue. Maximum: 6 months treatment. Do not inhale into lungs, puff as you would a pipe. Contraindicated for women with reactive airway disorder.

e. Lozenges 2 to 4 mg each lozenge. Maximum lozenges/day: 20 pieces. Allow to slowly dissolve (20 minutes), do not chew or swallow. Change position to different areas of the mouth. No food or beverages for 15 minutes during or 15 minutes after the lozenge is dissolved. Taper off as appropriate. Maximum duration for use is usually 12 weeks. May cause sensation of warmth or tingling.

f. Oral medication

   i. Bupropion hydrochloride (Zyban or Wellbutrin SR) 150 mg every day for 2 days, then 150 mg twice a day for 7 to 12 weeks. If longer period is necessary, Wellbutrin XL 300 mg daily may be initiated for convenience. Initiate medication 1 week prior to starting date. This week allows the patient to initiate behavioral interventions and prepare psychologically for quitting. Bupropion hydrochloride is an antidepressant that acts as an inhibitor of the neuronal uptake of norepinephrine, serotonin, and dopamine. The mechanism of action in smoking cessation is unknown, but it may serve to mimic the neurochemical effects of nicotine that serve as the pathway to addiction.

     a) Contraindications

       1) History of seizure disorder

       2) Prior diagnosis of eating disorder

       3) Concurrent use of monoamine oxidase inhibitor

b) Possible adverse reactions
1) Rash
2) Nausea
3) Agitation
4) Migraine
c) Cautionary note
1) Neuropsychiatric events such as depression, suicidal ideation, and suicide attempt or completion have been linked to the use of this medication. Their effects may be complicated by the coexisting symptoms of nicotine withdrawal.
2) All patients using bupropion for smoking cessation should be monitored regularly for changes in behavior, such as hostility, agitation, depressed mood, and suicide-related thinking or events.
3) Patients should be told to report any changes to their clinician.
ii. Varenicline (Chantix) acts on receptor sites by activating them and blocking nicotine from attaching to them. Dosage days: three white tablets (0.5 mg) one orally every day for days 4 to 7; one white tablet (0.5 mg) orally twice a day (morning and evening) starting from day 8 to end of treatment; one blue tablet 1 mg orally twice a day (morning and evening).
a) Important facts
1) Patients with kidney problem or undergoing dialysis treatment may need lower dose (see package insert).
2) Should be taken after meals with full glass of water.
3) If a dose is missed, it should be taken as soon as remembered. If it is close to time of next dose, skip missed dose, take regular dose on time.
4) Patients taking other medications such as blood thinner, insulin, and asthma medication may need to have dosages altered after cessation of smoking.
b) Cautionary notes
1) All patients taking varenicline should be closely monitored for changes in behavior, hostility, agitation, depressed mood, and suicidal ideation, attempts, or gestures
2) Patients with preexisting psychiatric disorders should be given varenicline after all other avenues have been exhausted and then only with caution and close monitoring
3) Patients and members of their family need to be advised that if the aforementioned symptoms present themselves, then varenicline should be stopped immediately and the prescribing clinician notified

        4) Varenicline should be avoided by persons operating aircraft, driving buses, or using machinery where a lapse in alertness could have serious consequences. Clinicians should be aware of emerging information regarding increased risk of heart disease with Chantix use.

    c) How to start

        1) Choose a quit date.

        2) Begin taking Chantix 7 days before the quit date. This allows Chantix to build up in the body. Patients can continue to smoke during this time.

        3) Most patients will take Chantix for up to 12 weeks. If medication has been successful, another 12 weeks may be prescribed to help patient remain cigarette-free.

    d) Patients may join Get Quit by calling (877) 242-6849

  iii. Nortriptyline (Pamelor; tricyclic antidepressant) 25 mg daily × 4 days, 50 mg daily × 4 days, then 75 mg daily × 12 weeks. For best results, start medication 14 days prior to quit date.

  iv. Citrol (dietary citric acid supplement). Spray 2 to 4 times directly on back of throat to reduce desire to smoke for approximately 1 hour. Use as needed.

  g. Hypnosis

  h. Acupuncture

  i. Plastic "cigarettes"

IX. COMPLICATIONS

  A. Relapse—most people who return to smoking do so within a month of quitting. The longer persons have abstained, the more likely they are to continue to do so.

    1. Patient may be doing well when a situation or stressor makes smoking too enticing to resist

    2. Patient may experience side effects from product used and may lose resolve

X. CONSULTATION

  A. Question regarding possible medical contraindication to use of nicotine replacement or bupropion hydrochloride

  B. Referral to intensive group sessions such as those offered by Nicotine Anonymous, American Cancer Society, American Lung Association, or a local hospital

XI. FOLLOW-UP

  A. Telephone call to patient within 1 to 2 weeks of quit date

  B. Office follow-up at 1 and 3 months

C. If relapse occurs
  1. Discuss and review problems and stressors that contributed to relapse
  2. Review and reinforce strategies that smoker can use to meet future challenges
  3. Renew smoker's commitment to total abstinence
  4. Review why patient wishes to quit; contract with patient to set another quit date
  5. Reassure patient that success is often achieved only after five to six repeated attempts; success may take several years

See Appendix I for a patient information sheet for photocopying or adapting.
See Bibliographies.
Websites: http://www.smokefree.gov; http://www.nida.nih.gov; http://www. cdc.gov/tobacco; http://www.surgeongeneral.gov/tobacco; http://www.cancer.org; http://www.americanheart.org; http://www.lungusa.org; http://www.ctcinfo.org; http://www.tobacco.org; http://www.quitnet.com http://www.atmc.wisc.edu

NOTE

1. Fagerstrom Test for Nicotine Dependence: http://www.ncbi.nlm.nih. gov/pubmed/1932883.

Weight Management

5

I. DEFINITION

Obesity is an excess of body fat. The most commonly used method for measuring body composition is the body mass index (BMI; *see Appendix H*). BMI is expressed as weight in kilograms divided by height in meters squared (kg/m^2). Normal weight is defined as a BMI of 18.5 to 24.9 kg/m^2; overweight as a BMI between 25 and 29.9 kg/m^2; mild obesity as a BMI between 30 and 34.9 kg/m^2; moderate obesity, 35 to 39.9 kg/m^2; and morbid obesity, greater than 40 kg/m^2. Health risks begin to surface with a BMI greater than 25 kg/m^2; the risk increasing as the BMI increases.

Increasingly, a subset of obese patients is being identified with insulin resistance syndrome. This syndrome is a cluster of conditions that can lead to an increased risk of cardiovascular disease and diabetes. Criteria for diagnosis include:

A. Obesity
   1. BMI greater than 30 kg/m^2
   2. Increased visceral adipose tissue, with a waist circumference of greater than 35 inches in women
   3. A small number of persons not meeting the criteria for obesity but present with laboratory values that identify them as metabolically obese
B. Dyslipidemia
   1. Hypertriglyceridemia 150 mg/dL or greater
   2. Decreased HDL-C levels less than 50 mg/dL in females
   3. LDL-C levels may be normal.
C. Elevated blood pressure
   1. New Advanced Technology Program III guidelines define elevated blood pressure as 130/85 mm Hg or greater (see website at www.atp.nist.gov/atp/psag-co.htm)
D. Impaired glucose function
   1. Fasting blood glucose of greater than 100 mg/dL
E. Increased fasting insulin levels
F. Polycystic ovary syndrome is not included in the criteria for diagnosis, but is present in a great percentage of women with metabolic syndrome

II. EPIDEMIOLOGY

Obesity is among the most serious and prevalent health problems in the United States; second only to cigarette smoking. More than 97 million Americans are defined as having a weight problem. Of these, 58 million are obese.

Prevalence continues to rise in the past decade, rising from 25% to 35%. Researchers have shown that prevalence varies greatly by sex, age, race, and socioeconomic status. More than 55% of the population defined as obese are women. Obesity in women is twice more common in lower socioeconomic groups than in women with higher socioeconomic status. Obesity itself is an independent risk factor for many medical conditions and negatively contributes to others.

III. ETIOLOGY

A. Obesity is a multifactorial disorder. Based on both genetics and behavior occurring because of an imbalance between energy expended and food consumed and with other contributing factors such as:

1. Metabolic (<1% of obese)
   a. Hypothyroidism
   b. Cortisol excess (Cushing's syndrome)
   c. Stein-Leventhal syndrome (polycystic ovary disease)
2. Medication
   a. Antidiabetics
   b. Antipsychotics
   c. Antidepressants
   d. Antiepileptics
   e. Adenergic antagonists
   f. Serotonin and histamine antagonists
   g. Steroids
3. Food consumption
   a. Portion size
   b. Selection of foods
      i. Foods high in fat
      ii. Foods and beverages high in sugar and complex carbohydrates
4. Lifestyles
   a. Sedentary/lack of physical activity
   b. Lack of calorie-burning (aerobic) exercise
   c. Use of food for comfort and to reduce stress
5. Other
   a. Of lesser contribution
      i. Endocrine
      ii. Deviant eating patterns (i.e., binge eating, night eating)

IV. RISKS ASSOCIATED WITH OBESITY

A. Obesity is associated with increased morbidity and mortality. It has been associated with more than 30 illnesses, among them are:

1. Type 2 diabetes
2. Hypertension
3. Stroke
4. Coronary artery disease
5. Dyslipidemia
6. Gallstone formation
7. Osteoarthritis
8. Gastrointestinal (GI) disorders
9. Sleep apnea
10. Breast inflammation
11. Respiratory diseases

12. Obesity has been implicated in some cancers, such as breast, colon, and endometrial
13. Increased risks in pregnancy, such as miscarriage, pre-eclampsia, gestational diabetes, infertility and, possibly, fetal anomalies, such as neural tube defects
14. Gouty arthritis
15. Pickwickian syndrome

V. HISTORY
A. Risk assessment
  1. Overweight and obese patients may not present with the stated desire to lose weight
  2. Presenting complaints are, most commonly, those associated with the risk factors listed in *Risks Associated With Obesity*, **IV.A**
  3. A weight loss assessment should be part of an annual exam
  4. Weight loss assessment
    a. Patient's recognition of need for weight reduction
    b. Patient's readiness to change
    c. Previous attempts at weight loss
    d. Dietary assessment
      i. Type and amounts of food typically consumed
      ii. Patterns of eating
      iii. Meals
      iv. Snacks
      v. Spontaneous eating
    e. Alcohol consumption
      i. Amount
      ii. Frequency
    f. Physical activity
      i. Type
      ii. How often, for how long
    g. Obesity-related problems
    h. Family history of weight and weight-related problems
    i. Signs and symptoms of depression
    j. Medications: prescribed, over the counter (OTC), including herbals, homeopathics, and nutritional supplements
    k. Smoker/nonsmoker

VI. PHYSICAL EXAM
A. As indicated by known problem or presenting complaint, or to rule out a secondary cause of obesity
B. Regardless of previous statement, exam should include:
  1. Height
  2. Weight
  3. Blood pressure
C. Head and neck examination for:
  1. Moon facies
  2. Hirsutism

3. Goiter
4. Buffalo hump
D. Skin
1. Striae
2. Hirsutism
3. Edema
4. Dryness
E. Calculation of BMI
1. BMI may be calculated by dividing the weight in pounds by the square of the height (square inches) and multiplying the result by 703
2. BMI may also be assessed by consulting a BMI table (*see Appendix H*)
F. Waist circumference measurement
1. Waist circumference of >35 cm on women

VII. LABORATORY EXAM
A. As indicated by known history or physical exam
B. The following should be considered if no underlying physical problem is indicated:
1. Lipid profile
2. Thyroid stimulation hormone (TSH), free thyrozine 4 (T^4)
3. Fasting blood sugar; 2-hour postprandial
4. Complete blood count (CBC)
5. Baseline electrocardiogram
6. Sleep studies if indicated
C. If insulin resistant syndrome is to be ruled out
1. Lipid levels
2. Fasting blood sugar; 2-hour postprandial
3. Fasting insulin level
4. Laboratory workup specific for polycystic ovary syndrome (PCOS) (*see Chapter 19*)

VIII. TREATMENT
A. Intervention needs to be multifaceted and tailored to meet the patient's needs and readiness for change
B. The need for weight loss should be presented to the patient in a nonjudgmental, nonconfrontational manner. Approach the problem as a partnership in an endeavor that will help the patient to enjoy a longer, healthier life.
C. Assessment of patient's willingness to make a change includes the following:
1. Patient may not be interested in making a change despite the identified risk and potential consequences
2. Patient may be interested, acknowledge the risk factors, but may not yet be ready to take action
3. Patient is ready to take on the challenge of weight loss

D. Assessment of the amount of weight to be lost based on physical findings and risk factors
E. Plan
   1. Assessment of caloric intake
   2. Assessment of energy expenditure and level of physical activity
   3. Assessment of limitations and/or existing factors
      a. Physical limitation
      b. Medications (alternatives may be considered)
      c. Financial limitations
      d. Cues or stimuli that affect eating
   4. Set realistic goals and expectations regarding the amount of weight to be lost
      a. Short term
         i. 5% to 10% loss in initial weight at 1 to 2 lbs/week rate
      b. Long term
         i. Realization of ideal weight
        ii. Maintaining ideal weight
   5. Contract with patient a framework for realization of goals
F. Interventions
   1. Diet, with emphasis on long-range behavior changes
      a. Nutritionist for evaluation and plan
      b. Self-help
         i. Weight Watchers
        ii. Take Off Pounds Sensibly (TOPS)
        iii. Overeaters Anonymous
        iv. Community-based programs
        v. Meal-replacement programs
        vi. Books, magazine articles
        vii. Website weight-loss programs
   2. Education in food selection and change in eating patterns (NHLBI/NIDDK guidelines are a good source of information—see website: www.nhlbi.nih.gov)
      a. Low fats, increase omega-3 fatty acids
      b. Moderate use of complex carbohydrates
      c. Decrease consumption of simple carbohydrates (i.e., sugary drinks, candy)
      d. Moderate use of low-fat protein
      e. Decrease in portion size
      f. Omit late-night eating
      g. Eating more slowly (20 minutes should pass between first and last bites of a meal)
      h. Drinking 8 (8 oz) glasses of water a day
      i. Use of daily food diary to keep track of consumption
   3. Physical activity
      a. Activity needs to be tailored to the patient's needs and limitation. CDC guidelines for appropriate physical activity according to age and limitations can be found at www.cdc.gov/physicalactivity/everyone/guidelines/adults.html

b. A general guideline of 30 to 40 minute/day of aerobic exercise, 3 to 4 times a week for strenuous exercise; 4 to 5 times a week for moderate exercise. This may be done at divided times (i.e., three 10-minute sessions).
c. Moderate-intensity physical activity provides significant health benefits, but needs to be done more often
d. Aerobic exercise may include (according to patient's ability):
   i. Running/jogging
   ii. Brisk walking (3 mph)
   iii. Swimming
   iv. Bicycling more than 10 mph for strenuous exercise; less than 10 mph for moderate exercise
   v. Cross-country skiing
   vi. Rowing
e. Flexibility, resistance/strength training are important components of an exercise program and provide additional health benefits. Activities include the following:
   i. Light weight lifting
   ii. Resistance bands
   iii. Pilates
   iv. Yoga
4. Pharmacotherapeutic options
a. Pharmaceutic intervention may be helpful in patients with a BMI of greater than 30 kg/m^2. This may also be helpful in patients who are slightly less obese (i.e., BMI of 27–29.9 kg/m^2), but who have a comorbidity.
   i. Orlistat (Xenical), a pancreatic lipase inhibitor
     a) How it works
       1) Blocks absorption of about 30% of ingested dietary fats
       2) Not an appetite suppressant
       3) Improves comorbid conditions related to obesity, especially hyperlipidemia and diabetes
     b) Dosage
       1) 120 mg orally, 3 times a day, taken just prior to a meal
       2) In patients with side effects, medication may be started by taking one 120-mg tablet with the largest fat-containing meal of the day and gradually titrating up to advised dosage as patient adjusts
     c) Side effects (are directly related to amount of fat in meal consumed)
       1) Soft stools
       2) Diarrhea (may be explosive and foul smelling)
       3) Anal leakage
     d) Additional information
       1) A daily multiple vitamins should be recommended, because Orlistat inhibits absorption of fat-soluble vitamins

e) An OTC preparation, Alli, is now available and U.S. Food and Drug Administration (FDA) approved; dosage is 60 mg, 3 times a day

ii. Phentermine (Adipex-P)

a) How it works

1) Appetite suppressant

2) FDA approved for short-term use (up to 12 weeks) in adults only

b) Dosage/administration: 37.5 mg, 3 times a day

1) Best taken on an empty stomach 1 hour prior to a meal

2) If a dose is missed, take as soon as possible. Patient should never take two doses to make up for missed dose

c) Side effects

1) Blurred vision

2) Dry mouth

3) Sleeplessness

4) Irritability

5) Stomach upset

6) Constipation

Note: These side effects may occur in the first few days of use. The patient should be advised to call her prescriber if these symptoms persist.

7) Chest pain, nervousness, pounding heart, difficulty urinating, mood changes, or breathing problems; the patient should be instructed to call her prescriber immediately

d) Precautions

1) Women with high blood pressure, hyperthyroidism, glaucoma, diabetes, or mental health problems should not be prescribed Adipex-P

2) Alcohol should not be used when taking Adipex-P. Alcohol can increase side effects, especially dizziness.

3) Should not be taken in pregnancy or while breastfeeding

4) Overdose symptoms may include confusion, diarrhea, nausea, rapid breathing, restlessness, GI symptoms (nausea, vomiting). If these symptoms are present, the patient should be instructed to call her local poison control center or hospital emergency room immediately.

iii. Diethylpropion hydrochloride (Tenuate)

a) How it works

1) Appetite suppressant

2) FDA approved for short-term use (up to 12 weeks) in adults only

        3) Recommended for use in patients with an initial BMI of greater than 30 kg/m^2 who have not responded to a diet and/or exercise regimen

        4) Not for use with another weight loss medication

    b) Dosage/administration

        1) Conventional tablets: 25 mg, 3 times daily, taken 1 hour prior to meals

        Note: An additional 25-mg dose may be taken midevening if necessary to overcome hunger

        2) Extended release tablets: 75-mg tablet taken mid-morning; must be taken whole

    c) Side effects

        1) Dizziness

        2) Headache

        3) Sleeplessness

        4) Blurred vision

        5) Overstimulation

        6) GI complaints, constipation, vomiting

        7) Rash

    d) Precautions

        1) Should not be taken when pregnant or nursing

        2) Should not be prescribed to patients who have arrhythmias, hypertension, epilepsy, glaucoma, arteriosclerosis, history of drug abuse, known heart murmur, or valvular disorder

        3) Potential for abuse, psychological dependence is possible. Use with caution in patients who have known mental health issues.

        4) Prescribe and dispense in smallest feasible quantities to minimize possibility of overdosage

        5) Should not be used within 14 days of monoamine oxidase (MAO) inhibitor therapy

        6) Alcohol should not be used while taking Diethylpropion HCl

        7) Should not be used concomitantly with other appetite suppressant preparations, including herbal and OTC preparations

        8) Mental alertness and physical coordination may be impaired. Patients should not operate machinery or drive until effect of drug on patient is unknown.

iv. Phendimetrazine (Obezine, Bontril PDM, Plegine, and Anorex to name a few)

    a) How does it work?

        1) Appetite suppressant

        2) FDA approved for short-term use, up to 12 weeks

        3) Recommended for use in patients with an initial BMI of greater than 30 kg/m^2, who have not responded to diet and/or exercise regimen

b) Dosage/administration
   1) 35 mg (immediate release tablets), taken 3 times daily in 4-hour intervals
   2) 105 mg (extended release tablets) are classified by the Drug Enforcement Administration as a Schedule III controlled substance. Extended release capsule is taken in the morning (30–60 minutes before morning meal).
c) Side effects
   1) Insomnia
   2) Nervousness/restlessness/agitation
   3) Dizziness
   4) Blurred vision
   5) Dryness of mouth
   6) GI symptoms, nausea, diarrhea, constipation, stomach pain
   7) Palpitations/tachycardia
   8) Elevated blood pressure
   9) Urinary frequency, dysceria
   10) Overdose symptoms include confusion, belligerence, hallucinations, and panic attack and should be handled as an emergency in a hospital emergency room setting
d) Precautions
   1) Should not be used in pregnancy or lactation
   2) Should not be used concomitantly with other appetite suppressant preparations, including herbal and OTC preparations
   3) Should not be prescribed to patients who have hypertension, diabetes, hyperthyroidism, glaucoma, known heart murmur, or valvular disease and to agitated patients or patients with a history of substance abuse. Alcohol use should be avoided.
   4) Should not be used for patients on MAO inhibitors or within 14 days of discontinuing use
   5) Because mental alertness and physical coordination may be impaired, patients should not drive or operate machinery until effect of drug is known
   6) Potential for dependence. Abuse may be associated with intense psychological dependence and severe social dysfunction. Patients exhibiting these symptoms should be seen in a hospital emergency room setting. Overdose can result in convulsions, coma, and death.
e) Other medications have been associated with weight loss pharmacology. They include:
   1) Bupropion (Wellbutrin), an antidepressant
   2) Topiramate (Topamax), an antiseizure medication

      3) Zonisamide (Zonegran), an antiseizure medication

      4) Metformin, a diabetes treatment

     Note: We have not elaborated on these as first-line weight-loss pharmaceuticals, because their use is off label.

5. Herbal or alternative medications
   a. Currently not recommended as alternative medications
      i. Not under any regulation
      ii. Ingredients (i.e., Ma Hung) possess the potential for serious side effects
6. Behavioral
   a. Stimulus control
      i. Identifying factors contributing to overeating and under-exercising
      ii. Identify ways in which contributory factors may be eliminated.
      iii. Structuring mechanism for elimination of the negative stimuli
   b. Stress management
      i. Meditation, progressive relaxation
      ii. Guided imagery
   c. Cognitive restructuring
      i. Identification of inner dialogue (i.e., self-talk, distorted/negative self-image)
      ii. Replacement of these negative and self-defeating cognitions with more positive ones
   d. Social support
      i. Seek out support/educational groups as noted in *Treatment VIII.F.1*
      ii. Join and participate in exercise groups and other recreation programs geared toward physical well-being and body conditioning
      iii. Seek support systems within family or peer group
      iv. Daily journal
7. Surgical
   a. May be considered for patients who have failed trials of diet, lifestyle changes, pharmacotherapy
   b. Most often used for patients younger than age 55 and in good health, with a BMI greater than 40 kg/m^2, and possessing a significant cofactor
   c. Prior to surgery, patient should undergo assessment by multidisciplinary team. Assessment should include the following:
      i. Medical
      ii. Surgical
      iii. Psychological
      iv. Nutritional
   d. Patient should be well motivated and well informed about potential benefits and risks

    e. Types of procedures
        i. Gastric banding—restricting gastric volume
        ii. Roux-en-Y gastric bypass, in addition to restricting volume, also alters digestion
    f. Success rates
        i. Regardless of procedure, most patients lose one-half to two-thirds their excess weight within 18 months
    g. Risks/side effects
        i. Postoperative wound infection
        ii. Atelectasis
        iii. Dehiscence
        iv. Deep vein thromboembolism
        v. Anastomotic leaks
        vi. Marginal ulcers
        vii. Pouch and distal esophageal dilation
        viii. Persistent vomiting
        ix. Cholecystitis
        x. Development of dumping syndrome
        xi. Vitamin deficiencies (i.e., B12, folate, iron)
8. Other
    a. Preconception counseling
    b. Preconception weight stabilization
    c. Counseling of pregnant women regarding micronutrient and vitamin supplementation, and close monitoring for appropriate weight maintenance and weight gain

IX. CONSULTATION

    A. BMI >40 kg/m^2 (morbidly obese)
    B. Psychiatric disorder (bulimia/depression)
    C. Sleep apnea
    D. Uncontrolled cofactor
        1. Hypertension
        2. Diabetes
        3. Heart disease
    E. Assessment and treatment for insulin resistance syndrome (consider endocrinologist)
    F. Medication

X. FOLLOW-UP

    A. Weight checks on regularly scheduled contracted schedule—4 weeks, if no adverse events and weight loss is being achieved
    B. Measurements as part of above
    C. Review and reassessment of goals on regular schedule
    D. Review of food and exercise diaries
    E. Review and assessment of problems, concerns, and side effects associated with pharmaceutical interventions

Guidelines for Assessing Victims of Abuse and Violence

6

ASSESSMENT FOR ABUSE AND/OR VIOLENCE

I. DEFINITION

Abuse and/or violence in a relationship is said to occur when one person physically, sexually, verbally, and/or emotionally abuses, or economically abuses/controls another person and/or destroys the property of the person. Experiencing fear for one's person in a relationship is characteristic of an abusive situation, regardless of whether or not there is physical violence. Fearing physical harm is enough to consider the relationship abusive. Power or control by one person over another in a relationship can constitute abuse; power and control in a relationship are hallmarks of abuse. Constant degradation damages ego, self-esteem, and confidence. Dating violence affects an estimated one in five adolescents and domestic violence affects one in four to one in 10 women.

II. HISTORY

Consider each woman in any setting as abused until proven otherwise
  A. What the patient may present with
    1. Description of abuse or violence in the relationship
    2. Unexplained symptoms or injuries such as bruises or fractures inconsistent with any disease pathology
    3. Numerous psychosomatic complaints with no physical evidence
    4. Vague physical complaints
    5. The woman's partner gives history and answers questions directed toward the woman
    6. Delay between presenting injury or problem and seeking care
    7. Woman seems embarrassed or evasive in giving history
    8. Woman seems fearful, withdrawn, does not name friends or family members as resources
  B. Additional information to be considered (*see questions on the Abuse Assessment Screen and the Danger Assessment in Appendices B and C, respectively*)
    1. Psychiatric, alcohol, and/or drug abuse by patient and/or partner
    2. Suicide gestures or attempts—suicidal ideation
    3. Many accidents in medical record, repeated visits to emergency department
    4. Any gynecologic or gastrointestinal complaints
    5. Level of anxiety the woman demonstrates over the visit or the physical exam

III. PHYSICAL EXAMINATION
  A. Unexplained bruises; whip-like injuries consistent with shaking; erythematous areas consistent with slapping; lacerations, burn marks, fractures, and/or multiple injuries in various stages of healing

B. Injuries on body hidden by clothing and injuries inconsistent with common accidents such as on the genitals, breasts, chest, head, face, and abdomen
C. Injuries at the back of arms consistent with a defensive posture
D. Evidence of sexual abuse such as lacerations on breasts, labia, urethra, perineum, and anal area
E. Healed fractures or scars
F. Fractures inconsistent with story of accident
G. Apprehensive during examination and injuries and other findings are inappropriate to her story or inexplicable
H. Abuse can have no symptoms: a well woman without visible injuries

IV. LABORATORY EXAMINATION
A. As indicated by physical findings
B. May include X-rays for evidence of new, healing, or old fractures

V. INTERVIEWING THE WOMAN
A. Provide a safe place alone and private where partner/spouse/abuser cannot hear
B. Assure her of confidentiality and safety
C. Phrase questions in a nonthreatening way, conveying empathy such as, "I noticed you have some bruises. Can you tell me how they happened? Have you been hit by someone? Has anyone hurt you in any way? When was the last time you cried?" (*see also questions on Abuse Assessment Screen* [AAS] *in Appendix B*).
D. Assess for current danger and for emotional and/or physical injuries (*see Danger Assessment tool in Appendix C*)

VI. DOCUMENTING EVIDENCE
A. Collect data from medical records and those of other health care providers
B. Record the most recent, as well as past incidents
C. Record any witnesses to abuse
D. Quote the woman's statements of abuse with, "Patient states . . . "
E. Protect patient by deleting any statements such as, "He hurt me so much; I wanted to kill him"
F. If the woman denies any abuse, record your assessment and suspicions for possible future use
G. Record any injuries or symptoms in detail about size, location, duration, onset, age, and pattern. Make a body map and locate injuries in as much detail as you can. Indicate any evidence of sexual abuse or restraint marks on skin.
H. Collect physical evidence of injuries and label after obtaining with the woman's written permission to do so
I. Photograph all evidence of injuries with the woman's written permission

VII. TREATMENT

A. Assure the woman that she is not alone
B. Assure the woman of confidentiality and that only she can authorize the release of evidence to the police, the release of her records, and your verbal testimony
C. Provide support that she does not deserve abuse and that no person should perpetrate any kind of abuse or violence on her
D. Show her the documentation in her record and indicate that its purpose is to protect her
E. Provide resources for her safety and for escape if she decides to do so; empower her to make her own plans and choices
F. Teach her about the patterns of violence and the laws in your state concerning abuse and violence in relationships; have copies of the state laws available
G. If she chooses to remain in the relationship, you can offer her emergency numbers of police, any domestic violence units or special forces, local emergency room(s), and shelters; help make a safety plan (money, car keys, important documents, where to go); for undocumented immigrant women who need counseling, give phone numbers of culturally sensitive programs

VIII. REFERRALS/CONSULTATION

A. Medical consultation as appropriate for treatment of injuries
B. Police, if woman chooses to file a complaint or police report
C. Shelters, special services for women in abusive/violent relationships
D. Mental health consultation if you believe the woman is suicidal or if the woman wishes to speak with a mental health clinician
E. Substance abuse or alcohol abuse treatment programs as appropriate and desired by the woman

IX. FOLLOW-UP

A. Plan a return visit so the woman has another opportunity for contact with you. Women may seem fine but may be degraded, depressed, afraid, or subjugated by a powerful partner who may control finances, children's money and welfare, and may be occasionally rewarding and caring.
B. As appropriate for care of injuries, presenting concerns, contraceptive needs, treatment of STDs, vaginitis, or gynecologic conditions

Appendix B's Abuse Assessment Screen and Appendix C's Danger Assessment may be photocopied or adapted for your patients.
See Bibliographies on abuse and violence.
Website: http://www.nnvawi.org

Part

II

Guidelines for Contraception and Preconception Care

Methods of Contraception and Family Planning

7

BARRIER METHODS

Diaphragm

I. DEFINITION/MECHANISM OF ACTION
A diaphragm is a shallow rubber or silicone cap with a flexible rim that is placed in the vagina to cover the cervix. It serves as both a mechanical barrier and a receptacle for (contraceptive) spermicidal cream or jelly, which must be used to ensure effectiveness.

II. EFFECTIVENESS AND BENEFITS
    A. Method: 97% effectiveness rate
    B. User: 80% to 85% effectiveness rate
    C. May be inserted up to 4 hours prior to intercourse
    D. May have some protective effects against transmission of certain sexually transmitted diseases
    E. Effective form of contraception for women who have infrequent intercourse or in whom there are contraindications for other methods

III. SIDE EFFECTS AND COMPLICATIONS
    A. Allergic reaction of patient or her partner to rubber (a silicone diaphragm is available) or to the spermicidal agent (a variety exists)
    B. Inability to achieve satisfactory fitting
    C. Inability of patient to learn the correct insertion and/or removal technique
    D. Use may be associated with an increased incidence of urinary tract infection because of upward pressure of the rim of the diaphragm against the urethra
    E. Pelvic discomfort, cramps, pressure on the bladder or rectum can occur if:
        1. Diaphragm is too large
        2. Patient has chronic constipation
    F. Toxic shock syndrome: Severe cases occurring immediately after use have been reported in diaphragm users during menses (although these appear to be related to damage to vaginal walls during scanty flow by tampon use rather than diaphragm use per se)
    G. Foul-smelling vaginal discharge may occur if the diaphragm is left in too long

IV. TYPES (REPRESENTATIVE OF SEVERAL MANUFACTURERS)
    A. Arcing spring
        1. Sturdy rim with firm spring strength (spiral, coiled spring)

2. Firm construction allows diaphragm to be kept in place despite rectocele, cystocele, mild pelvic relaxation, and uterine retroversion
3. Folds in an arc shape
B. Coil spring
1. Spring in rim is spiral, coiled, and sturdy
2. Best suited for women with good vaginal tone and no uterine displacement
3. Folds flat for insertion
C. Wide seal
1. Cuff inside rim
2. Available in arcing and coil spring, also in silicone

V. FITTING
A. Most diaphragms are available in sizes ranging from 50 or 55 mm to 95 or 100 mm (available sizes in 5-mm gradations)
B. Fit should be snug between the posterior fornix, pubic symphysis, and lateral vaginal walls but should cause no pressure or discomfort
C. The patient may review and sign informed consent form (*see Appendix A*)
D. After a diaphragm has been fitted, instructions have been given, and the patient has demonstrated her ability to insert and remove it, she may be given an appointment for a follow-up visit in 1 week. During this week, the patient is instructed to practice wearing the diaphragm at least for 8-hour intervals. (In many settings, the 1 week follow-up may be unrealistic, so diaphragm fitting and use will be taught at one visit, and the patient is given the prescription or kit.) It is helpful for the patient to be given a phone number and a schedule to call about any concerns or problems.
E. At the optional follow-up appointment:
1. Diaphragm is checked for fit and proper insertion
2. Instructions are again reviewed and patient is given an opportunity to ask questions
F. If the previous criteria are met, patient is then given a prescription for a diaphragm
G. Yearly diaphragm check is recommended, but the patient should return for recheck sooner if:
1. Diaphragm does not seem to fit well or can be displaced; this can occur with weight gain or loss of >15 lbs (6.8 kg)
2. The woman has any pelvic surgery
3. The woman has a miscarriage, abortion, or wishes to resume using diaphragm after giving birth
4. The woman is having problems with use

Appendix A may be photocopied and used as an informational handout on the diaphragm as well as a consent form for your patients.
See Bibliographies.

FemCap

I. DEFINITION/MECHANISM OF ACTION
The contraceptive FemCap is a prescription-only contraceptive device that is used to hold spermicide and to provide a partial barrier to sperm when placed over the cervix

II. EFFECTIVENESS AND BENEFITS
A. 96% to 98% effective
B. May be inserted before intercourse and left in place for up to 48 hours
C. Latex free
D. Reusable for more than a year

III. SIDE EFFECTS AND DISADVANTAGES
A. Vaginal irritation from the device
B. Vaginal irritation from the spermicide used with the device
C. Sensation of something in the vagina
D. Requires a prescription and pelvic examination

IV. CONTRAINDICATIONS
A. Allergy to spermicide
B. Allergy to the material the device is made of
C. Partner allergy to the device or spermicide
D. Device is expelled repeatedly during use
E. Cannot be used during menses
F. Known or suspected uterine or cervical cancer
G. History of toxic shock syndrome
H. Current infection of vagina or cervix, pelvic inflammatory disease (PID)
I. Cannot be used during postpartum or after an abortion for 6 weeks
J. Adhesions between cervix and vaginal walls
K. Third-degree uterine prolapse
L. Cut or tear in vagina or cervix noted on pelvic examination

V. TYPES
A. Available in three sizes: 22 mm for women who have never been pregnant, 26 mm for women who have been pregnant, and 30 mm for women who have delivered a full-term infant vaginally

VI. FITTING
A. A pelvic examination is needed to rule out anatomical or pathologic contraindications and to evaluate size and position of cervix
B. Select size based on the woman's history and examination findings: small for nulligravidas; medium for those with history of abortion or cesarean section; large for women with one or more vaginal deliveries

C. Follow up for any concerns or problems; annual examination
D. Website for FemCap information: http://www.femcap.com

Lea's Shield*

I. DEFINITION/MECHANISM OF ACTION
Lea's Shield is a contraceptive device that is used to hold spermicide and to provide a partial barrier to sperm when placed over the cervix

II. EFFECTIVENESS AND BENEFITS
A. 85% effective—limited data
B. May be inserted before intercourse and left in place for up to 48 hours
C. Latex free
D. Reusable for more than a year

III. SIDE EFFECTS AND DISADVANTAGES
A. Vaginal irritation from the device
B. Vaginal irritation from the spermicide used with the device
C. Sensation of something in the vagina
D. Difficulty in removing
E. Requires prescription

IV. CONTRAINDICATIONS
A. Allergy to spermicide
B. Allergy to the material the device is made of
C. Partner allergy to the device or spermicide
D. Device is expelled repeatedly during use
E. Cannot be used during menses
F. Known or suspected uterine or cervical cancer
G. History of toxic shock syndrome
H. Current infection of vagina or cervix, PID
I. Cannot be used during postpartum or after an abortion for 6 weeks
J. Adhesions between cervix and vaginal walls
K. Third-degree uterine prolapse

V. TYPES
A. Available in one size

VI. FITTING
A. A pelvic examination is needed to rule out anatomical or pathologic contraindications and to evaluate size and position of cervix
B. Follow up for any concerns or problems; annual examination

Discontinued in the United States, available at http://www.barriermethods.com

Vaginal Contraceptive Sponge

I. DEFINITION/MECHANISM OF ACTION
The Today vaginal contraceptive sponge looks like a small doughnut with a hollow area in the center. The hollow area fits over the cervix. The sponge measures about 1.75 in (4.45 cm) in diameter. Across the bottom is a string loop to provide for easy removal. The sponge is polyurethane and contains the spermicide nonoxynol-9. It provides a barrier between sperm and the cervix, traps sperm within the sponge, and releases spermicide to inactivate sperm for more than 24 hours. The Today sponge is the only one available in the United States.*

II. EFFECTIVENESS AND BENEFITS
    A. 89% to 90.8% effective
    B. May be inserted before intercourse and left in place for up to 24 hours
    C. Latex free
    D. Over the counter
    E. No need to add extra spermicide within 24 hours

III. SIDE EFFECTS AND DISADVANTAGES
    A. Vaginal irritation from the sponge
    B. Vaginal irritation from the spermicide in the sponge
    C. Sensation of something in the vagina
    D. Difficulty in removing
    E. May have a relationship to the development of toxic shock syndrome if not used as directed
    F. Frequent use of nonoxynol-9 can cause genital irritation and increase the risk of HIV and other sexually transmitted diseases (STDs)

IV. CONTRAINDICATIONS
    A. Allergy to spermicide
    B. Allergy to sponge material
    C. Partner allergy to sponge or spermicide
    D. Cannot be used during menses
    E. History of toxic shock syndrome
    F. Current infection of vagina or cervix, PID

V. HOW TO USE
    A. Patient should read instructions carefully prior to using the sponge
    B. The sponge can be left in place for up to 24 hours and offers protection for each act of intercourse

VI. FOLLOW-UP
Yearly physical examination including Papanicolaou (Pap) smear is recommended per the ASCCP guidelines

    Website: http://www.todaysponge.com; available online and over the counter in pharmacies

CONTRACEPTIVE SPERMICIDES AND CONDOMS

Spermicides

I. DEFINITION
Spermicides are substances used alone or with a vaginal barrier to prevent sperm from reaching the uterus. All contain an inert base or carrier substance and an active ingredient, most commonly the surfactant nonoxynol-9, which disrupts the integrity of the sperm cell membrane.

II. EFFECTIVENESS AND BENEFITS
  A. Method: 96% effectiveness rate
  B. User: 60% effectiveness rate
  C. Inexpensive and readily available

III. SIDE EFFECTS AND DISADVANTAGES
  A. Local irritation from spermicide or allergy to spermicide or carrier substance
  B. Can necessitate interruption of intercourse for application
  C. Emotional reaction to touching or inserting a substance into one's own body

IV. TYPES
  A. Creams, jellies, gels (some are flavored and nontoxic if ingested, some are colored)
  B. Foams
  C. Foaming tablets
  D. Suppositories
  E. Vaginal contraceptive film
  F. Bioadhesive gel
  G. Water-soluble lubricant with spermicide

V. HOW TO USE
  A. Instructions should be read carefully prior to using any spermicide. Method of insertion, time of effectiveness, time needed prior to intercourse, and other instructions vary with each type. Concentration of the spermicide varies among products.
  B. A new insertion of spermicide is needed before each act of intercourse
  C. Wash the applicator with soap and water after each use
  D. When the woman uses a spermicide alone, the partner should always use a condom
  E. Frequent use of nonoxynol-9 can cause genital and rectal lesions and increase the risk of HIV and other STDs

VI. FOLLOW-UP
Yearly physical examination including a Pap smear is recommended per the ASCCP guidelines

See Appendix I for patient handout on spermicides and condoms, and Bibliographies for references.

Condoms

I. DEFINITION
Condoms are thin sheaths, most commonly made of latex and also made of sheep intestine or polyurethane, that prevent the transmission of sperm from the penis to the vagina. The female condom (vaginal pouch) is made of polyurethane.

II. EFFECTIVENESS
  A. Method: 97% to 98% effectiveness rate
  B. User: 70% to 94% effectiveness rate; 85% for female condom (range 74%–91.1%)
  C. Inexpensive and readily available
  D. Offer protection against sexually transmitted diseases, including the AIDS virus (HIV)
  E. Encourage male participation with birth control (conventional male condom)
  F. Female condom is polyurethane (fewer allergic reactions as compared with latex)
  G. Use of both vaginal spermicides and condoms has an effectiveness rate in the high 90s when both methods are used correctly

III. SIDE EFFECTS AND DISADVANTAGES
  A. Allergic reactions to latex (rare) or lubricant or spermicide on products with either of these in place
  B. Use necessitates interruption of intercourse for application
  C. May decrease tactile sensation
  D. Psychological impotency may occur
  E. Only latex condoms can be considered effective protection against the AIDS virus (HIV); the polyurethane vaginal pouch (female condom) is twice as thick as latex, and viral permeability may be less than latex
  F. Polyurethane male condoms are more likely than latex to break or slip off, but they are useful for persons who do not like latex condoms or are latex sensitive

IV. TYPES
Condoms (male) vary in color, texture (smooth, studded, or ribbed), shape, size, and price. They come lubricated or nonlubricated, impregnated

with spermicide, flavored, or plain. Some are extra strength, some are sheerer and thinner, and some are uniquely shaped or scented. The new eZ•on male condom is made of polyurethane, a thin, strong, 100% latex-free material. It is designed to go on in either direction and has no reservoir tip.

V. HOW TO USE
A. Male condom
 1. The male condom should always be put on an erect penis before there is any sexual contact and used in every act of intercourse
 2. The male condom should not be pulled tightly over the end of the penis; about 1 in (2.54 cm) should be left for ejaculation fluid and to avoid breakage; some condoms have a reservoir tip
 3. The penis should be withdrawn before it becomes limp, and the open end of the male condom should be held tightly while withdrawing to prevent spilling the contents
 4. The partner should always use a contraceptive spermicide when a male condom is used
 5. Condoms should be used only once
B. Female condom (comes prelubricated)
 1. Pinch ring at closed end of pouch and insert like a diaphragm, covering the cervix; adding one or two drops of additional lubricant makes insertion easier and decreases or eliminates squeaking noise and dislocation during intercourse
 2. Adjust other ring over labia
 3. Can be inserted several minutes to 8 hours prior to intercourse
 4. Remove after intercourse before standing up by squeezing and twisting the outer ring and pulling out gently

VI. FOLLOW-UP
Annual examination, Pap smear per ASCCP guidelines

Appendix I has information on contraceptive spermicides and condoms that you may wish to photocopy for distribution to your patients.
See Bibliographies.
Website: http://www.asccp.org

EMERGENCY CONTRACEPTION

I. DEFINITION
Emergency contraception (EC), often known as the "morning-after pill," is a pharmacologic or mechanical intervention after exposure to the possibility of conception with no or uncertain contraceptive protection.

Such intervention is based on inhibiting fertilization or implantation. The means for intervention are either mechanical (an intrauterine device [IUD]) or hormonal (high-dose, short-term oral contraceptives [OCs], or progestational agents).

II. ETIOLOGY
   A. Disruption of fertilization or of implantation beginning within 120 hours after unprotected intercourse is based on several theoretical premises
      1. Progestational agents will change or interfere with sperm migration or the capacity of a sperm to penetrate the egg
      2. Progestational agents are thought to inhibit motility of the fallopian tubes—also to affect follicle growth and development of the corpus luteum
      3. Estrogen, specifically ethinyl estradiol (EE), is thought to reduce plasma level of progesterone and may, therefore, interfere with the function of the corpus luteum or, possibly, the function of luteinizing hormone, thereby disrupting ovulation
      4. Progestational agents and estrogen (estradiol) are known to shorten the luteal phase of the cycle
      5. Intrauterine contraceptive devices (IUCDs), specifically copper-bearing devices, are thought to interfere with the enzyme systems of the endometrium, and perhaps alter the permeability of the endometrial microvasculature, which perhaps interferes with implantation

III. EFFECTIVENESS
Used within 120 hours, hormonal EC reduces the risk of pregnancy by 75% for those women who would have become pregnant (8 of 100), so 2 of 100 will become pregnant. The sooner EC is used after unprotected intercourse, the more effective it is.

IV. HISTORY
   A. What the patient presents with
      1. Last act of unprotected intercourse within the past 120 hours
      2. Desire to inhibit fertilization or implantation
   B. Additional information to be obtained
      1. Cycle history and any previous use of contraceptives
      2. Estimated day(s) of exposure to sperm without any protection or with known method failure (e.g., condom broke or slipped off; IUD [IUCD] expelled; cap, shield, or diaphragm displaced; missed seven or more combination of OCs in the past 2 weeks or missed two or more progestin-only OCs)
      3. Contraindications to hormone or IUD (IUCD) use
      4. Circumstance of unprotected exposure—rape, possible STD exposure, teratogen exposure
      5. Other acts of unprotected intercourse during this cycle

V. PHYSICAL EXAMINATION
A. Pelvic exam—speculum and bimanual—if appropriate
B. Collect specimens per rape/sexual assault guidelines in practice setting as necessary/desired by the woman; complete assessment for evidence

VI. LABORATORY DIAGNOSIS
A. Pregnancy test
B. STD testing as warranted by history

VII. DIFFERENTIAL DIAGNOSIS
A. Consider alternatives should the woman desire to keep a pregnancy if one should occur
B. Sexual assault—consider rape counseling
C. Pregnancy already established prior to current exposure with unprotected intercourse

VIII. TREATMENT
A. Combination OCs (Yuzpe method) and progestin-only OCs must be initiated within 72 hours of exposure. See individual package inserts for use.
B. Plan B (levonorgestrel): Treatment must be initiated within 120 hours[1] (causes less nausea and vomiting); one white pill then one more white pill 12 hours later, or both pills at the same time. Plan B is now available over the counter in some parts of the United States (check individual state regulations).
C. ellaOne: 30-mg tablet of ulipristal acetate (a synthetic progesterone) protects when taken up to 5 days after unprotected intercourse (approved by the U.S. Food and Drug Administration [FDA] in July 2010)
D. Mechanical agents
   1. ParaGard or Mirena insertion within 5 to 7 days of exposure with precautions for IUD (IUCD) use, STD exposure, risk factors for IUD (IUCD) use; some guidelines specify prophylactic antibiotics with insertion

IX. EXPLANATION OF METHOD
A. Education: For each woman specific for postcoital intervention method, including side effects of intervention and danger signs; if IUD (IUCD) is inserted, instructions about IUD (IUCD) use, danger signs, and complications and potential for 5 or 10 years of protection against pregnancy
B. Education about resumption of menses: Based on the woman's cycle history, if hormones are taken during follicular phase, menses will follow at about Day 21; if during ovulation, around Day 26; and if in the luteal phase, about Day 29

X. COMPLICATIONS AND SIDE EFFECTS

A. Pelvic infection with IUD (IUCD) use (*see guideline for PID in Chapter 17*)

B. Ectopic pregnancy: possible increased risk with hormone use (up to 100% of pregnancies); copper IUD (IUCD) use will not inhibit tubal implantation (*see information on ectopic pregnancy in the guideline on acute pelvic pain in Chapter 17*)

C. Pregnancy
   1. Decision making regarding continuation or termination of pregnancy

D. Nausea and vomiting
   1. Drink a glass of milk or eat a snack with each oral dose to reduce risk of nausea and vomiting.
   2. Compazine 25-mg rectal suppository every 12 hours or 10 mg orally 4 times a day
   3. Tigan, 200-mg suppository every 12 hours
   4. Meclizine hydrochloride (Antivert, Dramamine II) 25 mg 1 hour before EC pills
   5. Give extra tablets of OCs in the event of vomiting dose; instruct the woman to take repeat dose if vomiting occurs within 1 hour after taking the dose and pills are visible in vomitus

XI. CONSULTATION AND REFERRAL

A. For pregnancy exposure as the result of sexual assault/rape, refer to rape crisis center, rape counseling, or to a setting with a sexual assault nurse examiner (SANE)

B. For complications of postcoital intervention as necessary

XII. FOLLOW-UP

A. No menses within 3 weeks after intervention, return for evaluation for continued pregnancy (failure of EC or preexisting pregnancy) to rule out ectopic pregnancy

B. For a contraceptive method chosen by the woman for use following the EC
   1. Immediate use: condoms, diaphragm, spermicides, sponge, quick-start OCs
   2. With next menses
      a. OCs—Sunday start or first day quick start; injectable, contraceptive patch, vaginal ring
      b. IUDs—insert with or after menses
      c. Natural family planning (NFP)—initiate with menses
   3. Sterilization anytime

The Emergency Contraceptive Hotline, 1-800-NOT-2-LATE, is a 24-hour toll-free service offered in English and Spanish. Callers can get names, phone numbers, and location of three local clinicians. Internet access: http://not-2-late.com; www.go2planB.com.

See Appendix A and Bibliographies.

HORMONAL CONTRACEPTION

I. TYPES OF HORMONAL CONTRACEPTION
A. Oral contraceptives
1. Definition
OCs (also known as birth control pills) are pills that when taken by mouth produce systemic changes that prevent conception
a. Types of pills
   i. A combination of synthetic estrogen and synthetic progestin
   ii. Progestin only (also known as mini-pills)
   iii. Formulations with additives such as folic acid and iron
   iv. Most formulations are to be swallowed whole; one combination of synthetic estrogen and progestin is available in chewable form
   v. OC formulations and regimens vary across products (e.g., type of synthetic progestin and estrogen; combination pills followed by estrogen-only pills; pills with active ingredients followed by pills with inactive or other ingredients; monophasic, biphasic, triphasic, extended use, and continuous use patterns; short hormone-free interval, estrogen added during placebo week)
2. Directions for use
a. Risks outweigh benefits for women with a body mass index (BMI) of ≥35; contraindicated for women with a BMI of ≥40
b. The combination pill is typically taken for 21 to 24 days and a placebo pill; some with another ingredient (or no pill) is taken for 4 to 7 days, during which time withdrawal bleeding should occur; some packets have 21 OC pills only, so the woman then takes no pills for 7 days
c. Consecutive use, 12 weeks or more, of a monophasic pill (e.g., Seasonale, an 84-combination pill regime) may be considered in certain situations, or EE and levonorgestrel (e.g., Lybrel) taken continuously including
   i. Headaches regularly occurring during withdrawal weeks
   ii. Heavy withdrawal bleeding
   iii. Endometriosis after workup
   iv. Patient's preference
3. Directions for use (progestin only): Progestin-only pills are taken continuously
a. Indications for using a progestin-only pill
   i. A good choice in situations when estrogen is contraindicated
   a) Smokers
   b) Lactation

        c) History of or current deep vein thrombosis/pulmonary embolism

        d) Surgery with immobilization

        e) Valvular heart disease

        f) Severe headaches including migraine without focal neurologic symptoms

        g) Gallbladder disease

        h) Seizure disorders

      ii. Elevated blood pressure (BP) of ≥140/90

  b. Other considerations for progestin-only methods (benefits may outweigh risks)

      i. Undiagnosed breast cancer

      ii. Gallbladder disease while on combination method

     iii. Diabetes without vascular involvement (Type 1 or 2)

     iv. Diabetes with nephropathy, retinopathy, and/or neuropathy

      v. History of current ischemic heart disease

     vi. Peripartum cardiomyopathy more or less than 6 months

    vii. Moderately or severely impaired cardiac function

   viii. Rheumatoid arthritis—with or without immunosuppressive therapy

     ix. History of bariatric surgery

      x. Endometrial hyperplasia

     xi. Inflammatory bowel disease

    xii. Solid organ transplantation—complicated or uncomplicated

   xiii. History of cerebrovascular accident

   xiv. Severe headaches, including migraines, with focal neurologic symptoms

    xv. Mild cirrhosis (uncompensated)

   xvi. Undiagnosed hypertension (not hypertension in pregnancy)

   xvii. HIV-positive women (IUD, IUCD)

  c. Women who fit the previous criteria after appropriate screening and physical exam may be candidates for progestin only, bearing in mind that irregular bleeding may present a major clinical problem. Because the number of pills varies with the manufacturer, carefully review instructions on use and pill pack.

4. Procedure for pill-related bleeding problems (e.g., amenorrhea, scant menses, breakthrough bleeding)

  a. Rule out the following

      i. Faulty OC taking (review packet)

      ii. Pregnancy

     iii. Uterine or cervical pathology—leiomyomata, polyp, cancer

     iv. Pelvic or vaginal infection

      v. Drug interference

       vi. Gastrointestinal problems
      vii. Endometriosis
     viii. Thyroid disorder

  b. Based on the information gained, treatment is as follows
      i. Amenorrhea or scant menses
        a) Reassure the woman
        b) Consider method change
      ii. Breakthrough bleeding
        a) During the first 3 months of hormone use, reassure only
        b) Consider method change
        c) Consider STD testing
        d) If treatment for A or B is unsuccessful and symptoms persist, consult with gynecologist or other collaborating physician.
     iii. For hormonal amenorrhea
        a) Pregnancy test
        b) If amenorrhea continues after 6 months and pill has not been changed, change pill; if no withdrawal bleeding, discontinue pill and consider progestin challenge; if still with no withdrawal bleeding, refer to amenorrhea protocol for workup
     iv. If a woman is on any medication that decreases contraceptive effect, she should be offered the option of back-up contraception, such as condoms and/or spermicidal protection. Decisions about hormonal contraceptive use with medications should be individualized. If there is any question regarding drug interaction and interference of method with other drugs, consult with gynecologist, other collaborating physicians, or pharmacist.

5. Explanation of method: Ways in which OCs are taken[2]
  a. Start OC on Day 1 (first day of menses) *or* start taking first pill on the first Sunday after the menstrual period begins *or* quick start taking the first pill at the time of the office or clinic visit regardless of the cycle day (with the caveat that if this is after the seventh cycle day, the patient could be pregnant at that time or become pregnant if a backup method is not used for the first 7 days)
  b. OC ideally should be taken at the same time of day (within an hour either way)
  c. Backup contraception is necessary for 7 days (first cycle only) if OCs started later than the fifth cycle day
  d. In case of missed pills
      i. One pill missed: woman to take pill when she remembers, and then take scheduled pill at regular time.
      ii. Two pills missed in first 2 weeks: take two pills at regular time for 2 days. Use backup contraception for the remainder of the cycle.

      iii. Two or more pills missed in third week, take two OCs daily until all OCs are taken; restart OC cycle with one pill daily within 7 days; use backup contraception until OCs are restarted with a new packet and for the first 7 days of that packet.

      iv. Three or more pills missed any time in cycle, restart OCs within 7 days with one pill daily. Use a backup method for 7 days of that cycle.

      v. If one or more pills are missed, no backup contraception is used, and no withdrawal bleed occurs, the woman should be instructed to call to discuss possible pregnancy test.

B. Transdermal contraceptive: Contraceptive patch Ortho Evra[3]

  1. Definition

    The contraceptive patch is a three-layer transdermal polyethylene/polyester device about the size of a matchbook, with an adhesive on one side. It is impregnated with norelgestromin (NGMN), a synthetic progestin, and EE, a synthetic estrogen, and releases 150 µg of NGMN and 20 µg of EE every 24 hours.

  2. Directions for use

    a. Women weighing >198 lbs (>90 kg) are at an increased risk for pregnancy. An alternative method is recommended.

    b. Patch is changed weekly for 3 weeks, then off for 1 week.

  3. Explanation of method

    a. Ways in which the patch is used

      i. Apply the patch on the first day of menses or on the first Sunday after bleeding begins; postpartum nonnursing women, 4 weeks or with resumption of menses.

      ii. Apply to clean, dry, healthy skin on buttocks, abdomen, upper outer arm, or upper torso. Patch should not be applied to the breasts. If applied to the pubic area, it may result in genital swelling.

      iii. Instruct the woman not to use lotions, cosmetics, creams, powders, or other topical products in area of the patch or area where the patch will be applied.

      iv. Instruct the woman to press down firmly on the patch for at least 10 seconds and then check if the edges adhere.

      v. Instruct the woman to check the patch daily.

      vi. If the patch detaches, instruct the woman to immediately apply a new patch. Supplemental tapes or adhesives should not be used.

      vii. Apply a new patch the same day of the week 7 days after first patch. Repeat this in Week 3.

      viii. No patch is applied in Week 4.

      ix. Begin a new cycle on the same day of the week for Week 1 and repeat cycle of 3 weeks on and 1 week off.

      x. Withdrawal bleed will occur during the fourth week.

    xi. If the woman forgets to apply a new patch and less than 48 hours have passed, she should apply a new patch as soon as she remembers and then apply the next patch on the usual renewal day.

   xii. If more than 48 hours have elapsed, the woman should stop the current cycle and immediately begin a new 4-week cycle by applying a new patch. The day for patch renewal will now change. Instruct her to use backup contraception for 1 week.

  xiii. If missed change day occurs at the end of the 4-week cycle, instruct the woman to remove the patch and apply a new patch on the usual change day to begin a new cycle.

C. Intravaginal contraceptive: Contraceptive vaginal ring NuvaRing
  1. Definition

The contraceptive vaginal ring is flexible, transparent, colorless, and about 2 in (5.08 cm) in diameter. It is impregnated with etonogestrel, a synthetic progestin, and EE, a synthetic estrogen, and releases 120 μg of progestin and 15 μg of EE every 24 hours over a period of 3 weeks. *Note:* A new vaginal ring with Nestorone and EE is in clinical trials.

  2. Explanation of method and ways in which the ring is used
    a. Insert ring into vagina between Day 1 and Day 5 of the menstrual cycle
    b. Keep ring in place for 3 weeks in a row
    c. Remove ring for 1 week for withdrawal bleeding
    d. If the ring is removed and is out of the vagina for more than 3 hours, backup contraception is required for the next 7 days, except for the hormone-free week
    e. Offers symptom relief form menorrhagia, dysmenorrhea, polycystic ovary syndrome (PCOS)

D. Intramuscular contraceptive: Injectable contraceptive (Depo-Provera)[4]
  1. Definition

The synthetic hormonal substance in Depo-Provera (depot medroxyprogesterone acetate or DMPA) that acts by blocking gonadotropin, thus preventing ovulation from occurring. This injectable decreases sperm penetration through cervical mucus and causes endometrial atrophy preventing implantation. It is injected intramuscularly (IM) every 12 weeks into the muscle of the upper arm or buttocks.

  2. Explanation of use

Depo-Provera is injected IM (in gluteal or deltoid muscle) or subcutaneously (SC) in the first 5 days of the menstrual cycle (after onset of menses), within 5 days postpartum, or, if breastfeeding, at 4 to 6 weeks postpartum. For women with additional risk factors for loss of bone mineral density (BMD)—cigarette smokers, chronic corticosteroid use—consider supplemental use of menopausal doses of estrogen (or another method if risk factors for estrogen use exist).

The injection consists of one 150-mg dose administered IM or one SC injection of 104 mg of DMPA every 12 weeks for as long as contraceptive effect is desired. If time between injections is greater than 13 weeks, do pregnancy test before administration. Inject IM with a 1.5-inch needle or up to 3-inch needle (depends on the size of the woman because it needs to be administered deep IM), or subcutaneously with a 1-in needle, and do not rub the site because rubbing breaks up the microcrystals and increases absorption. Depo-Provera is available in 150 mg/ml and 104 mg/0.65 ml prefilled syringes, as well as in single- and multiple-dose vials.

Visit every 12 weeks for injection. Counsel the woman about age-appropriate calcium and vitamin D intake.

Note the black box warning about the effects on BMD; the Society for Adolescent Medicine noted benefits outweigh risks; loss of BMD is reversible.

E. Contraceptive implant: Implanon
  1. Definition
  Single-rod, implantable polymer contraceptive device impregnated with 68 mg of etonogestrel. It is effective for up to 3 years.
  2. Explanation of use
    a. Inserted subdermally on the inner side of the woman's upper arm; the device releases a low, steady dose of the synthetic progestin etonogestrel

II. PHYSICAL CHANGES OCCURRING WITH HORMONAL CONTRACEPTION
  A. Ovulation is suppressed
  B. The endometrium becomes deciduous, making it unreceptive to implantation
  C. The cervical mucus is altered, so it is hostile to sperm
  D. Transport of the ovum may be altered
  E. Possible luteolysis
  F. Possible inhibition of capacitation of sperm

III. EFFECTIVENESS
  A. 99.6% effectiveness rate for combination pill
  B. 97% effectiveness rate for progestin-only pill
  C. 98% to 99% effectiveness rate for vaginal contraceptive ring
  D. 99% effectiveness for contraceptive patch
  E. +99% effectiveness for contraceptive injectable
  F. +99% effectiveness for contraceptive implant

IV. CONTRAINDICATIONS
  A. Absolute contraindications to hormonal contraception (may vary with method):[5]
    1. Thromboembolic disorder (or history thereof) including deep vein thrombosis, pulmonary embolism, or thromboembolism; stroke

2. Thrombotic cerebrovascular accident (or history thereof)
3. Coronary artery disease (or history thereof), or multiple risk factors for arterial cardiovascular disease; current angina pectoris; structural heart disease complicated by pulmonary hypertension; atrial fibrillation; valvular heart disease with complication
4. Known or suspected carcinoma of the breast
5. Major surgery with prolonged immobility or any surgery on the legs
6. Known impaired liver function at present time, liver problems, hepatic adenoma, liver cancer or history of active viral hepatitis, severe cirrhosis, benign or malignant liver tumor with prior OC use or other estrogen product
7. Known or suspected estrogen-dependent neoplasm (or history thereof) including endometrial carcinoma
8. Older than 35 years of age and currently a smoker
9. Triglyceride level greater than 350 mg/dl; hypercholesterolemia (Type 2 hyperlipidemia)
10. Known or suspected pregnancy
11. Chronic hypertension and smoking, or uncontrolled hypertension; vascular disease
12. Undiagnosed abnormal vaginal/uterine bleeding
13. History of hormonal contraception-related cholestasis or cholestatic jaundice of pregnancy
14. Leiden Factor V mutation
15. Allergic reaction to any components of the ring, patch, or Depo-Provera, or any of its ingredients (check allergic reaction to local anesthetics for dental or other procedures—the carrier substance is the same for local anesthetics and Depo-Provera)
16. Migraines with aura at any age
17. Diabetics with nephropathy/retinopathy/neuropathy or diabetes of >20 years duration
18. Breastfeeding <6 weeks postpartum

B. Relative contraindications
1. Severe headaches or common migraines, which start or worsen with initiation of hormonal contraception use especially in women 35 years or older
2. Hypertension with resting diastolic BP of 90 or more, or resting systolic BP of 140 or more on three or more separate visits, or an accurate measurement of 110 diastolic BP or more on a single visit
3. Impaired liver function (i.e., acute phase mononucleosis, medication-induced changes)
4. Hypertriglyceridemia; worrisome low density lipoprotein (LDL):high density lipoprotein (HDL) ratio
5. Gallbladder disease: medically treated, current biliary tract disease

C. Other considerations (advantages of hormone contraception generally outweigh disadvantages):
   1. Diabetes: without vascular disease
   2. Congenital hyperbilirubinemia (Gilbert's disease)
   3. Failure to have established regular menstrual cycle (without prior workup; *see amenorrhea guideline in Chapter 16*)
   4. Conditions likely to make it difficult for the woman to use the method correctly and consistently (learning disability, major psychiatric problems, alcoholism or other drug abuse, history of repeatedly taking OCs or other medications incorrectly)
   5. Major surgery with no prolonged immobilization
   6. Undiagnosed breast mass
   7. Cervical cancer awaiting treatment; cervical intraepithelial neoplasia (CIN)
   8. Use of drugs affecting liver enzymes (altering absorption of the medication): phenytoin, carbamazepine, barbiturates, topiramate, primidone, rifampin, rifabutin, griseofulvin
   9. Younger than 35 years of age and heavy smoker (>15 cigarettes per day)
   10. Use in breastfeeding not yet approved for NuvaRing and Ortho Evra
   11. Skin disorder that may predispose to application site reactions
   12. Risk factors for low BMD (cigarette smoking, corticosteroid use)
   13. Weight of >198 lbs (>90 kg; BMI of >30); weight may decrease efficacy with some pills

V. ADVERSE DRUG INTERACTIONS
A. All women prior to starting hormonal contraception and on a yearly follow-up basis should review and re-sign the informed consent for method of choice—emphasizing drug interaction and knowledge of danger signs.
B. If a woman is on any medications that decrease contraceptive effect, she should be offered the option of a backup contraception such as condoms and/or spermicidal protection. Decisions about hormonal contraceptive use with medications should be individualized. If there is any question regarding drug interaction and interference of the method with other drugs, consult with a gynecologist or pharmacist.
C. Drug interactions with oral contraception: Some drugs can decrease the effectiveness of OCs by decreasing the available level of hormones. This can result in pregnancy. Drugs that may decrease the effectiveness of OCs include:
   1. Antibiotics
      a. Cephalosporins
      b. Chloramphenicol
      c. Macrolides
      d. Penicillins
      e. Tetracyclines
      f. Sulfas

2. HIV protease inhibitors
   a. Amprenavir
   b. Nelfinavir mesylate
   c. Ritonavir
   d. Modafinil
3. Rifamycins
   a. Rifampin
4. Antiseizure medications
   a. Barbiturates
   b. Carbamazepine
   c. Phenytoin
   d. Primidone
   e. Topiramate
5. St. John's wort

VI. LABORATORY
A. Lipid screen
   1. Lipid screen prior to using hormonal contraception; significant immediate family history
      a. Younger than 50 years of age—stroke, coronary, or sudden death
         Do a lipid screen. If levels are abnormal, consult with a physician before starting hormonal contraception. If levels are normal, start hormonal contraception and repeat test in 2 years.
   2. Lipid screen is strongly advised if parents or siblings have hypertension, vascular disease, myocardial infarction, arteriosclerotic heart disease, and/or hyperlipidemia before the age of 50, or are on medication for hypertension
B. Monitor carefully any prediabetic and diabetic women using hormonal contraception. Consider screening with fasting blood sugar and/or 2-hour postprandial blood sugar if parents or siblings are diabetic, or if the woman is otherwise at an increased risk of developing diabetes.
C. Liver profile if the woman has had mononucleosis or mono-like illness within the past year, or if the patient has a history of hepatitis or other liver disease or drug or alcohol history
D. In combination hormonal methods, Leiden Factor V for women with a personal or family history of venous thromboembolism

VII. FOLLOW-UP
A. For all methods of hormonal contraception:
   1. BP check as needed
   2. Smoking cessation counseling
   3. Review of side effects and danger signs
B. For injectables:
   1. Depo-Provera
      a. Revisit every 12 weeks

b. If more than 13 weeks has passed since the last injection, use a very sensitive pregnancy test prior to injection

See Appendix A for consent form and informational handout on OCs for patients. See other appendices for informational handouts on other hormonal methods. See Bibliographies.
Website: http://www.implanon-usa.com

INTRAUTERINE DEVICES/INTRAUTERINE CONTRACEPTIVE DEVICES

I. DEFINITION/MECHANISM OF ACTION
A. A sterile foreign body placed in the uterus to prevent pregnancy. This is accomplished through several mechanisms:
  1. A local sterile inflammatory response to the foreign body (i.e., IUD, IUCD) causes a change in the cellular makeup of the endometrium; with the copper devices, there is an effect on the endometrium of interfering with the enzyme systems, and with the progesterone device, an effect over time of a less well-developed endometrium
  2. A possible increase in the local production of prostaglandins that may increase endometrial activity
  3. Alteration in uterine and tubal transport
  4. IUDs (IUCDs) probably exert an antifertility effect beyond the uterus and interfere with fertility before an ovum reaches the uterus
  5. Alteration of cervical mucus causing a barrier to sperm penetration (progesterone IUD)
  6. Ovulation suppression on the first year with levonorgestrel intrauterine system (LNG IUS) Mirena. Releases 20 μg/day of levonorgestrel.
  7. Possible protective effect against endometrial cancer in obese women (treatment)
  8. Levonorgestrel-releasing IUD (IUCD) treatment for endometrial hyperplasia and to protect endometrium in women with breast cancer treated with tamoxifen
B. The exact mechanisms of action are not completely understood. One thing that has become clear is that the IUD (IUCD) does not act as an abortifacient.
C. Different types of IUDs (IUCDs) use varying mechanisms of action to prevent pregnancy.
D. World Health Organization Category 3 (risks outweigh advantages for HIV-positive women):[6] For HIV-positive women on antiretroviral therapy, both copper-bearing and LNG-releasing IUDs can be used.

II. EFFECTIVENESS
A. Theoretically: 92% to 99.9% effectiveness rate
B. User: 92% to 99% effectiveness rate
The range is close because the patient's participation is low and, therefore, there is little possibility of patient error.

III. CONTRAINDICATIONS
A. Absolute contraindications
1. Active pelvic infection (acute or subacute), including known or suspected gonorrhea or *Chlamydia*
2. Known or suspected pregnancy
3. Recent or recurrent pelvic infection; postpartum endometritis; postabortion infection (past 3 months)
4. Purulent cervicitis; untreated acute cervicitis or vaginitis
5. Undiagnosed genital bleeding
6. Distorted uterine cavity (bicornuate; severely flexed)
7. History of ectopic pregnancy
8. Allergy to copper (known or suspected), or diagnosed Wilson's disease (ParaGard only); hypersensitivity to any part of Mirena
9. Abnormal Pap smear, cervical or uterine malignancy, or pre-malignancy (endometrial hyperplasia, CIN, or cancer), unless used as therapy for endometrial hyperplasia
10. Impaired responses to infection (diabetes, steroid treatment, immunocompromised patients)
11. Presence of previously inserted IUD (IUCD)
12. Genital actinomycosis
13. Acute liver disease or liver tumor (Mirena)
14. Known or suspected breast cancer (Mirena)
15. Malignant gestational trophoblastic disease
16. Known pelvic tuberculosis
B. Relative contraindications (benefits usually outweigh risks)
1. Multiple sexual partners or partner has multiple partners
2. Emergency treatment difficult to obtain should complications occur; this would primarily be a problem in very rural areas or developing countries
3. Cervical stenosis
4. Impaired coagulation response (idiopathic thrombocytopenic purpura [ITP], anticoagulant therapy, etc.)
5. Uterus sounding less than 6 cm or more than 10 cm
6. Endometriosis
7. Leiomyomata
8. Endometrial polyps
9. Severe dysmenorrhea (Mirena may be therapeutic)
10. Heavy or prolonged menstrual bleeding without clinical anemia; consider oral iron or nutritional alterations to prevent with IUD (IUCD; Mirena may be therapeutic)
11. Impaired ability to check for danger signals

12. Inability to check for IUD (IUCD) string
13. Concerns for future fertility
14. History of PID (with subsequent intrauterine pregnancy, risk decreased)

IV. INSERTION TECHNIQUE
A. Procedure
  1. The woman is scheduled for appointment for insertion only during menses or within 7 days of onset of menses (Mirena) and after
     a. Negative Pap smear (within 6 months)
     b. Negative gonorrhea/*Chlamydia* testing
     c. Appropriate medical and menstrual history is obtained
  2. Patient should be instructed to eat before coming to an appointment
  3. Take oral analgesic or nonsteroidal anti-inflammatory 30 to 60 minutes before procedure
  4. IUD (IUCD) consent form (*see Appendix A*) and minor surgical consent form must be reviewed and signed at the time of an IUD (IUCD) consultation and evaluation after discussion of
     a. Procedure
     b. Mechanism of the device
     c. Side effects and complications
     d. Relationship to a woman's needs
  5. Atropine 0.5 mg should be available at the time of insertion for severe vasovagal response
  6. An anxious woman, or a woman for whom it is deemed necessary to perform a paracervical block and/or use IV atropine (to decrease likelihood of vasovagal reaction), should be referred to a gynecologist for insertion
  7. Insertion under sterile technique
     a. Bimanual examination to determine uterine position and size; insert warmed speculum
     b. Cleanse the vagina, cervix, and endocervical canal with iodine solution (unless allergic to iodine)
     c. Xylocaine gel or hurricane spray could be used to decrease discomfort of tenaculum
     d. Use tenaculum to straighten the uterine body and cervical canal
     e. Sound the uterus (depth less than 6 cm or more than 10 cm is a contraindication)
     f. Insert specific IUD (IUCD) as instructed by manufacturer
     g. Spasm of the internal cervical os may occur; it is usually relieved by simply waiting. *Never* force entry of the sound or applicator.
     h. After insertion, observe the patient for weakness, pallor, diaphoresis, either bradycardia or tachycardia, hypotension, and syncope, which may occur (check BP several times following insertion)

    i. If patient has mild cramping, the following may be used:
        i. Nonaspirin analgesic 650 mg every 4 hours, or
       ii. A prostaglandin inhibitor (nonsteroidal anti-inflammatory drug [NSAID]) such as Motrin 400 mg orally 4 times a day
    j. Explain to patient that the IUD (IUCD) is effective immediately. In some settings, it is recommended that the patient abstain for 1 day because of the disruption of the cervical mucus barrier.
    k. Instruct patient to check for presence of IUD (IUCD) string postmenstruation or after unusual cramping prior to relying on device for continued contraception effect
    l. Follow up with appointment in 6 weeks to 3 months; at that time, be sure that the woman can feel the IUD (IUCD) strings

V. COMPLICATIONS FOLLOWING INSERTION AND WHAT TO DO ABOUT THEM

  A. Immediate, severe vasovagal response
    1. Notify physician
    2. Place patient in shock position
    3. Monitor pulse and BP until stable
    4. Administer oxygen as needed
    5. Atropine 0.4 mg SC or IM may be administered if appropriate
  B. Severe immediate cramping: remove IUD (IUCD)
  C. Excessive pain or bleeding is often a sign of perforation (fundal); consult physician for management
  D. Side effects or later complications
    1. Two or more missed periods: recommend a serum pregnancy test (e.g., ParaGard). With Mirena, irregular, little, or no bleeding is normal. Missed menses: 2 of 10 women have no menses after 1 year of Mirena. Pregnancy is rare, but when this happens, there is a 50% chance of miscarriage. If IUD (IUCD) is removed, this drops to 25%.
    2. Pregnancy occurring while IUD (IUCD) is in place: it is now recommended that, because of the risk of infection, the IUD (IUCD) should be removed at the time of diagnosis whether the pregnancy is continued or terminated. There should be consultation with a gynecologist prior to removal of the IUD (IUCD) by the gynecologist or nurse practitioner.
    3. Breakthrough bleeding related to IUD (IUCD): use the following guidelines for removal:
      a. Bleeding is associated with endometritis
      b. Hematocrit falls 5 points
      c. There is a hematocrit of 30% to 32% or lower
      d. The IUD (IUCD) is partially expelled
      e. The patient wants the IUD (IUCD) removed

4. Cramping and pelvic pain
   a. Rule out ectopic pregnancy
      i. Obtain a serum pregnancy test
      ii. Consider ultrasound and surgical consult (physician consult)
   b. Pain or cramping caused by or associated with
      i. Partial expulsion of IUD (IUCD)
         a) Remove IUD (IUCD)
      ii. PID (a long-standing, foul-smelling discharge in an IUD [IUCD] wearer is presumed to be PID until proven otherwise)
         a) Remove IUD (IUCD)
         b) Treat infection, culture, and sensitivity at time of removal and adjust treatment as indicated
         c) Consult a physician prior to inserting another IUD (IUCD; some sources advise waiting a year)
      iii. Spontaneous abortion
5. Migraine headache
   a. First time or focal migraine with asymmetrical vision loss or other symptoms of transient cerebral ischemia, consult with a physician
6. Expulsion
   a. Objective findings when the cervix is visualized
      i. The IUD (IUCD) is seen at the cervical os or in the vagina
      ii. The IUD (IUCD) string is lengthened (partial expulsion)
      iii. The IUD (IUCD) string is absent (complete expulsion)
      iv. The IUD (IUCD) cannot be located using various methods of probing (physician consult)
      v. The IUD (IUCD) is absent on ultrasound of abdomen
   b. Removal and reinsertion of IUD (IUCD)
      i. If partial expulsion occurs, IUD (IUCD) should be removed. IUD (IUCD) may be reinserted immediately if there is no infection or possibility of pregnancy, or with the next menses.
      ii. If completely expelled, a new IUD (IUCD) may be reinserted as outlined previously.
7. Lost IUD (IUCD) strings
   a. Referrals for locating IUD (IUCD) include
      i. Exploration of canal with gentle probing; if not found, then,
      ii. Ultrasound,
      iii. Flat plate of abdomen, or
      iv. Hysterosalpingogram
8. Difficulty in removing IUD (IUCD)
   The following techniques may help in the removal of IUD (IUCD):
   a. Remove only during menses

    b. Employ gentle, steady traction; remove IUD (IUCD) slowly. If IUD (IUCD) does not come out easily, physician consult is in order.

    c. If IUD (IUCD) strings are not visible, nurse practitioner may probe for them in the cervical canal with narrow forceps.

  9. Uterine perforation (fundal or cervical), embedding of the IUD (IUCD)

    a. Objective findings include

      i. Absence of IUD (IUCD) string

      ii. Inability to withdraw IUD (IUCD) if string is still present

      iii. Demonstration of displaced IUD (IUCD) by ultrasound, hysteroscopy, or X-ray

    b. If perforation or embedding is suspected, referral to physician is in order

    c. Reinforcement of education that multiple partners increase the risk of infection, including HIV infection

VI. FOLLOW-UP

  A. Yearly Pap smear per ASCCP guidelines and pelvic examination with removal and reinsertion as the particular IUD (IUCD) requires (Mirena: 5 years; ParaGard T 380A: 10 years)

  B. As needed for any of previously mentioned complications with physician consultation as necessary

Appendix A may be photocopied for your patients as an informational handout as well as a consent form for using an IUD (IUCD).

See Bibliographies.

Websites: http://www.paragard.com; http://www.mirena.com; http://www.asccp.org

NATURAL FAMILY PLANNING[7]

I. DEFINITION

Natural family planning is an umbrella term for methods that use naturally occurring fertility signs to determine the fertile and infertile days of the menstrual cycle

II. ETIOLOGY

Effects of hormones on basal body temperature, cervical mucus, the position of the cervix, the cyclical nature of the ovulatory and endometrial cycles, and the physical process of the release of an egg make possible knowledge of occurrence of ovulation

III. BACKGROUND FOR ELECTING THE METHOD

  A. What the patient presents with

    1. Motivation to learn natural signs and symptoms of ovulation for purposes of fertility regulation

    2. Often a history of previous use of other methods of family planning
    3. Failure, dissatisfaction, or lack of harmony in values with other methods
    4. Cultural, ethnic, religious values, and personal beliefs harmonious with natural family planning
    5. Medical contraindications to the use of one or more other methods
  B. Additional background information to be obtained from the patient
    1. Medical/surgical history
    2. Obstetrical history
    3. Gynecologic history including menstrual cycle history
    4. Family planning method currently being used
    5. The patient's knowledge about the female human body, especially the ovulation cycle
    6. Family history

IV. PHYSICAL EXAMINATION
  A. Vital signs
    1. Temperature
    2. Pulse
    3. BP
  B. Complete physical examination
  C. External examination of genitalia
  D. Vaginal examination using a speculum to observe position of cervix and mucus
  E. Bimanual examination, noting
    1. Adnexal pain
    2. Masses
    3. Tenderness

V. LABORATORY TEST
  A. Pap smear if none within past year; cultures, wet mount as appropriate or per protocol
  B. Mammography as recommended

VI. DIFFERENTIAL DIAGNOSIS
  A. Preference for other methods

VII. TEACHING ABOUT NATURAL FAMILY PLANNING
  A. Fertility awareness
  B. General introduction to natural family planning
  C. Basic information about natural family planning and methods
    1. Cervical mucus method
    2. Basal body temperature (BBT) method
    3. Symptothermal method
    4. Keeping and interpreting a chart

D. Interpersonal and intimate relationships and natural family planning methods

See Appendix I, Natural Family Planning to Prevent or Achieve Pregnancy.

VIII. COMPLICATIONS
A. Inability of patient to interpret signs and symptoms
B. Lack of acceptability of method to partner
C. Unplanned pregnancy

IX. CONSULTATION/REFERRAL
A. To specialist or program for teaching of natural family planning

X. FOLLOW-UP
A. Annual examination and Pap smear per ASCCP guidelines
B. Evaluation of effectiveness of the method
C. Evaluation of patient satisfaction

See Appendix I and Bibliographies.
Websites: http://www.cyclebeads.com; http://www.asccp.org

STERILIZATION

I. DEFINITION
Sterilization in women is the purposeful occlusion of the fallopian tubes by surgical disruption or occlusion device. Several methods are practiced through closed laparoscopy, open laparoscopy, or suprapubic minilaparotomy. The method of tubal occlusion depends on the surgical route. These occlusion methods include excision of a portion of each tube and suturing of the ends; excision of the fimbriated end; excision of a portion and then suturing of the proximal end into the muscle of the uterus and the distal end in the broad ligament; banding with Silastic bands (Falope rings, Yoon band) or clips (Hulka-Clemens clip, Filshie clip); ligation of a loop of the tubes with nonabsorbable suture material; and occlusion by bipolar cautery. Another method is transcervical to place Essure tubal occlusion device.

II. BACKGROUND FOR ELECTING STERILIZATION
Decision by the woman to seek permanent sterilization through tubal ligation or occlusion as a means of fertility regulation

III. HISTORY
A. What the woman may present with
   1. History of use of one or more methods of contraception
   2. Dissatisfaction with available methods and/or method failure
   3. Experiencing problems with one or more methods and a decision not to have any more children

      4. Medical contraindications for use of one or more methods
      5. Psychosocial contraindications for use of one or more methods
      6. Desire to have no more children or no children at all; need or desire for permanent method
      7. Premenopause, less than 1 year without a period
  B. Additional information to be obtained
      1. Knowledge about all family planning methods used
      2. Psychosocial and cultural aspects: size of family desired, beliefs about sterilization, family attitudes
      3. Knowledge about the sterilization procedures available and beliefs about reversibility
      4. History of any previous pelvic surgery, partial or total hysterectomy, oophorectomy, salpingectomy, laparoscopy, assisted reproductive procedures, or plastic surgery such as tubal reconstruction
      5. Medical/surgical history, present use of medications
      6. Type of anesthesia for previous surgeries, any untoward effects
      7. Gynecologic and obstetric history: pregnancies, live births, abortions, ectopic pregnancies, endometriosis, uterine anomalies, presence of adhesions, uterine leiomyomas (fibroids)
      8. Menstrual history to the present, last period, premenstrual syndrome (PMS), character of menses and menstrual cycle
      9. Contraceptive use to present and reasons for discontinuation

IV. PHYSICAL EXAMINATION
  A. Vital signs
      1. BP
      2. Pulse
  B. General physical exam: lungs, heart, neck, abdomen, breasts, extremities, thyroid
  C. Pelvic examination
      1. External: Skene's glands, Bartholin's glands, urethra, labia, fourchette
      2. Vaginal examination: walls, discharge, cervix; inspect for cystocele, rectocele, urethrocele
      3. Uterus: masses, tenderness, enlargement, possible pregnancy
      4. Adnexa: masses, tenderness, palpable ovaries or tubes, enlargement

V. LABORATORY (FOR PREOPERATIVE WORKUP ONLY OR FOR SYMPTOMS OF PROBLEM)
  A. Urinalysis, culture if signs of urinary tract infection
  B. Complete blood count
  C. Pregnancy test
  D. Gonorrhea culture
  E. *Chlamydia* test
  F. Pap smear

VI. DIFFERENTIAL
None

VII. TREATMENT
A. Teaching
 1. Methods of sterilization and possible failure
 2. Chance of future reversal; choice of method of sterilization related to this
 3. Information on informed consent
 4. Risks and benefits
 5. Discussion of regret
 6. Information on waiting period
 7. Postoperative implications (i.e., restrictions)
 8. Sexual adjustments following procedure
 9. Information on possible posttubal ligation syndrome

VIII. COMPLICATIONS
Conditions contraindicating procedure or choice of procedure such as previous surgery or extensive adhesions; allergy or untoward response to anesthesia

IX. CONSULTATION/REFERRAL
To clinician who performs tubal ligations if the procedure is not offered in the practice setting

X. FOLLOW-UP
A. Postoperative care

See Bibliographies.
Website: http://www.essure.com

Sterilization: Postoperative Care

I. DEFINITION
Follow-up care after the completion of sterilization by tubal ligation or occlusion; time of follow-up will vary depending on the procedure performed

II. ETIOLOGY
A. Transabdominal surgical procedure: ligation and resection, electro-
 coagulation
B. Laparoscopy and electrocoagulation, clips or rings
C. Transcervical tubal occlusion: Essure microplugs

III. HISTORY
A. Type of procedure done, date of the procedure, anesthesia used
B. Any sutures to be removed

    C. Menstruation: last menstrual period, character
    D. Resumption of sexual activity, response; change in sexual habits
    E. What patient may present with:
       1. Pain, fever, bleeding, or discharge from operative site
       2. Abdominal pain, pelvic pain, shoulder pain
       3. Vaginal discharge
       4. Urinary symptoms: frequency, dysuria, hematuria
       5. Any new symptoms/concerns with menstrual cycle not experienced prior to tubal ligation such as endocrine manifestations

IV. PHYSICAL EXAMINATION
    A. Vital signs
       1. BP
       2. Pulse
       3. Temperature
    B. Abdominal examination
       1. Inspection: incision site(s) if any
       2. Auscultation: bowel sounds, hyperactive, or hypoactive
       3. Palpation: tenderness, guarding, masses
    C. Pelvic examination
       1. Uterus: tender, enlarged, masses, fixed or mobile; pain on cervical manipulation
       2. Adnexa: masses, tenderness

V. LABORATORY
    A. Cervical culture if fever, uterine, or adnexal tenderness is present (gonorrhea, *Chlamydia*)
    B. Urinalysis and culture if there are signs of urinary tract infection
    C. Complete blood count (CBC), differential, sedimentation rate, and/or C-reactive protein if with fever, tenderness
    D. Pregnancy test if uterus is enlarged or with adnexal mass, signs of ectopic pregnancy present

VI. DIFFERENTIAL DIAGNOSIS
    A. Urinary tract infection
    B. Perforation of bowel
    C. Pelvic infection
    D. Salpingitis
    E. Peritonitis
    F. Tubal hemorrhage
    G. Problems with sexual expression; lack of libido, unresponsiveness

VII. TREATMENT
As indicated by symptoms and diagnosis

VIII. COMPLICATIONS
    A. Hemorrhage
    B. Increased risk of ectopic pregnancy

C. Perforation of bowel
D. Pelvic inflammatory disease
E. Urinary tract infection syndrome
F. Salpingitis
G. Infection of incision site(s)
H. Pelvic abscess
I. Peritonitis
J. Bladder damage burns with electrocoagulation
K. Uterine perforation
L. Posttubal ligation
M. Regrets

IX. CONSULTATION/REFERRAL
A. Consultation/referral to surgeon for differential diagnosis and treatment of any problem
B. Referral for mental health counseling if experiencing sexual maladjustment, regrets

X. FOLLOW-UP
A. Return for recheck after resolution of any complications
B. Age-appropriate annual exam including Pap smear per ASCCP guidelines

See Bibliographies.
Website: http://www.managingcontraception.com

NOTES

1. Emergency contraception is indicated for 120 hours; efficacy rates are based on pills taken within 72 hours.
2. Consult individual method package insert.
3. Some concerns have been raised about the patch because of higher exposure to estrogen as compared to most birth control pills. FDA labeling has been changed to indicate this. Clinicians should keep up to date with the American College of Obstetricians and Gynecologists (ACOG) news releases at www.acog.org/from_home/newsrel.cfm or check www.drugs.com/pro/depo-provera.html
4. U.S. Boxed Warning: Prolonged use of medroxyprogesterone contraceptive injection may result in a loss of bone mineral density (BMD). Loss is related to the duration of use, and may not be completely reversible on discontinuation of the drug. The impact on peak bone mass in adolescents should be considered in treatment decisions. U.S. Boxed Warning: Long-term use (i.e., >2 years) should be limited to situations where other birth control methods are inadequate. Consider other methods of birth control in women with (or at risk for) osteoporosis. Retrieved from http://www.rxlist.com/depo_provera-drug.htm

5. K. M. Curtis, D. J. Jamieson, H. B. Peterson, & P. Marchbanks (2010). Adaptation of the World Health Organization's medical eligibility criteria for contraceptive use for use in the United States. *Contraception, 82*(1), 3–9; M. E. Gaffield & K. R. Culwell (2010).
6. New recommendations on the safety of contraceptive methods for women with medical conditions: World Health Organization's medical eligibility criteria for contraceptive use, fourth edition. *IPPF Medical Bulletin, 44*(1), 1–5.
7. The natural family planning guideline was developed by the late Eleanor Tabeek, RN, PhD, CNM, and is used with her permission and that of her family. Updates for subsequent editions by Nancy Keaveney, RN, BS, and for this edition, by Mary Finnigan, BA, MA.

Preconception Care

8

I. DEFINITION
Advanced planning aimed at reducing maternal and perinatal mortality and morbidity[1]

II. ETIOLOGY
A. Reasons for promoting preconception care (PCC) include:
   1. Maximize healthy life for woman and baby
   2. Identify any medical condition or medications in either prospective parent
   3. Identify genetic disorders
   4. Review past gestational and pregnancy history
   5. Identify high-risk exposures (e.g., tobacco, drug, and alcohol use) and environmental hazards (e.g., toxins, chemicals, including pesticides, gases, foods)

III. HISTORY
A. Woman's medical and surgical history, including but not limited to:
   1. Diabetes
   2. Phenylketonuria (PKU)
   3. Cardiovascular, including elevated blood pressure
   4. Lung
   5. Thyroid
   6. Kidney
   7. Infectious diseases (e.g., HIV, hepatitis B and C, toxoplasmosis, rubella, varicella, tuberculosis [TB], sexually transmitted diseases [STDs], vaginosis, vaginitis)
   8. Autoimmune diseases
   9. Connective tissue disorders
   10. Eating disorders
   11. Metabolic conditions
   12. Psychiatric illness or mental health issues
   13. Epilepsy
   14. Thromboembolic episodes
   15. Any surgery
   16. Diethylstilbestrol (DES) exposure
   17. Allergies
B. Obstetric and gynecologic history
   1. Contraception
   2. Menstrual history
   3. Gynecologic history
   4. Pap smear history
   5. High-risk behaviors (including STDs)
   6. Pregnancy history, including spontaneous abortion and therapeutic abortion
C. Immune status: need to have documentation
   1. Rubella
   2. TB

3. Hepatitis A, B, and C
4. Varicella
5. Tetanus if $\geq$ 10 years
6. Polio
7. Influenza
D. Drug history
   1. Current prescription medications: Some medications have different safety periods between cessation and conception
   2. Current over-the-counter medications
   3. Current vitamin and botanical use
   4. "Street" drug–use history
E. Nutritional status
   1. Height and weight, body mass index (BMI)
   2. Eating habits; note especially fad diets, vegan
   3. Food allergies
   4. Caffeine and artificial sweetener intake
   5. History of being overweight or underweight: underweight BMI, less than 19.8 kg/m^2; overweight BMI, greater than 26.1–29.0 kg/m^2; and obese BMI, greater than 29.0 kg/m^2
   6. History of an eating disorder
   7. Current exercise habits and other physical activities
F. Genetic history
   1. May use a genogram to identify couples with a personal or family history of problematic diseases such as:
      a. Tay–Sachs disease
      b. Thalassemia
      c. Sickle-cell disease or trait
      d. PKU
      e. Cystic fibrosis
      f. Hemophilia
      g. Mental retardation
      h. Myotonic dystrophy
      i. Adult polycystic kidney disease
      j. Birth defects
      k. Other anemias
   2. Family background
      a. Related outside marriage
      b. Ethnic background: African American, Mediterranean, Ashkenazi Jew, and Asian
G. Exposure to teratogenic toxins; areas of concern include:
   1. Exposure to
      a. Metals (lead)
      b. Organic solvents
      c. Gases
      d. Ionizing radiation
      e. Pollutants (e.g., secondhand smoke)
      f. Pesticides, herbicides

      g. Lead paint
      h. Plastics, vinyl monomers
      i. Hyperthermia
    2. Consumption of
      a. Alcohol
      b. Cigarette smoke
      c. Street drugs
  H. Social history
    1. Age
    2. Marital/partner status
    3. Family structure; household composition
    4. Support systems
    5. Employment/financial status
    6. Cultural beliefs
    7. Child care issues
    8. Safety issues (e.g., spousal/partner abuse)
    9. Work history: exposure to chemicals, radiation, standing at work, and occupational risks such as not wearing respirator, mask, and special clothing
  I. Partner health history
    Thorough health/genetic/social history should be taken on prospective fathers. Little conclusive research has been done on how partner's exposures to chemicals/toxins/drugs may affect fetal development. Recent studies have indicated that alcohol consumption in the month prior to conception contributes to low spermatogenesis. Findings need to be integrated with maternal health history findings.

IV. PHYSICAL EXAMINATION
  A. Baseline height, weight, BMI, and vital signs
  B. General physical examination, including pelvic examination
  C. Comprehensive exam based on medical history

V. LABORATORY
  A. Pap smear as indicated per ASCCP guidelines
  B. Baseline studies may be considered, including
    1. Blood Rh and type
    2. Hemoglobin/hematocrit
    3. Urinalysis
    4. Rapid plasma reagin (RPR) test/venereal disease research laboratory (VDRL)
    5. Check status for
      a. Hepatitis B, C
      b. Varicella
      c. Rubella
      d. HIV
      e. TB

6. Based on history, check
   a. Toxoplasmosis
   b. Cytomegalovirus (CMV)
7. GC, *Chlamydia*, wet mount, mycoplasma, and ureaplasma

VI. EDUCATION
A. Begin at least 1 month prior to planned conception
   1. Avoid environmental toxins
   2. Cease smoking and alcohol consumption and use of street drugs
   3. Begin exercise program (e.g., walking, swimming, cycling): heart rate not to exceed 140 beats per second
   4. Bring immunizations up to date (if live vaccine is used, postpone conception at least one month; Centers for Disease Control and Prevention [CDC] recommendation)
   5. Eat a balanced diet
   6. Start vitamin therapy
      a. 0.4 mg orally of folic acid daily (increase dosage for women who are at increased risk for neural tube defects, or are obese, to 0.8 mg daily; some sources say 5 mg/day)
      b. Increase calcium intake to an equivalent of 1 quart of milk daily (or 1,200–1,500 mg/day)
   7. Avoid or at least decrease caffeine intake
   8. Consult with primary care provider regarding prescription medications (e.g., psychotropics, antihypertensives, anticonvulsants), botanicals, and vitamins
   9. If hemoglobin is < 12 g/dl, add iron to prenatal vitamins.
   10. Women with PKU should start a low phenylalanine diet
   11. Avoid hot tubs and saunas (bringing body temperature above 101 °F can damage the embryo)
   12. Do not empty cat litter box
   13. Do not consume raw meat or raw fish

VII. REFERRAL/CONSULTATION
A. For genetic consultation if indicated
B. Evaluation of prescriptive medication use with specialists
C. Substance abuse counseling if indicated
D. Nutritional counseling if indicated (e.g., obesity, gestational diabetes with prior pregnancies, vegetarian)
E. Community/federal programs for financial assistance if indicated
F. Domestic violence intervention

VIII. FOLLOW-UP
A. Refer for obstetric care if pregnancy occurs (if setting does not provide care)
B. If conception does not occur within 1 year, return for further evaluation/possible referral
C. Consider sooner if older than age 30

Appendix I may be photocopied or adapted for your patients.
See Bibliographies.
   Websites: http://www.cdc.gov/mmwr/preview/mmwrhtml/rr5506a1.htm; http://www.acog.org/departments/dept_notice.cfm?recno=20&bulletin=5155; http://www.marchofdimes.com/Pregnancy/getready_emotional.html

NOTE

1. Ideally, women should consider having a reproductive life plan. *See website*: March of Dimes Reproductive Life Plan at www.centralhealth-center.org/RLP.

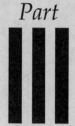

Guidelines for Managing Women's Health Conditions

Breast Conditions

9

ABNORMAL BREAST DISCHARGE

I. DEFINITION
A. Under certain conditions, an abnormal fluid may be expressed from the breast(s) or flow spontaneously
B. Up to 50% of women in their reproductive years may express discharge when the nipple is compressed
C. Most nipple discharge is associated with a benign process, but malignancy should be ruled out with all new onset of nipple discharge
D. Pathologic versus physiologic discharge
    1. Pathologic discharge is likely:
        a. Spontaneous
        b. From a single duct
        c. Persistent
        d. Contains gross or occult blood
    2. Physiologic discharge is likely:
        a. With compression only
        b. From multiple ducts
        c. Resolves when refraining from compression
        d. Nonbloody (milky, clear, green, brown)

II. ETIOLOGY
A. Physiologic causes
    1. Pregnancy, puerperium
    2. Intercourse
    3. Stimulation of the breast
    4. Chest wall surgery or trauma
    5. Exercise
    6. Emotional stress
    7. Sleep (affects measurable amounts of prolactin)
B. Pharmacologic causes
    1. Numerous psychotropic drugs
    2. Cimetidine
    3. Some antihypertensives
    4. Opiates
    5. Estrogens/oral contraceptives/progestins
    6. Antiemetics
    7. Alcohol (chronic abuse)
    8. Marijuana
    9. Danazol
    10. Isoniazid (INH)
C. Pathologic causes
    1. Benign intraductal papilloma
    2. Ductal ectasia
    3. Breast tumor
    4. Pituitary tumor

5. Hypothalamic tumor
6. Infections
7. Empty sella syndrome
8. Hypothyroidism
9. Polycystic ovarian syndrome (PCOS)

III. HISTORY
A. What the patient may present with
1. Breast discharge
2. Amenorrhea
3. Possibly pain
4. Possibly mass
5. Possibly localized heat and swelling
6. Possibly nipple retraction
7. Possibly no symptoms (discharge can be an incidental finding of breast exam)
B. Additional information to be considered
1. Elicited versus spontaneous
2. Unilateral versus bilateral
3. Number of ducts involved (one vs. multiple ducts)
4. Color of discharge
5. Duration of discharge
6. Last menstrual period
7. Headaches
8. Sexual activity
9. Birth control method, hormone therapy
10. Medications or illegal drugs currently being used
11. Medications recently taken
12. Recent pregnancy (within 1 year), regardless of outcome
13. Exercise program (e.g., jogging)
14. Nipple stimulation (e.g., fondling, sucking)
15. Recent trauma to chest or surgery
16. Chronic illness (e.g., thyroid disease, psychiatric illness)
17. Lifestyle changes (e.g., increased stress)
18. Alcohol consumption (chronic abuse)
19. Family history of breast disease
20. Breast pain or tenderness
21. Breast surgery (biopsy, reduction, augmentation, and implants)

IV. PHYSICAL EXAMINATION
A. Complete examination as described in the section on Breast Mass.
B. Closely examine the nipple
1. Palpate nipple by compressing nipple areola with thumb and index finger, gently milking the subareolar ducts from just outside the apex of the papilla. Repeat moving around the nipple in a clockwise direction. Pay close attention to the position of the duct(s) that produce discharge.

2. If discharge is expressed, note the following:
    a. Location of duct(s)
    b. Color
    c. Unilateral versus bilateral
    d. Guaiac test all discharge for occult blood
    e. Cytology of discharge is not recommended (likely to be inaccurate and may confuse workup).
C. Thyroid—palpate for nodes, size
D. Bimanual examination
    1. Ovarian irregularity or enlargement
    2. Uterine enlargement

V. LABORATORY EXAMINATION
A. Guaiac test all discharge for occult blood
B. Cytology of discharge is not recommended (likely to be inaccurate and may confuse workup)
C. Prolactin level: sample should be drawn between 8 and 10 a.m. (literature indicates prolactin level is lowest between 8 and 10 a.m. but not directly after gynecologic examination, intercourse, exercise, or breast stimulation including breast examination)
D. Thyroid panel
E. Mammogram from women older than age 30
F. Subareolar ultrasound
G. Serum pregnancy test if indicated

VI. DIFFERENTIAL DIAGNOSIS (*see Etiology, II*)

VII. TREATMENT
As needed according to laboratory report and etiology

VIII. COMPLICATIONS
Vary by individual, according to diagnosis

IX. CONSULTATION/REFERRAL
A. Refer to endocrinology
B. Refer subareolar ultrasound
    1. Abnormal lab results
    2. Lack of definitive diagnosis
C. Refer to breast specialist for consideration of biopsy or duct excision
    1. Abnormal imaging findings
    2. Additional suspicious clinical exam findings
    3. All spontaneous, unilateral, and/or bloody nipple discharge
    4. Lack of definitive diagnosis
D. When in doubt, consider referral to breast specialist

X. FOLLOW-UP
  A. Repeat laboratory work as indicated in *Abnormal Breast Discharge, V.*
  B. In the case of physiologic nipple discharge, encourage patients to stop squeezing/stimulating their nipples. Discharge may reduce with reduced stimulation.
  C. Reevaluate patient in 4 to 6 weeks to confirm stability of clinical exam findings. Refer women with persistent symptoms.

See Bibliographies.

BREAST MASS

I. DEFINITION
A breast mass is a thickening or lump that is felt in a woman's breast, which may or may not have the following characteristics:
  A. Nipple retraction
  B. Discharge from nipple
  C. Skin dimpling
  D. Inflammation or discoloration
  E. Skin thickening
  F. Palpable axillary or supraclavicular nodes
  G. Tenderness
  H. Change in the size of the breast

II. ETIOLOGY
  A. *Fibrocystic disease*—catch-all term for nonmalignant conditions
  B. Fibroadenoma
  C. Carcinoma
  D. Mammary duct ectasia
  E. Intraductal papilloma
  F. Normal premenstrual breast tissue (i.e., with tenderness and prominent breast tissue secondary to hormone levels—physiologic nodularity, mastoplasia)
  G. Mastitis (cellulitis, skin boils, abscess)
  H. Cysts
  I. Hematoma or fat necrosis
  J. Superficial phlebitis
  K. Phyllodes tumors—painless, solid, smooth, lobular, bulky, stromal hyperplasia

III. HISTORY
  A. Woman may present with
    1. Lump
    2. Pain
    3. Swelling
    4. Redness, edema

5. Bruised area that does not resolve
6. Discharge from nipple
7. Nipple retraction
8. Change in appearance of skin and areola
9. Dimpling, scaliness

B. Additional information to be considered

1. Last menstrual period (Has patient noticed a relationship to menses?)
2. History of previous breast lumps or breast disease, biopsy (type) or aspiration; breast surgery including reduction, enlargement, implants, and type
3. Recent trauma (may cause hematoma or fat necrosis)
4. Recent weight loss (significant weight loss may change the texture of the breasts because of reduced adipose tissue)
5. Birth control method(s) used: hormone therapy (type, dose, duration) and how soon after menopause
6. Recent pregnancy, lactation

C. Risk factors

1. Nonmodifiable risk factors
   a. Gender (breast cancer occurs 100 times more frequently in women than men)
   b. Age (risk increases as women age)
   c. Genetics
      i. 5% to 10% of breast cancers are thought to be hereditary.
      ii. BRCA1 and BRCA2 (most common cause of hereditary breast cancer is an inherited mutation in the BRCA1 and BRCA2 genes)
         a) Risk of breast cancer may be as high as 80% for some families
         b) Cancers tend to occur in younger women and, more often, affect both breasts
         c) Mutation carriers are more likely to develop other cancers, especially ovarian cancer
         d) Mutations are most common in families of Ashkenazi descent but can occur in any racial or ethnic group
      iii. In women who do not carry a mutation, breast cancer risk doubles with one first-degree relative with breast cancer and triples with two first-degree relatives with breast cancer
      iv. Risk increases with family history of male breast cancer
      v. Personal history of previous breast cancer
      vi. Race and ethnicity (risk varies by group)
      vii. Dense breast tissue on mammography
      viii. History of previous biopsy (especially showing proliferative lesions, lesions with atypia, and lobular carcinoma in situ)

      ix. Menstrual periods (early menarche—before age 12 and late menopause—after age 55—increase risk because of lifetime exposure to estrogen)

      x. Previous chest wall radiation (treatment for Hodgkin lymphoma or non-Hodgkin lymphoma as child or young adult significantly increases risk)

      xi. Diethylstilbestrol exposure (mothers have slightly increased risk)

  2. Modifiable risk factors

    a. Late childbearing (after age 30 or nulliparity)

    b. Recent oral contraceptive use (within past 10 years)

    c. Hormone therapy after menopause (especially combined hormone therapy)

    d. Breastfeeding (may slightly *lower* risk)

    e. Alcohol (risk increases with amount of alcohol consumed)

    f. Being overweight (excess adipose tissue produces excess estrogen), physical activity (risk *decreases* with increased activity)

IV. PHYSICAL EXAMINATION

  A. Breast physical examination

    1. Ideal time to examine breasts is 1 week after first day of menstrual cycle

    2. Examine in both upright and supine positions

    3. Include the neck, chest wall, both breasts, and axillae in examination

    4. Examine regional lymph nodes (axillary and supra/infraclavicular)

    5. Begin with inspection and then palpation

  B. Inspect for the following:

    1. New asymmetry of breasts

    2. Skin changes such as dimpling, retraction, erythema, or discoloration

    3. Nipple changes such as retraction, nipple scaling, excoriation, or spontaneous discharge

  C. Palpate for the following:

    1. Solitary or multiple lesion(s)

    2. Consistency of any mass (rubbery vs. firm)

    3. Boarders of any mass (smooth vs. irregular)

    4. Size of any mass (in centimeters)

    5. Tenderness of mass

    6. Movable or fixed on chest wall

    7. Displacement or retraction of nipple

    8. Retraction or dimpling of skin overlying mass

    9. Palpability of regional lymph nodes (axillary or supra/infraclavicular)

    10. Discharge expressed: color, amount, unilateral or bilateral, consistency

    11. Express breast for any discharge if none is noted on palpation

   C. Document findings
1. Symmetry of breasts (If there is an asymmetry, is it baseline or new?)
2. Appearance of skin (dimpling, retraction, or discoloration)
3. Appearance of nipple (retraction, scaling)
4. If present, describe nipple discharge (spontaneous vs. elicited, color, amount, unilateral or bilateral)
5. If present, describe palpable mass (position on breast using numbers on a clock, distance from nipple in centimeters, size of lesion in centimeters, and consistency and borders)

V. LABORATORY EXAMINATION
   A. Bilateral diagnostic mammogram (if older than age 30)
   B. Targeted ultrasound of area of concern
   C. If discharge is present, guaiac test all discharge for occult blood

VI. DIFFERENTIAL (*see Etiology, II*)

VII. TREATMENT
   A. Medication
1. Appropriate antibiotic for mastitis, abscess
   B. General measures
1. If a suspicious mass is identified, arrange consult with breast specialist (*see Consultation/Referral, IX*)
2. If a benign appearing mass is identified on imaging, consider consult with breast specialist for further guidance
3. If no discrete lesion is identified on clinical exam or imaging, have the patient return 1 week after next menses for reevaluation and possible referral (4–6 weeks for postmenopausal women).

VIII. COMPLICATIONS
May be grave and extensive if misdiagnosed

IX. CONSULTATION/REFERRAL
   A. The following lesions should be referred immediately to breast specialist for consideration of biopsy:
1. Any abnormal findings on imaging
2. Dominant mass despite negative imaging
3. Mass associated with nipple retraction or nipple discharge
4. Dimpling of skin; orange peel appearance to skin
5. Inflammation, swelling, scaling, or excoriation
6. Palpable axillary or supra/infraclavicular nodes
7. Cystic mass; for possible aspiration
   B. The following should be referred to breast specialist upon reevaluation:
1. Developing/increasing mass despite negative imaging
2. Increase in associated symptoms
   C. When in doubt, always refer

X. FOLLOW-UP
A. Appropriate to *Treatment*, **VII** and *Consultation/Referral*, **IX**

See Bibliographies.

BREAST PAIN

I. DEFINITION
A. Background
   1. Breast pain is the most common symptom among women seeking consultation
   2. Breast pain alone is rarely the presenting symptom in women diagnosed with breast cancer
   3. However, up to 7% of women with newly diagnosed breast cancer presented with breast pain as their only symptom
B. Cyclic breast pain
   1. Begins during luteal phase and resolves with menses
   2. Usually bilateral with no focal concern
   3. Most common in younger women
C. Noncyclic breast pain
   1. Does not correlate with menstrual cycle
   2. May be unilateral or focal
   3. More common in women ages 40 to 50
D. Referred pain
   1. Referred pain from sites outside the breast

II. ETIOLOGY
A. Cyclic breast pain
   1. Fibrocystic breast tissue (dense, cystic tissue)
   2. Hormonal fluctuations associated with the menstrual cycle
B. Noncyclic breast pain
   1. Breast mass
   2. Breast cyst
   3. Mastitis
   4. Weight gain
   5. Trauma (hematoma or fat necrosis may be present)
   6. Caffeine (controversial)
   7. Exogenous hormone use
   8. Dermal lesions
   9. Pregnancy
C. Extramammary (referred) pain
   1. Musculoskeletal
      a. Chest wall muscle pain (recent trauma; overuse from repetitive movement)
      b. Costochondritis
      c. Rib pain

  2. Nerve pain
  3. Cardiopulmonary origins (especially on left sided pain)

III. HISTORY
  A. What women may present with
  1. Pain
  2. Lump
  3. Swelling
  4. Redness—bruised area that does not resolve
  5. Discharge from nipple
  6. Nipple retraction
  7. Change in appearance of skin and areola
  8. Dimpling, scaliness
  B. Additional information to be considered
  1. Is the pain unilateral or bilateral?
  2. Is the pain focal or diffused?
  3. Does the pain correlate with the menstrual cycle?
  4. Is the woman perimenopausal?
  5. Does she feel a mass?
  6. Erythema, warmth, swelling, fever
  7. Was there any recent trauma?
  8. Has the woman gained weight?
  9. Exogenous hormone use
  10. Recent pregnancy or nursing

IV. PHYSICAL EXAM (*see Breast Mass, IV*)

V. LABORATORY EXAMINATION
  A. Diagnostic mammogram (if older than age 30)
  B. Targeted ultrasound of area of concern if pain is focal
  C. If discharge is present, guaiac test all discharge for occult blood

VI. DIFFERENTIAL (*see Etiology, II*)

VII. TREATMENT
  A. If clinical or imaging findings are suspicious, refer to breast specialist
  B. If a large cyst is seen, refer to breast specialist for aspiration
  C. If mastitis is present
  1. Trial of antibiotics
  2. Refer for incision and drainage if necessary
  3. Ultrasound for evaluation of potential fluid collection to be aspirated
  4. Cultures should be sent if infection is suspected
  D. If clinical exam and imaging are negative, offer reassurance (likelihood of malignancy is low)

E. For women with a negative workup, offer relief recommendations
1. Nonsteroidal anti-inflammatory drugs (NSAIDs)
2. Well-fitting bra (sports bra, wearing at night may be helpful)
3. Eliminate caffeine (may be placebo but helps with some women)
4. Weight reduction
5. Reduce/eliminate exogenous hormones
6. Vitamin E and evening primrose oil (inconclusive, likely placebo)
7. Medical treatment (danazol, tamoxifen) can be considered for severe persistent pain that interferes with daily activities but should be offered only under the guidance of a breast specialist

VIII. COMPLICATIONS
A. Anxiety related to breast pain
B. Pain may impact daily activities
C. Evaluation may result in identification of suspicious lesion

IX. CONSULTATION/REFERRAL
A. If clinical or imaging findings are suspicious, refer to breast specialist
B. If a large cyst is seen, refer to breast specialist for aspiration to reduce discomfort
C. All mastitis/cellulitis that do not resolve
D. Mastitis/cellulitis that is severe or extensive at presentation
E. Referral to plastic surgery for women with large breasts who are considering reduction
F. When in doubt, refer to breast specialist

X. FOLLOW-UP
A. Reevaluate patient after next menstrual cycle (or in 6 weeks for postmenopausal women) to confirm stability of exam findings and discuss benefit of relief measures
1. Refer patients who have a change in their clinical exam
2. Refer patients with significant persistent pain to breast specialist for further recommendations
B. Continue to follow all mastitis/cellulitis to resolution. Refer patients who do not respond quickly to antibiotics or who have extensive infection at presentation

See Bibliographies.

Cervical Aberrations

10

CERVICITIS

I. DEFINITION
A. Chronic or acute inflammation of the cervix that is visible to the clinician. Causes symptoms observed by the woman and/or by cytologic examination.
B. Mucopurulent cervicitis is characterized by mucopurulent exudate and easily induced cervical bleeding. Centers for Disease Control and Prevention (CDC) sexually transmitted disease (STD) guidelines: http://www.cdc.gov/std/treatment/2010

II. ETIOLOGY
A. Bacterial
1. *Neisseria gonorrhoeae*
2. Mycoplasmas such as *Mycoplasma genitalium*
3. Ureaplasmas
4. *Chlamydia trachomatis*
5. Bacterial vaginosis
B. Viral
1. Herpes simplex
2. Human papillomavirus (HPV)
C. Parasitic
1. *Trichomonas vaginalis*
D. Nonmicrobiologic
1. Inflammation in zone of ectopy
2. DES exposure
3. Chemical irritants
4. Frequent douching

III. HISTORY
A. What the patient may present with
1. No symptoms
2. Friable cervix
3. Postcoital bleeding
4. Erythema of cervix (if friable with first pass of swab)
5. Edematous cervix
6. Ulcerated or eroded cervix
7. Hypertrophied cervix
8. Ectropion
9. Cervical discharge; may be purulent or mucopurulent endocervical exudate on exam
10. Vaginal discharge
11. Leukoplakia on cervix
12. Endocervical bleeding
B. Additional information to be considered
1. Onset of symptoms
2. Partner with symptoms

3. History of sexually transmitted diseases
4. Sexual lifestyle; use of sex toys
5. Last Pap smear and results; any history of abnormal Pap smear result
6. Contraception past and present
7. Colposcopy, cone biopsy, cauterization of cervix, cryo, LEEP
8. Laceration of cervix: childbirth, abortion, dilation and curettage (D&C), biopsy, sex toys, partner with genital jewelry
9. Pregnancy history, infertility
10. Dyspareunia, pelvic pain
11. Urinary symptoms: frequency, urgency, dysuria
12. Menstrual history: last menstrual period
13. DES exposure

IV. PHYSICAL EXAMINATION
  A. Cervix
    1. Color
    2. Character of any discharge: green, yellow, opaque, white, clear, cloudy, purulent, mucopurulent, serous, pH
    3. Size
    4. Lesions
    5. Friability
    6. Hood
    7. Any polyps noted
  B. Vagina
    1. Color
    2. Erythema
    3. Lesions
    4. Discharge
  C. Bimanual exam
    1. Masses
    2. Tenderness
    3. Cervical motion tenderness
    4. Uterine enlargement
    5. Position of organs
  D. Adenopathy

V. LABORATORY EXAMINATION
  A. Gonorrhea culture
  B. *Chlamydia* smear
  C. Bacterial vaginosis
  D. Trichomoniasis
  E. Wet prep; saline, KOH; >10 WBCs/high power field associated with GC, *Chlamydia*
  F. Pap smear
  G. Culture for bacteria
  H. Gram stain >30 polymorphonuclear (PMN) leukocytes
  I. Serology test for syphilis

  J. Herpes culture, antibodies
  K. Viratyping
  L. HIV testing (this criterion may be helpful but not standardized)

VI. DIFFERENTIAL DIAGNOSIS
  A. Bacterial vaginosis
  B. Trichomoniasis
  C. Condyloma acuminata
  D. Chlamydia
  E. Gonorrhea
  F. Cervical cancer
  G. Cervical infection; bacterial, including mycoplasma, ureaplasma
  H. Ectropion
  I. Leukoplakia
  J. Herpetic exocervicitis
  K. Trichomonas
  L. Cervical ulceration (erosion) because of trauma; fingernail, cervical biopsy, postpartum, sex toys
  M. Pelvic inflammatory disease (PID)
  N. Infection secondary to trauma with sex toy
  O. Cervical polyp

VII. TREATMENT
  A. Medication
    1. As indicated by organism; *see section for gonorrhea,* Chlamydia, *herpes, condyloma, trichomonas, in Chapter 21 and PID in Chapter 17*
    2. Bacterial (mycoplasma, urea plasma); *see PID section in Chapter 17*
    3. Mucopurulent cervicitis (women meeting CDC criteria) without confirmed organism can be treated empirically for gonorrhea and *Chlamydia,* bacterial vaginosis, trichomoniasis
      a. Prevalance of these is high in patient population, such as women younger than or equal to 25 years of age
      b. New or multiple sex partners
      c. Unprotected sexual encounters
      d. Patient might be difficult to locate for treatment
    4. Presumptive treatment—azithromycin 1 g orally in single dose, or doxycycline 100 mg orally twice a day for 7 days, and consider treatment for gonorrhea, bacterial vaginosis, and trichomoniasis per CDC STD guidelines (*see Chapter 21*)
  B. Other measures
    1. Ectropion—evaluate Pap smear results and follow-up as indicated; document with diagram and description for later follow-up; with persistent friability, refer or evaluate with colposcopy and biopsy
    2. Leukoplakia—refer or evaluate with colposcopy and biopsy
    3. Cervical cancer—refer for medical evaluation and intervention; in suspected cases despite negative Pap smear, refer or evaluate with colposcopy and biopsy

4. Cervical ulceration, erosion—follow-up as indicated by extent and nature of trauma; consider referral for medical evaluation and intervention

5. Consider colposcopy for all women who do not meet CDC guidelines for mucopurulent cervicitis, have a negative STD screen, and negative Pap smear

6. Manage sex partners appropriate for identified or suspected STD

7. Patients and sex partners abstain from sexual intercourse for course of treatment 7 days after single-dose regimen or completion of 7-day regimen

VIII. COMPLICATIONS
Progression of condition to secondary or systemic infection (depending on organism) or PID; to metastatic disease; infertility; cervical stenosis

IX. CONSULTATION/REFERRAL
A. Unable to evaluate and diagnose
B. No response to treatment; persistent symptoms with poor response to treatment

X. FOLLOW-UP
A. Repeat testing of all women with positive *Chlamydia* or gonorrhea in 3 to 6 months
B. As indicated by condition and treatment
C. Return for reevaluation if symptoms persist

See Bibliographies.
Website: http://www.mayoclinic.com/health/cervicitis/DS00518

PAP SMEAR AND COLPOSCOPY

I. DEFINITION
The Pap smear is collected from exfoliated cells in the endocervix and on the portia to detect preinvasive lesions (e.g., dysplasia, carcinoma in situ), as well as invasive lesions
A. History
1. DES exposure in utero
2. Smoking; exposure to passive smoke
3. Previous abnormal Pap smear; cervical treatment
4. HPV, other sexually transmitted diseases
5. Sexual practices, partners (number, partner[s] had previous partner[s] with abnormal Paps, partner's sexual history)
6. Family history of cervical cancer; personal history of cancer
7. Age of beginning sexual activity
8. Immunosuppressive therapy; immunosuppression
9. HIV/AIDS or risk

10. Hormone use
11. Per American College of Obstetricians and Gynecologists (ACOG), American Cancer Society, or guidelines for practice setting

III. TECHNIQUE

A. Cytologic specimens may be obtained prior to the bimanual pelvic exam; a nonlubricated speculum must be used (speculum can be warmed with water)
B. May do a palpation of the vagina and cervix to locate the cervix and identify the position of the os
C. The cervix and vagina must be fully visible when the smear is obtained to see entire squamocolumnar junction
D. Vaginal discharge, when present in large amounts, should be carefully removed with a large swab prior to obtaining the smear. Small amount of blood should not preclude cytologic sampling.
E. Both liquid-based and conventional methods of cervical cytology screening are acceptable for screening. Exfoliated cells are collected from the transformation zone of the cervix, and may be transferred to a vial of liquid preservative that is processed in the laboratory to produce a slide for interpretation—the liquid based technique—or may be transferred directly to the slide and fixed using the conventional method.
   1. With the liquid-based technology, ThinPrep Pap test, the sample is collected on a broom-type cervical sampling device. Rotate this device 5 times in the same direction while applying soft pressure on the cervix. Detach the broom head and deposit into the liquid solution. Alternatively, a plastic spatula is applied to the entire cervix to include the entire squamocolumnar junction. A cyto brush is inserted into the endocervix and rotated half turn, removed, and both are rinsed in a vial of preserving solution and discarded. The vial is capped, labeled, and sent to the laboratory.
   2. Liquid based technology, SurePath, CytoRich, is preformed the same as in *E.1*, except the devices are left in the solution, snapping off the handles. The vial is capped, labeled, and sent to the laboratory.
   3. Conventional method technology is preformed the same as *E.1*, except the spatula and cyto brush are used, and the material is rolled onto the slide, without clumping both sides of the spatula, roll brush on the slide with immediate fixation (within 10 seconds) to prevent drying, is required (spray 9"–12" away). In some settings, the handle of the spatula is used to sample the vaginal pool prior to sampling the cervix.
F. For DES-exposed women, additional slides are prepared using smear taken from the upper two-thirds of the vagina at its circumferences. Gentle wiping of the vaginal wall mucosa initially to remove discharge increases the diagnostic accuracy.

IV. BETHESDA 2001 TERMINOLOGY FOR PAP SMEARS
  A. Specimen adequacy
   1. Satisfactory for evaluation (note endocervical/transformation zone component)
   2. Unsatisfactory for evaluation (specify reason)
   3. Specimen rejected/not processed (specify reason)
   4. Specimen processed and examined, but unsatisfactory for evaluation of epithelial abnormality because of (specify reason)
  B. General categorization
   1. Negative for intraepithelial lesion or malignancy
   2. Epithelial cell abnormality
   3. Other
  C. Interpretation/result
   1. Negative for intraepithelial lesion or malignancy
   2. Organisms
      a. Trichomonas vaginalis
      b. Fungal organisms morphologically consistent with Candida species
      c. Shift in flora, suggestive of bacterial vaginosis
      d. Bacteria morphologically consistent with *Actinomyces* genus
      e. Cellular changes consistent with herpes simplex virus
      f. Other non-neoplastic findings
      g. Reactive cellular changes associated with inflammation (includes typical repair) radiation
      h. Intrauterine contraceptive device
      i. Glandular cells status posthysterectomy
      j. Atrophy
   3. Epithelial cell abnormalities
      a. Squamous cell
      b. Atypical squamous cells (ASC) of undetermined significance (ASC-US) cannot exclude HSIL (ASC-H).
   4. Low-grade squamous intraepithelial lesion (LSIL)
      a. Encompassing: HPV/mild dysplasia/cervical intraepithelial neoplasia (CIN) 1
   5. High-grade squamous intraepithelial lesion (HSIL)
      a. Encompassing—moderate and severe dysplasia, carcinoma in situ; CIN 2 and CIN 3
      b. Squamous cell carcinoma
   6. Glandular cell
      a. Atypical glandular cells (AGC; specify endocervical, endometrial, or not otherwise specified [AGC-NOS])
      b. Atypical glandular cells, favor neoplastic (specify endocervical or not otherwise specified)
      c. Endocervical adenocarcinoma in situ (AIS)
      d. Adenocarcinoma
   7. Other (list not comprehensive)
      a. Endometrial cells in a woman older than 40 years of age

D. Automated review and ancilllary testing (include as appropriate)
   1. Educational notes and suggestions
      a. The 2001 Bethesda System, *Journal of the American Medical Association*, *287*, 2114–2119. Retrieved from http://www.cancer.gov/cancertopics/factsheet/detection/Pap-test

V. TERMINOLOGY

A. AutoPAP computer-driven cytosmear evaluation technique approved by U.S. Food and Drug Administration (FDA) for selection of 10% of Pap smears to be manually rescreened; selects 10% most likely to exhibit abnormalities
   1. Consider offering to patients when available in lab used; can increase cost
B. PAPNET computerized system is programmed to recognize cellular abnormalities on Pap slides prepared in the conventional way
   1. Consider offering to patients when available; can add to cost of Pap smear
C. Adjunctive screening
   1. Speculoscopy; combines with conventional Pap smear
      a. Pap smear is obtained
      b. Cervix is washed with vinegar solution, and then illuminated with a chemiluminescent light attached to the upper blade of the speculum (SpecULite) assists clinician in visualizing aceto-white areas of cervix

VI. 2006 CONSENSUS GUIDELINES

A. ASC-US
   1. Repeat cervical cytology testing (Pap) at 6 and 12 months, if both tests negative, return to routine screening, if ASC on either result, refer for colposcopy OR
   2. Do HPV DNA testing (preferred) if liquid-based cytology or co-collection is available
   3. If positive for HPV DNA, refer for colposcopy; if CIN positive on biopsy, manage per ASCCP guidelines. If HPV DNA negative, repeat cytology in 12 months. If ASC or HPV positive, repeat colposcopy; if negative, return to routine screening.
B. ASC special population
   1. Adolescent women with ASC-US or LSIL (females 20 years and younger) should repeat cytology at 12 months. If HSIL, repeat cytology at 12 months, if negative return to routine screening. If ASC, refer for colposcopy. If HSIL, refer for colposcopy. HPV DNA testing and colposcopy are unacceptable for adolescents with ASC-US. If HPV testing is inadvertently performed, the results should not influence management.
   2. Immunosuppressed women with ASC-US should be managed the same as women in the greater population.
   3. Pregnant women older than 20 years old with ASC-US are identical to nonpregnant women with the exception that it is acceptable

to defer colposcopy until at least 6 weeks postpartum. Endocervical curettage is unacceptable in pregnant women.
C. ASC cannot exclude high-grade SIL (ASC-H)
1. Refer for colposcopy; if no CIN 2,3, repeat cytology at 6 and 12 months or HPV DNA testing at 12 months. If ASC or HPV positive, refer for colposcopy. If negative, return to routine screening. If positive CIN 2,3, manage per ASCCP guidelines.
D. LSIL
1. Refer for colposcopy (endocervical sampling is preferred) if non-pregnant and no lesion is identified or unsatisfactory colposcopy examination or satisfactory colposcopy and lesion identified.
   a. If no CIN 2,3, repeat cytology at 6 and 12 months or HPV DNA testing at 12 months
   b. If ASC-US or HPV positive, refer for colposcopy. If cytology negative, return to routine screening OR
   c. If endocervical sampling or biopsy CIN 2,3, manage per ASCCP guideline
2. LSIL special population
   a. Adolescent women with LSIL, follow up with annual cytologic testing is recommended. At 12 months follow-up, only adolescents with HSIL or greater should be referred for colposcopy. At the 24-month follow up, those with ASC-US or greater, refer for colposcopy. HPV DNA testing is unacceptable for adolescents with LSIL. If HPV DNA testing is inadvertently performed, results should not influence in management.
   b. Pregnant women with LSIL: colposcopy is preferred for pregnant, non adolescent women. If no CIN 2,3 identified, postpartum follow up recommended. If CIN 2,3 is identified, manage per ASCCP guidelines. Endocervical curettage is unacceptable in pregnant women. Deferring initial colposcopy until at least 6 weeks postpartum is acceptable. Additional colposcopic and cytologic examinations during pregnancy are unacceptable for these women.
E. High-grade squamous intraepithelial lesion
1. Immediate loop electrosurgical excision (LEE) OR
2. Colposcopy with endocervical assessment
3. No CIN 2,3 with negative endocervical sampling and satisfactory colposcopy
   a. Diagnostic excisional procedure OR
   b. Repeat colposcopy and cytology at 6-month intervals for 1 year OR
   c. Review material, change in diagnosis, manage per ASCCP guidelines
4. If HSIL at either visit, refer for diagnostic excisional procedure
5. Other results—manage per guidelines
6. Diagnostic excisional procedure if unsatisfactory colposcopy at either visit
7. If negative cytology at both visits, return to routine screening

F. HSIL special population
 1. Adolescents with HSIL
   a. Colposcopic examination (immediate loop electrosurgical excision is unacceptable)
     i. If no CIN 2,3, observation with colposcopy and cytology at 6-month intervals up to 2 years is preferred, provided that the colposcopic exam is satisfactory, and endocervical sampling is negative
     ii. If other results, manage per ASCCP guidelines
     iii. If HSIL persists for 24 months with no CIN 2,3 identified, refer for excisional procedure
     iv. If high-grade colposcopic lesion or HSIL persists for 1 year, perform biopsy
     v. If CIN 2,3 manage per ASCCP guideline for adolescents with CIN 2,3
     vi. If two consecutive negative Pap smears and no HSIL colposcopic abnormality, return to routine screening
     vii. If unsatisfactory colposcopy or CIN of any grade on endocervical assessment, diagnostic excisional procedure
 2. Pregnant women with HSIL
   a. Colposcopy is recommended for HSIL. Biopsy of lesions suspicious for CIN 2,3 or cancer is preferred; biopsy of other lesions is acceptable. Endocervical curettage is unacceptable in pregnant women.
   b. Reevaluation with cytology and colposcopy is recommended no sooner than 6 weeks postpartum for pregnant women with HSIL with negative CIN 2,3
G. Atypical gladular cells
 1. Initial workup
   a. All subcategories of AGC or AIS, except atypical endometrial cells
     i. Colposcopy with endocervical sampling and HPV DNA testing and endometrial sampling (if older than 35 years or at risk for endometrial neoplasia)
   b. Atypical endometrial cell endometrial and endocervical sampling (if no endometrial pathology, refer for colposcopy)
 2. Subsequent management for women with atypical glandular cells (AGC)
   a. Initial Pap screening of AGC-NOS
     i. If no CIN and no glandular neoplasia
     ii. If HPV status is unknown, repeat cytology at 6-month intervals 4 times
     iii. If HPV DNA status is negative, repeat cytology and HPV DNA testing at 12 months; if negative, return to routine screening
     iv. If HPV DNA positive, repeat cytology and HPV DNA testing at 6 months. If both tests are negative, return to routine screeenting.

      v. If ASC or HPV positive, refer for colposcopy

     vi. If CIN, but no glandular neoplasia, manage per ASCCP guideline

    vii. If glandular neoplasia irrespective of CIN, manage per ASCCP guidelines

  b. Initial Pap of AGC favors neoplasia or AIS

    i. No invasive disease—diagnostic excisional procedure

H. Other forms of glandular abnormalities

  1. Benign-appearing endometrial cells

    a. Asymptomatic premenopausal women with benign endometrial cells, endometrial stromal cells, or histiocytes—no further treatment

    b. Postmenopausal women with benign endometrial cells—endometrial assessment is recommended regardless of symptoms

    c. Post hysterectomy women with a cytologic report benign glandular cells—no further evaluation

I. AGS special population

  1. Pregnant women—initial evaluation of AGC refer to nonpregnant women guideline, except endocervical curettage and endometrial biopsy are unacceptable

J. Recommended management, different cobinations of results

  1. General recommendations

    a. HPV DNA testing target only high-risk (oncogenic) HPV types

    b. Women 30 years and older, who have a cytology result of intraepithelial lesions or malignancy, but test positive for HPV, repeat cytology and HPV testing at 12 months preferred. If positive, repeat colposcopy is recommended.

VII. CLINICAL MANAGEMENT GUIDELINES FOR CERVICAL CANCER SCREENING (ACOG RELEASE NOVEMBER 2009)

A. Initial Pap screening at age 21 years old

B. Screen every 2 years between 21 and 29 years of age

C. Screen only every 3 years between 30 and 65 to 70 years old in low-risk women, screen for women at high risk more frequently and as indicated

D. Continue to have annual well women exam/women treated in the past for cervical precancerous lesions or cancer; continue annual screening for at least 20 years

E. Consider stopping screening at age 65 to 70 for women with 3 or more consecutive, documented negative pap tests and no abnormal pap tests within 10 years

F. Cease screening after hysterectomy for documented benign disease, continue to screen after hysterectomy for cervical precancerous lesions or cancer and those without documentation or any lesions

G. If using cotesting (Pap and HPV test) for women older than 30 years of age, only do every 3 years if pap negative and HPV negative

VIII. A NEW OPINION FOR THE 2009 RECOMMENDATIONS (PUBLISHED BY ACOG, 2010)

A. Pap smears should begin at age 21, but cases exist, whereas Pap testing should begin earlier, but continue to advise against HPV DNA testing

B. Adolescents with HIV be screened at 6-month interval in first year after diagnosis, then annually

C. Adolescents with compromised immune systems (organ transplant; long-term steroids) screen at onset of sexual activity, and screen at 6 months and 1 year, then yearly

D. Any adolescent who was screened prior to age 21, with one or more normal results, rescreen at age 21

E. Adolescents with low- to high-grade lesions, manage through periodic observation. When screening results show regression of abnormal cells, rescreening may be delayed until age 21

F. If CIN 3, refer to 2006 *Consensus Guidelines, VI*

IX. FOLLOW-UP FOR ANY ABNORMAL PAP TEST FINDING

A. Follow up as indicated in *VI*

B. Procedures for follow-up (one example)

1. If report recommends repeat test or treatment, the patient is notified by letter and perhaps by telephone as well; also, it may be useful to have a stamp with "Pap letter sent" on it to stamp the lab result sheet, and the clinician can also sign and date this sheet. This procedure can be modified to electronic medical records (EMR) available in many clinical sites.

2. Either a file card is filled out with the patient's name or ID number, the clinician's initials, and the date and results of the test or the information can be entered into the EMR in a recall system using the same information.

3. At the end of each month, using the site-specific retrieval system, overdue patients are identified and the information is given to the clinician who performed the test or the person responsible for following up. A letter is sent to the patient, reminding her that her Pap smear is overdue. Following the same procedure the following month, a second letter is sent to the patient. If the Pap results were LSIL or lower, the clinician's responsibility ends. If the results were greater than LSIL, and no response from patient to the second letter, a registered letter with this information is sent to the patient. All letters and visits should be documented.

4. If test results show no abnormal cells, but indicate reactive and reparative changes, inflammation, a letter should be sent to the patient, stating that the laboratory findings for malignancy were negative, but that there is evidence of a possible infection, and that an infection check is recommended if no check was done at the time of the Pap test. No follow-up letters are necessary.

X. INDICATIONS FOR COLPOSCOPY
  A. As indicated by Pap test; algorithm with *2006 Consensus Guidelines, VI*
  B. History of physical examination that revealed possible diethyl-stilbestrol exposure
  C. Any obvious lesions of the cervix
  D. Lesions in vagina or vulva that are a diagnostic problem
  E. If deemed necessary by physician or nurse practitioner

XI. COLPOSCOPY REFERRAL PROCEDURE
  A. Refer woman to physician of her choice or one available at same setting or to nurse practitioner or nurse midwife (increasingly being trained in colposcopy)
  B. Instruct woman that she will probably be billed for procedure, which is generally covered by insurance; make any arrangements possible if she has no insurance
  C. When patient chooses an outside clinician, a signed release form will be sent with referral sheet, so a copy of the referral visit report can be returned to the original facility

XII. USE OF COLPOSCOPE BY NURSE PRACTITIONERS
  A. Use of colposcopy examination with HPV treatment
    1. A colposcopy examination of vulva, vagina, and cervix is done on all women and found to have vulvar HPV lesions prior to beginning treatment
      a. Vulvar warts: treat according to protocol
      b. Cervical warts: refer to gynecologist or treat per clinician preparation
    2. Colposcopy examination may be done at each visit. If warts are still present after 8 to 12 treatments, consult with gynecologist
    3. Colposcopy examination may be done when warts appear to have resolved to verify treatment
  B. Use of colposcope as a diagnostic tool
    1. Used at discretion of clinician for closer inspection of vulva, vagina, and/or cervix
  C. Procedure for colposcopy examination
    1. Explain procedure to patient
    2. Complete all necessary lab work
    3. Prepare area
      a. Swab entire vulva and vagina with acetic acid (white vinegar), applying generously
    4. Examine with colposcope
    5. Perform any biopsies indicated based on Pap findings

XIII. FOLLOW-UP
Per guidelines of setting, based on Pap test findings, colposcopy follow-up protocol; follow-up guidelines for other evaluation methods

Appendix I contains information about colposcopy that you may wish to photocopy or adapt for your patients.

See Bibliographies.

Websites: http://cancernet.nci.nih.gov; http://www.asccp.org/consensus/ histological.shtml; http://www.asccp.org/consensus.shtml; http://nih.techriver.net

Emotional and Mental Health Issues

11

Authors' note: Increasingly, clinicians practicing in primary care settings and gynecologic settings are finding themselves in the position of needing to prescribe and provide follow-up monitoring for women needing psychotropic medication management. This chapter will provide both education and guidelines for such instances. We hope that it will prove helpful.

APPROPRIATE FOR ASSESSMENT AND TREATMENT IN WOMEN'S HEALTH CARE SETTING

I. DEFINITION
An alteration in mood or behavior resulting in discomfort to a woman. These changes may place the woman in chronic or acute distress. Attempting to cope with this distress may alter her ability to function, causing family relationship or workplace disturbances, as well as somatic manifestations that may contribute to morbidity and mortality.

II. PSYCHIATRIC CONDITIONS COMMONLY SEEN IN WOMEN'S HEALTH CARE SETTING
    A. In this guideline, one asterisk (*) indicates a condition appropriate for assessment by a clinician in an office setting, two asterisks (**) indicate a condition appropriate for referral for further assessment and treatment, and three asterisks (***) indicate a condition appropriate for immediate referral to a hospital emergency room or other immediate care settings
    B. Mood disorders
        1. Bipolar disorder**
        2. Dysthymia*
        3. Mild situational depression*
        4. Secondary depression**
          a. Caused by underlying medical disease
          b. Caused by medication
        5. Major depression**
        6. Postpartum depression (PPD)* or **
        7. Premenstrual dysphoric disorder (PMDD)*
        8. Seasonal affective disorder (SAD)*
    C. Anxiety disorders
        1. General anxiety disorder (GAD)*
        2. Obsessive–compulsive disorder (OCD)* or **
        3. Panic disorder**
        4. Posttraumatic stress disorder (PTSD)**
        5. Social phobia*
    D. Eating disorders
        1. Anorexia**
        2. Bulimia**

E. Personality disorders
   1. Borderline personality disorder**
   2. Narcissistic**
   3. Avoidant**
   4. Dependent**
   5. Self-defeating*
F. Cognitive disorders
   1. Dementia**
   2. Delirium***
G. Psychotic disorders
   1. Schizophrenia***
   2. Other psychotic disorders***
      a. Delusional thought disorders
      b. Hallucinations
      c. Disordered thought process
      d. Disorganized behaviors
H. Sexual dysfunction* OR **
   1. Sexual desire disorders
      a. Hypoactive sexual disorder
      b. Sexual aversion disorder (sexual phobia)
      c. Sex addiction
   2. Sexual arousal disorders
   3. Orgasmic disorders
   4. Pain disorders
I. Sleep disturbances* OR **
   1. Insomnia
      a. Psychophysiologic—may occur at any time, usually time-limited condition that may begin with a stressor and become a learned behavior. Usually present for at least a month, if chronic or long term, should be assessed for other causative factors (i.e., depression/anxiety).
      b. Restless/wakeful sleep
      c. Early morning awakening with inability to resume sleep
   2. Narcolepsy
      a. Excessive daytime sleepiness
   3. Obstructive sleep apnea**
      a. A patient may misinterpret this disorder as insomnia, but, in fact, it is characterized by loud, irregular snoring which causes sleep interruption
   4. Substance-dependent sleep disorders**
   5. Restless legs syndrome—characterized by fragmented sleep and increased involuntary movements of the legs (may also involve other limbs)
   6. Sleep disorders associated with medical disorders—including, but not limited to, sleep-related asthma, pain syndrome, gastroesophageal reflux disorder, fibromyalgia, and menopause

7. Parasomnias**
   a. Sleep walking
   b. Night terrors, not the same as nightmares (usually only seen in children)
J. Substance abuse disorders**
   1. Alcohol
   2. Nicotine
   3. Medications
      a. Antianxiety drugs such as benzodiazepines
      b. Prescribed opiates
   4. Drugs of abuse such as cocaine, heroin, hallucinogens, and marijuana in larger quantities
K. Suicidal threats or ideation***
   1. Depressed patients should always be asked about suicidal thoughts and/or plans
      a. Are you having any thoughts that life is not worth living?
      b. Do you think about harming yourself?
      c. Have you ever thought about taking your life?
      d. Do you have a thought about killing yourself? If yes, what is your plan?
      e. Have you ever made an attempt to end your life?
   2. Patients who appear to be at risk need an immediate referral to a psychiatrist/clinic or hospital emergency room
L. Somatoform disorders* OR **
   1. Body dysmorphic disorder (BDD)*
   2. Hypochondriasis*
   3. Conversion disorder**
   4. Somatization disorder*
   5. Factitious disorder**
   6. Malingering**
   7. Pain disorder**

III. RESPONSIBILITIES OF CLINICIANS
A. Knowledge of signs and symptoms indicating a psychiatric condition or a psychiatric component in a medical condition
B. Screening and assessment
C. Intervention
   1. Treatment
   2. Referral for further assessment
   3. Emergency intervention if condition warrants

IV. HISTORY
A. What the patient may present with
   1. Stomach pain
   2. Back pain
   3. Pain in arms, legs, joints

    4. Mood changes associated with menses
    5. Loss of libido
    6. Headaches
    7. Chest pain
    8. Dizziness
    9. Rapid/pounding heart
   10. Shortness of breath
   11. Gastrointestinal complaints: pain, diarrhea, constipation, nausea, vomiting
   12. Fatigue and/or low energy
   13. Sleeping difficulties
   14. Feeling edgy or nervous
   15. Excessive worry
   16. Difficulty swallowing or "lump in throat"
   17. Feelings of sadness without known cause

B. Additional information to be considered
    1. Generalized feeling of sadness or hopelessness
    2. Weight loss or weight gain: what was patient's weight 6 months/ 1 year ago?
    3. Alcohol consumption/use of prescription or illicit drugs
    4. Has partner or close associates commented on alcohol or prescriptive/illicit drug consumption?
    5. Does patient feel guilty about drinking?
    6. Does patient avoid social situations?
    7. Changes in interest in sex or responsiveness during intimacy
    8. History of depression or other psychiatric problem or dementia in biological family
    9. Number of visits to health care provider in the past year
   10. Has patient found it difficult to concentrate or been easily distracted, finding it hard to find words, forgetting things?
   11. Changes in work or family environment
   12. Suicidal assessment
   13. Seasonal pattern
   14. Prescription, over-the-counter (OTC) medicine, or herbal or other complementary and alternative medicine (CAM) used currently
   15. Information on any of the problems listed in *II* if not spontaneously volunteered

C. Interview techniques
    1. Nonverbal messages are important in obtaining a reliable psychiatric history
      a. Patient and clinician should be seated at equal height with no furniture between them (i.e., desk)
      b. Establish eye contact
      c. Put pen down, give patient your full attention
      d. Ask clear, open-ended questions
      e. Allow patient to talk
      f. Be supportive

      g. Be watchful for important subtexts (i.e., changing the subject, avoidance, careless, or exaggerated responses, inability to maintain eye contact)

      h. Maintain a nonjudgmental attitude; however, be open to challenge contradictory statements

V. PHYSICAL EXAM

  A. Appropriate to physical complaint or symptomatology

  B. In addition to appropriate physical exam, clinician should be alert for the following physical manifestations of emotional distress:

    1. Appearance of sadness

    2. Gross anxiety

    3. Elevated respiratory rate and pulse

    4. Excessive perspiration

    5. Coldness and dampness of hands

    6. Tremor

    7. Inability to make eye contact

    8. Unkempt appearance

  C. If indicated by information and observation mentioned previously, a general mental status exam or a mini-mental status exam should be conducted

    1. Mini-mental status exam

      a. Appearance

        i. Grooming

        ii. Clothing: dirty, clean, appropriate to seasonal condition, revealing

      b. Behavior

        i. Are mannerisms and gestures appropriate?

      c. Attitude

        i. Is patient aggressive, angry, guarded, cooperative?

      d. Mood

        i. Anxious

        ii. Depressed

        iii. Manic or hyperactive

        iv. Alternating moods

      e. Speech

        i. Quantity and quality

        ii. Speed, pressure

      f. Cognitive functions

        i. Concentration

        ii. Memory

      g. Affect

        i. Normal variety of facial expression

        ii. Blunted, flat, or immobilization of facial features

VI. DIFFERENTIAL DIAGNOSIS

  A. Mental and physical disorders are frequently overlapping; the challenge presented in diagnosis is consideration of both dimensions at the same time and ability to differentiate between the two; by the way in which both entities may be present and contributing to the symptomatology

1. Hypothyroidism
2. Hyperthyroidism
3. Hypoglycemia
4. Mitral valve prolapse
5. Ménière syndrome/vestibular neuronitis
6. Esophageal tumors or other obstructions
7. Asthma
8. Caffeine abuse
9. Coronary artery disease
10. Alzheimer's disease or senile dementia
11. Irritable bowel syndrome
12. Crohn's disease
13. Brain tumors
14. Valvular diseases
15. Cardiac arrhythmias

B. Signs and symptoms of conditions indicated in *II* as suitable for diagnosis and treatment in a primary women's health care setting

1. Dysthymia—milder form of depression, symptoms are not disabling but chronic, typically lasting for many years. These symptoms may be so much a part of an individual's life that they are taken for granted and patient does not complain to provider.
   a. Depressed mood/chronic sadness lasting more than a year
   b. Poor appetite
   c. Insomnia
   d. Hypersomnia
   e. Low energy/fatigue
   f. Low self-esteem
   g. Poor concentration
   h. Difficulty making decisions
   i. Feelings of hopelessness

2. Mild situational depression. Symptoms present for not more than 2 months after the event; generally associated with loss of a loved one. May also be associated with loss of a job.
   a. Functional impairment—inability to carry on with life
   b. Exaggerated guilt (i.e., "It should have been me." "I should have done more.")
   c. Preoccupation with feelings of worthlessness
   d. Psychomotor retardation

3. PPD. A self-limiting period of affective lability occurring within a few days to a week or so after childbirth. Many times, PPD goes without diagnosis, which may leave the woman with lifelong feelings of guilt, fear, and inadequacy. The following symptoms (a) through (d) indicate a nonpsychotic PPD and (e) through (i) may indicate a psychotic illness. The psychotic

and/or delusional mother may be at risk to herself and/or her child. Evaluation by a mental health professional is indicated. Women who have experienced one episode of PPD are at greater risk for another. Women with inadequately treated psychotic symptoms are at greater risk for future mental health illness.

a. Sleeplessness
b. Weeping
c. Sadness
d. Guilt
e. Agitation
f. Prolonged sleeplessness
g. Lack of personal hygiene
h. Anorexia
i. Preoccupation with concerns or delusions about the infant
j. If left untreated, the preceding symptoms may contribute to lack of bonding and has been implicated in lifelong problems for mother and infant

4. PMDD. A cluster of symptoms regularly presenting during the last week of the luteal phase, beginning to remit within a few days of the follicular phase. Symptoms are always absent in the week following the menses. Symptoms are not present prior to the last week of the luteal phase. Symptoms are of comparable severity, but not duration, to those displayed in a major depressive episode, including:

a. Sadness
b. Hopelessness
c. Anxiety/tension/feeling on edge
d. Mood instability with tearfulness
e. Persistent irritability
f. Increased anger
g. Increased interpersonal conflicts
h. Binge eating
i. Insomnia
j. It is helpful in making a diagnosis if the patient maintains a daily diary, charting symptoms over a 2-month period

5. SAD
a. Essential feature is that symptoms of a depressive episode occur seasonally, during fall or winter, remitting during spring

6. GAD. An essential feature is excessive anxiety and worry occurring more days than not during a period of 6 months. Other symptoms include:

a. Restlessness
b. Easy fatigue
c. Difficulty concentrating
d. Irritability
e. Muscle tension

      f. Disturbed sleep patterns

      g. Fearfulness

      h. Somatic complaints (i.e., cold hands, lump in throat, etc.)

      i. Social phobia

7. BDD. An essential feature of BDD is preoccupation with a defect in appearance. This preoccupation must cause significant distress or impairment in lifestyle and in other areas of function. Complaints commonly include:

      a. Hair thinning

      b. Acne

      c. Wrinkles

      d. Scars

      e. Vascular markings

      f. Paleness or redness of complexion

      g. Facial asymmetry or disproportion

      h. Excessive hair on face

      i. Preoccupation with a bodily part

8. Panic disorder. A discrete period of intense fear and/or discomfort. Onset is rapid, without warning, symptoms mild then rapidly crescendo, generally within 10 minutes. Symptoms include:

      a. Fear that something terrible is about to happen, maybe as intense as feeling death is imminent

      b. Patient may feel that she is detached from herself

      c. Somatic symptoms may include palpitations, diaphoresis, respiratory distress, chest discomfort, nausea, and paresthesia

9. OCD. Characterized by recurrent, unbidden thoughts or images (obsessive). To control this, the patient begins a pattern of compulsive, repetitive behaviors, which serve to control the obsessive thoughts. Symptoms include:

      a. Unreasonable fear of something

      b. Unreasonable fear of losing control and doing something violent or harmful

      c. Waxing and waning of obsessions and compulsions

      d. Phobic avoidant behaviors

10. PTSD. Exposure to an event or events that involved threatened death or life altering loss resulting in intense fear or horror. The patient then goes on to reexperience the event by thinking, dreaming, or imagining that is recurring (flashback). Symptoms may occur at any time, although often shortly after the events. Symptoms may include:

      a. Intrusive thinking

      b. Nightmares

      c. Hypervigilance

      d. Excessive startle response

      e. Avoidance of people, situations which may serve as a reminder

VII. LABORATORY EXAMINATION
A. The following may be considered according to presenting complaint and symptomatology
1. Complete blood count (CBC)
2. Urinalysis
3. Electrolytes
4. Blood glucose levels
5. Thyroid function tests
6. Liver enzymes
7. Hormone levels
8. Electrocardiogram (EKG)
9. Electroencephalogram (EEG)
10. Drug screen if indicated

VIII. TREATMENT
A. Medication. All of the conditions listed, as suitable for office treatment, usually respond well to the use of an antidepressant or antianxiety medication. Most antidepressants are effective in treating anxiety as well as depression. Included subsequently are those medications that can be most effectively and safely used in a general practice setting. When a patient does not respond well to one choice she or he may do better with another. When switching medications, do not stop initial drug abruptly prior to starting a new one, instead cross taper over a few weeks. For pregnant women, only Prozac, Zoloft, and Wellbutrin are currently recommended. Only Paxil has specific warnings against use in pregnancy.
1. Antidepressant/antianxiety medications
   a. Selective serotonin reuptake inhibitors (SSRIs)
      i. Citalopram hydrobromide (Celexa)—starting dose: 10 to 20 mg/day; usual daily dose: 20 to 60 mg/day
      ii. Fluoxetine hydrochloride (Prozac/Sarafem)—starting dose: 10 to 20 mg/day; usual daily dose: 20 to 60 mg/day. Sarafem is used for PMDD and is generally given for 2 weeks prior to menses. Usual dose: 20 to 40 mg/day.
      iii. Fluvoxamine maleate (Luvox)—starting dose: 50 mg/day; usual daily dose: 50 to 300 mg/day
      iv. Paroxetine hydrochloride (Paxil)—starting dose: 10 to 20 mg/day; usual daily dose: 20 to 60 mg/day
      v. Sertraline hydrochloride (Zoloft)—starting dose: 25 to 50 mg/day; usual daily dose: 50 to 200 mg/day
      vi. Escitalopram oxalate (Lexapro)—starting dose: 10 mg/day; usual daily dose: 10 to 20 mg/day
   b. Major side effects of SSRIs include:
      i. GI disturbances
      ii. Sexual side effects
      iii. Restlessness
      iv. Insomnia
      v. Headaches

   vi. Orgasmic dysfunction
   vii. Activation of mania in patients with bipolar disorder
   viii. Avoid use of paroxetine, fluoxetine, and sertraline in
        women on tamoxifen because of CYP2D6 metaboliz-
        ing in the liver—resulting in decreased absorption of
        tamoxifen
 c. Norepinephrine–dopamine reuptake inhibitors (NDRIs)
   i. Bupropion hydrochloride (Wellbutrin)—starting dose:
      100 mg/day; usual daily dose: 100 mg 3 times a day
   ii. Bupropion hydrochloride sustained release (Wellbutrin
      SR)—starting dose: 100 mg or 150 mg/day; usual daily
      dose: 300 mg/day (150 mg twice a day)
   iii. Bupropion hydrochloride Wellbutrin XL 150 mg to 300 mg—
      starting dose: 150 mg daily × 7 days; usual daily dose:
      300 mg daily in the morning. Useful in SAD—start in
      autumn, taper, and stop in early spring.
   iv. Desvenlafaxine (Pristiq) extended release. Starting dose
      50 mg/day
   v. Major side effects of DNRIs
      a) Seizures possible with high dose (450 mg/day and his-
         tory of eating disorder or seizure disorder)
      b) Nausea and vomiting with SR formulation
      c) Headaches
      d) Psychosis (use cautiously in psychotic disorders)
 d. Serotonin–norepinephrine reuptake inhibitors (SNRIs)
   i. Venlafaxine (Effexor)—starting dose: 37.5 mg/day; usual
      daily dose: 7.5 mg twice a day
   ii. Venlafaxine extended release (Effexor XR)—starting
      dose: 37.5 mg/day; usual daily dose: 75 to 225 mg/day
   iii. Duloxetine hydrochloride (Cymbalta) 20 mg, 30 mg, or
      60 mg
   iv. Major side effects with SNRIs
      a) Hypertension
      b) Nausea
      c) Activation
      d) Sexual dysfunction
      e) Not recommended for women with increased daily
         alcohol ingestion
 e. Serotonin modulators (SMs)
   i. Nefazodone (Serzone)—starting dose: 50 mg daily; usual
      daily dose: 150 to 300 mg/day
   ii. Trazodone (Desyrel)—starting dose: 50 mg daily; usual
      daily dose: 75 to 300 mg/qd in divided doses twice a day
   iii. Major side effects of SMs
      a) Orthostatic hypotension
      b) Anticholinergic symptoms
      c) Sedation
      d) Priapism (trazodone in males)

  f. Norepinephrine-serotonin modulators (NSMs)
    i. Mirtazapine (Remeron)—starting dose: 15 mg daily; usual daily dose: 15 to 45 mg daily
    ii. Major side effects of NSMs
      a) Anticholinergic symptoms
      b) Weight gain
      c) Sedation
      d) Increase in cholesterol levels
      e) Agranulocytosis (discontinue medication)
 2. Antianxiety Medication
  a. Benzodiazepines should be used for short-term only (i.e., specific situation known to cause anxiety/panic or sleeplessness, plane flights, recent loss). This category of drugs is habit forming and can quickly lead to dependence. Use with caution, if at all, in patients with past or present alcohol dependence or abuse.
    i. Alprazolam (Xanax)—usual dose: 0.5 mg 3 times a day
    ii. Clonazepam (Klonopin)—usual dose: 0.5 mg twice a day
    iii. Diazepam (Valium)—usual dose: 10 mg twice a day
    iv. Lorazepam (Ativan)—usual dose: 1 mg 3 times a day
    v. Oxazepam (Serax)—usual dose: 15 mg 3 times a day
    vi. Most common side effects of Benzodiazepines
      a) Frequent: drowsiness, ataxia
      b) Occasional: confusion, amnesia, disinhibition, depression, dizziness
      c) Withdrawal symptoms: delirium/convulsions (with abrupt discontinuation), rebound insomnia, or excitement
      d) Discontinue by tapering dose, no more than 25% per week decrease in dose
  b. Other treatment
    i. Psychotherapy
      a) Cognitive therapy
      b) Interpersonal therapy
      c) Behavioral therapy
    ii. Exposure therapy
    iii. Biofeedback therapy
  c. Other medications
    i. Buspirone hydrochloride (BuSpar)—starting dose: 5 or 10 mg daily; usual daily dose: 10, 15, or 30 mg twice a day.
    ii. Most common side effects:
      a) Frequent: headaches, dizziness, nausea
      b) Occasional: nausea, paresthesias, diarrhea
      c) Rare: psychosis, mania
  d. Insomnia medication/interventions
    i. Sleep hygiene should first be used
      a) Avoid caffeine, tobacco, and alcohol in the evening
      b) Establish consistent pattern for bedtime and waking

    c) Establish regular exercise program, but do not exercise in late evening

    d) Avoid daytime napping or limit to no more than 20 minutes in the morning and afternoon

    e) Establish a good sleep environment. Comfortable bed, pillow, and covering; consistent, comfortable temperature with good ventilation.

    f) Avoid eating or watching TV in bed

    g) If you cannot fall asleep, get up and do something in another room

  ii. Medications—non-benzodiazepine hypnotics

    a) Zalepion (Sonata)—usual dose: 5 to 10 mg at bedtime, 5 mg in the elderly

    b) Zolpidem (Ambien)—usual dose 5 to 10 mg at bedtime, 5 mg in the elderly

    c) Zolpidem controlled release (Ambien CR)—usual dose 6.25 to 12.5 mg at bedtime, 6.25 mg in the elderly

    d) Eszopiclone (Lunesta)—usual dose 2 to 3 mg at bedtime, 1 to 2 mg in the elderly

    e) Medications listed previously should be used for short-term use or episodic use only, ideally 6 to 8 weeks. Persistent insomnia after short-term treatment should be referred for psychiatric evaluation.

    f) Side effects of medications listed previously include:

      1) Unpleasant taste

      2) Central nervous system (CNS) effects

      3) Complex sleep-related behaviors such as sleepwalking

      4) Dry mouth

      5) GI upsets

      6) Use with caution in patients with alcohol or other CNS dependent use

e. Complementary therapy

  i. St. John's wort (hypericum perforatum)—usual daily dosage: 300 mg 3 times a day or 450 mg twice a day for use in depression. Interaction with all medications listed previously. Serotonin syndrome of nausea, diarrhea, and headache may occur if used simultaneously.

  ii. Essential fatty acids are increasingly used for mood stabilization

  iii. Meditation/relaxation therapy

  iv. Regular exercise program

  v. Regulation of sleep/wake patterns

  vi. Dietary changes, including decrease or elimination of caffeine

  vii. Light therapy with seasonal affective disorder

  viii. Yoga

IX. COMPLICATIONS
A. Untreated
1. Increased risk for suicide or harm to others
2. Increased risk for other impulsive and acting-out behavior
3. Loss of friends, job
4. Decrease in family harmony
5. Exacerbation of any of the symptoms previously mentioned
B. Treated
1. Behaviors and somatic problems listed previously
C. SSRI/SNRI discontinuation syndrome
1. Abrupt discontinuation of an SSRI/SNRI antidepressant has the potential for a withdrawal effect known as "antidepressant discontinuation syndrome."
2. Discontinuation syndrome has been linked to all SSRI/SNRI antidepressants, especially those with the shortest half-life elimination. Discontinuation syndromes are variable in their incidence and severity. Onset of symptoms generally occurs within hours to a day.
3. Common symptoms include a range of somatic complaints. Included are headache, restlessness, dizziness, anxiety, irritability, mood lability, decreased concentration, insomnia, and panic attacks. The GI system may also become involved. Common symptoms include nausea, cramping, and occasional vomiting.
4. The causative factor is considered to be the sudden removal of excess serotonin after neuronal adaptation. Other related issues are related to the removal of inhibitor serotonin effect on noradrenergic and cholinergic neurons: this may lead to transient hypotension, which may account for the headaches associated with the discontinuation syndrome.
5. Although discontinuation syndrome may occur with any SSRI/SNRI, those most commonly implicated are listed subsequently. Medications are listed in order of the rapidity of elimination (half-life).
   a. Effexor
   b. Pristiq
   c. Cymbalta
   d. Paxil
   e. Zoloft
   f. Lexapro
   g. Celexa
   h. Prozac
6. Dosage tapering or substitution may minimize the discontinuation syndrome. Patients should be advised to wean off medication by pill splitting or capsule opening, in a minimum of 1-week steps. Patients should be urged to taper in one half to one fourth dosage per week steps, over a week period. If symptoms reoccur, the patient should be directed to go back to the last step on alternating days for a week or two.

7. An alternative method requires to have the patient go to the end of second week of weaning and then take two 10 mg Prozac daily for 2 days, then one 10 mg Prozac daily if the symptoms reoccur.
8. There are rare patients who continue to exhibit symptoms. These ongoing symptoms most frequently occur with Paxil and Effexor. Patients who continue to experience uncomfortable somatic complaints should be referred for a psychiatric evaluation.

X. CONSULTATION
A. All conditions indicated previously
B. Failure to improve
C. Collaboration for an appropriate medication
D. Medication use in pregnant and lactating women

XI. FOLLOW-UP
A. Monitor response, mood relief from symptoms
B. Follow-up appointment in 3 to 6 weeks to monitor response to treatment and adverse reactions

See Bibliographies.
Websites: http://www.nimh.nih.gov; http://www.adaa.org; http://www *.cognitivetherapy.com; http://www.apa.org; http://www.mentalhealth.today* *.com/dep/dsm.html; http://www.allaboutdepression.com*

Genitourinary Tract Conditions

12

INTERSTITIAL CYSTITIS/PAINFUL BLADDER SYNDROME

I. DEFINITION
Interstitial cystitis (IC) is a chronic, inflammatory, noninfectious disorder of the bladder with no associated histologic changes affecting both men and women. IC is more common in women than in men. Of the 1 million Americans with IC, up to 90% are women and 15% of those are of Jewish heritage.

II. ETIOLOGY
    A. The exact pathogenesis and etiology of IC remains unclear; they are thought to be multifactorial
        1. Abnormal bladder epithelial permeability and inflammation including fibrosis and discrete bleeding ulcers
        2. Neurogenic abnormalities
        3. Autoimmune disorders
        4. Allergic reactions
        5. Infectious etiologies
        6. May present as part of a more visceral pain syndrome
    B. Genetics
    Researchers have found a higher than expected prevalence of IC among first-degree relatives of index IC cases

III. HISTORY
    A. What a patient may present with
        1. Urinary urgency and urinary frequency; voiding as often as 15 times a day, sometimes every hour, including nocturia
        2. Dyspareunia
        3. Pressure, pain (can be worse during menstruation) and tenderness around bladder, pelvis, and perineum
    B. Additional information to consider
        1. Treatment of urinary tract infection (UTI) with no response to antibiotics
        2. Pain worse with menses
        3. Pain influenced by diet, medications, and supplements
        4. Feeling of depression or anxiety
        5. Decreased quality of life

IV. PHYSICAL EXAMINATION
    A. Thorough medical history
    B. Pelvic exam essential to rule out pelvic inflammatory disease (PID), vaginitis, vaginosis, or sexually transmitted disease (STD)
    C. Abdominal exam, tenderness, and mass
    D. Vital signs

V. LABORATORY EXAMINATION
    A. Urinalysis and culture
    B. Urine cytology
    C. Vaginal and cervical cultures

D. Bladder diagnosis
Potassium sensitivity test may be done in office as a minimally invasive procedure that involves the instillation of a potassium chloride solution into the bladder to determine the degree of the patient's pain or urgency response
E. Cystoscopy with biopsy
F. Patient assessment questionnaire

VI. DIFFERENTIAL DIAGNOSIS
A. Endometriosis
B. Irritable bowel syndrome
C. UTI
D. Vulvodynia
E. Nonbacterial prostatitis (males)
F. Fibromyalgia
G. Coexisting depression and anxiety
H. Bladder cancer
I. Kidney disorders
J. STDs
K. Neurologic or rheumatologic disorders

VII. TREATMENT
A. Bladder distention—researchers are not sure why bladder distention helps, but some believe that it may increase capacity and interfere with pain signals transmitted by nerves in the bladder
B. Bladder instillation (bladder wash or bath)—the bladder is filled with a solution that is held on average of 10 to 15 minutes before being emptied
C. Dimethyl sulfoxide (DMSO, RIMSO-50) treatments are given every week or two for 6 to 8 weeks and repeated as needed. Most people who respond to DMSO notice an improvement 3 to 4 weeks after the first 6- to 8-week cycle of treatment.
D. Oral drugs
1. Pentosan polysulfate sodium (Elmiron) 100 mg 3 times a day
2. Analgesic medications
3. Tricyclic antidepressants
4. Antihistamines
5. Antispasmodics
6. Anticholinergics
E. Transcutaneous electrical nerve simulation
F. Diet—there is no scientific evidence linking diet to interstitial cystitis/painful bladder syndrome (IC/PBS), but many health care providers and patients find that the following may contribute to bladder irritation and inflammation:
1. Alcohol
2. Tomatoes
3. Spices
4. Chocolate

5. Caffeinated beverages
6. Citrus beverages and fruits
7. Highly acidic foods
8. Artificial sweeteners
G. Eliminate smoking—many patients feel that smoking makes their symptoms worse
H. Exercise—gentle stretching exercises may help relieve IC/PBS symptoms
I. Bladder training methods vary but, basically, patients void at designated times and use relaxation techniques and distractions to keep to the schedule
J. Physical therapy and biofeedback

VIII. COMPLICATIONS
A. Missed diagnosis
B. Depression (rare cases), suicidal ideation

IX. CONSULTATION
A. Consult with a physician regarding the appropriate testing
B. Refer to a physician for appropriate testing
C. Refer to a urologist or IC specialist

X. FOLLOW-UP
A. 1 to 2 weeks after initial workup and evaluation
B. 4 to 6 weeks after starting any treatment
C. Initially as needed to adjust treatment measures and symptoms—this may take months
D. Regular follow-up visits to monitor symptoms and progress

Websites: http://www.ichelp.org; http://www.ic-network.com; http://www .mayoclinic.com/health/interstitial-cystitis/ds00497

URINARY TRACT INFECTION

I. DEFINITION
An infection of the urethra, bladder (cystitis), ureters, or kidneys.

II. ETIOLOGY
A. Specific causes
1. Bacteria: *Escherichia coli*, 75% to 90% of all acute uncomplicated infections. *Staphylococcus saprophyticus*, second most commonly isolated organism; formerly thought to be a contaminant; now thought to be of causative significance, especially in women aged 16 to 25 years old. Others in descending order of implication: *S. saprophyticus, Klebsiella, Proteus mirabilis, Enterobacteriaceae, Citrobacter freundii, Enterococcus*, and others including

Serratia, Providencia, Pseudomonas, Group B *Streptococcus, Staphylococcus aureus, Staphylococcus epidermidis, Mycoplasma,* and *Chlamydia.*
2. Fungi, especially in diabetes and patients with catheters; immunocompromised persons
3. Viruses that cause viruria—measles, mumps, herpes simplex, cytomegalovirus, adenovirus, varicella zoster leading to hemorrhage in bladder, and cystitis
B. Mechanism: most commonly ascending infection
   1. In females: gastrointestinal flora (*E. coli*)
   2. In males: prostate plays a role in harboring infection, constricting urethra causing urine retention
C. Other predisposing factors
   1. Size of inoculum
   2. Virulence of organism
   3. Incomplete or infrequent bladder emptying
   4. Urinary tract abnormalities: obstruction, calculi, congenital defects, prostatic hypertrophy
   5. Use of catheters
   6. Newly sexually active (honeymoon cystitis)
   7. Chemical contamination secondary to spermicidal, barrier methods of contraception
   8. Possibly being postmenopausal with estrogen deficiency
   9. Family history of UTI

III. HISTORY
A. What the patient may present with
   1. Dysuria
   2. Frequency, urgency
   3. Suprapubic pain, ache, pressure, scorched feeling after urination
   4. Back pain, ache or pressure in genitals
   5. No systemic symptoms except, occasionally, a low grade fever of less than 101°F
   6. Gross hematuria
   7. Vague abdominal discomfort
B. Additional information to consider
   1. Any previous cystitis or pyelonephritis; when was the last treatment, how it was treated, and response to treatment
   2. Previous urologic workup
   3. Any vaginal discharge, character, and onset
   4. Any chronic condition, diabetes, paraplegia, quadriplegia, cerebral palsy, meningomyelocele, and spina bifida
   5. Duration of symptoms
   6. Possible pregnancy with high-risk complications or use of contraindicated drugs
   7. Sexual activity, especially 24 to 48 hours postvaginal intercourse
   8. Method of contraception

IV. PHYSICAL EXAMINATION
A. Vital signs: temperature
B. Abdomen: any tenderness, masses
C. Back: any costovertebral angle tenderness or pain
D. Pelvic examination essential to rule out PID, vaginitis, vaginosis, or STD

V. LABORATORY EXAMINATION
A. Urinalysis: clean catch midstream urine; pyuria ≥ 5 white blood cells (WBC) per high-power field
B. Culture alone is sufficient on first time ever with UTI with no risk factor; all others should have culture and sensitivities
   1. Culture and sensitivities typically >100,000 organisms felt to be diagnostic
   2. If between 10,000 and 100,000, it would probably be significant if the clinical symptoms support the diagnosis
C. *Note:* Urine may be stored at room temperature for 1 hour or may be refrigerated for up to 72 hours
D. In acute, uncomplicated cystitis (nonpregnant woman), use dipstick if the patient is positive both for nitrates and leukocyte esterase; or if microscopic examination of urine shows an increase in WBCs (10 in high-powered field), consider treating presumptively

VI. DIFFERENTIAL DIAGNOSIS
A. Upper tract disease: pyelonephritis
B. Urethritis caused by:
   1. *Chlamydia*
   2. Bacteria from urethral manipulation causing irritation; thought to be early cystitis
C. Vaginitis
D. PID
E. STD
F. Interstitial cystitis
G. No recognized pathology (honeymoon cystitis)
H. Pregnancy
I. Hormonal urethral changes
J. Urologic cancer
K. Overactive bladder

VII. TREATMENT
A. Antibiotics
   1. For the first episode of UTI in women without risk factors, institute treatment with any of the following, provided that the woman is not allergic to the drug
      a. Nitrofurantoin (Macrodantin) 50 mg 4 times a day for 7 days and, depending on repeat culture results, possibly 25 mg 4 times a day for 7 more days or Macrobid 100 mg twice a day for 7 days

    b. For uncomplicated first or second episodes, trimethoprim (160 mg) and sulfamethoxazole (800 mg); take two Septra DS or Bactrim DS STAT or one twice a day for 3 days; or trimethoprim 100 mg twice a day for 3 days

    c. Cipro (ciprofloxacin HCl) 100 to 250 mg twice a day for 3 days; or ciprofloxacin extended release 500 mg once a day for 3 days; or Floxin (ofloxacin) 200 mg twice a day for 3 days; or gatifloxacin 400 mg once a day for 3 days or a single 400-mg dose; or Augmentum (amoxicillin 400 mg/clavulanic acid 125 mg) one twice a day for 3 days; or Noroxin (norfloxacin) 400 mg twice a day for 3 days; or Maxaquin (lomefloxacin) 400 mg once a day for 3 days (these drugs should be reserved for complicated UTIs and in areas where local resistance rates to trimethoprim/sulfamethoxazole are high)

    d. Monurol (fosfomycin) 3 g in a single dose mixed in 3 to 4 oz of cold water (not recommended for patients younger than 18 years of age)

2. For reinfection or UTI in women without risk factors, treatment is the same as for the first episode. It is important to distinguish reinfection from relapse. Reinfection occurs within weeks to months of preceding episode, and is often caused by a new organism. Relapse is a recurrence of symptoms and infection after finishing a medication course, and is caused by the same organism as the original infection.

3. For relapse in women
    a. Consider retreatment with same medication, with a test of cure 24 to 48 hours after the completion of medication
    b. Consider change of medication with a test of cure 24 to 48 hours after the completion of medication
    c. For second relapse, consult with a physician

4. For patients with risk factors (past history of pyelonephritis, known urinary tract abnormality, use of catheter, diabetes), consider referral to a physician

B. For pregnant women
  1. The causative pathogen in pregnant women is usually *E. coli*. Do culture before treatment; do sensitivity only if no improvement from medication.
    a. First choice: Ampicillin 250 mg one 4 times a day for 10 days (caution of increasing antibacterial resistance among urinary *E. coli*)
    b. Second choice: Nitrofurantoin (Macrodantin) or Macrobid (pregnancy Category B); note caution of use near time of labor and delivery
    c. In areas with high resistance of *E. coli*, consider fosfomycin (pregnancy Category B)
    d. Do not use Sulfa, Septra, or Bactrim (trimethoprim), or ciprofloxacin (pregnancy Category C)

C. Pain relief: Phenazopyridine hydrochloride (Pyridium, AZO Standard, Baridium, diazo, Phenazo, Urodine) 200 mg 3 times a day for 24 hours; Uristat (phenazopyridine HCl 95 mg) two tablets 3 times a day for no more than 2 days (available over the counter [OTC]; not recommended in pregnancy)

D. General measures
1. Advise voiding before and after sex
2. Advise adequate lubrication for sex
3. Teaching about hygiene, contamination
4. Treat as mentioned previously (*see Treatment, VII.A*) if bacteria is present
5. Consider treatment with Pyridium, AZO Standard (phenazopyridine hydrochloride), Uristat, or other such product only if the patient is symptomatic in the absence of pathogenic organism
6. Cranberry juice; 6 to 8 glasses of water a day; cranberry juice capsules; AZO 450 mg cranberry juice concentrate one to four capsules per day with meals; CranXact urinary formula (tannins in cranberries prevent *E. coli* from attaching to urinary tract)
7. Decrease bladder irritants such as caffeine, smoking, and artificial sweeteners
8. Wear cotton underwear, avoid tight-fitting garments
9. Consider topical or vaginal estrogen in postmenopausal woman with recurrent cystitis as adjunct

VIII. COMPLICATIONS
A. Pyelonephritis

IX. CONSULTATION/REFERRAL
A. Consider physician consult on:
1. Women with relapsed infections
2. Women who are symptomatic after 3 days of treatment
3. Women who have more than three episodes in a year
4. Complicated UTIs
5. Pregnant women especially those who are close to term

X. FOLLOW-UP
A. Follow-up culture if symptoms do not resolve after treatment
B. Consider test of cure up to 1 week after completion of medication

Appendix I, Cystitis, may be photocopied or adapted for your patients.
See Bibliographies.

Infertility

13

I. DEFINITION
Inability to conceive after 1 year or more of unprotected intercourse

II. ETIOLOGY
A. Factors in male infertility: faulty sperm production; reproductive tract anomaly; physical and chemical agents (coal tar, radioactive substance, orchitis, other infection, etc.); endocrine disorders; general state of health; blocked vas deferens; testicular infection; injury to reproductive organs/tract; nerve damage; impotence; lifestyle factors (smoking, alcohol, street drugs, etc.); incompatible immunologic factors for sperm—anti-spermatozoa antibodies
B. Factors in female infertility: blocked fallopian tubes; anovulatory cycles; anatomical anomalies; hormonal imbalance; polycystic ovary syndrome (PCOS); obstruction of vaginal, cervical, and/or uterine cavity; hostile cervical mucus; ovarian cyst or tumor; pituitary tumor; endometriosis; previous sexually transmitted diseases (STDs), vaginitis, vaginosis, pelvic inflammatory disease (PID), septic abortion, history of and drug treatment for thyroid disease, depression, asthma; lifestyle factors (alcohol, smoking, street drugs, etc.)
C. Factors in couple infertility: improper technique for intercourse; infrequent intercourse; emotional state; male and female factors contributing to infertility

III. HISTORY
A. What the patient presents with
   1. History of failure to conceive for period with no use of contraception
   2. Desire for pregnancy
B. Additional information to be obtained
   1. Complete medical and surgical history, including immunizations; family history
   2. Complete menstrual history, including menarche, character of menses, frequency, duration, last menstrual period, post-menarche amenorrhea
   3. Gynecologic history: anomalies; problems; infections; surgery; abnormal Pap smears, including loop electrosurgical excision procedure (LEEP); diethylstibestrol (DES) exposure; endometriosis; fibroids; previous treatment for menstrual disorders related to PCOS
   4. Contraceptive history to the present, including post method amenorrhea
   5. Obstetric history: any previous conceptions; number of children, abortions, stillbirths; complications
   6. Partner's reproductive history; medical, surgical history
   7. Employment history: exposure to radiation, viruses, other substances known to cause sterility; teratogens

8. Sexual history: techniques, frequency, and timing of intercourse in relation to the menstrual cycle; use of lubricants, douches, sex stimulants; trauma
9. Report of any previous infertility testing, workups; diagnoses; interventions; genetic evaluation
10. Lifestyle history: use of recreational (street drugs, prescription drugs, alcohol, running); stress tobacco, caffeine, eating habits, saunas or hot tubs, exercise (including biking)
11. Age of patient/partner may determine timing of intervention

IV. PHYSICAL EXAMINATION
A. Vital signs
   1. Temperature
   2. Pulse
   3. Blood pressure
B. Complete physical examination; observation of secondary sex characteristics; signs/symptoms of PCOS
C. External examination (careful observation for signs of infection, lesions, or anomalies)
   1. Clitoris
   2. Labia
   3. Skene's glands
   4. Bartholin's glands
   5. Vulva
   6. Perineum
D. Pelvic examination
   1. Length of vagina
   2. Position and character of cervix
   3. Any anomalies
E. Bimanual examination (examine for palpable masses, tenderness, anomalies, signs of trauma)
   1. Uterus
   2. Ovaries
   3. Adnexa

V. DIFFERENTIAL DIAGNOSIS
A. Partner infertility or sterility
B. Sterility
C. Anomaly, absence of reproductive organs

VI. LABORATORY/PRELIMINARY
A. Pap smear, maturation index; mammogram as appropriate
B. *Chlamydia* smear; *Neisseria gonorrhea* culture; rapid plasma reagin (RPR) status (syphilis), TB status, HIV, hepatitis status, rubella titer, varicella titer
C. Pregnancy test in amenorrhea
D. Complete blood count; erythrocyte sedimentation rate

E. Serum progesterone level days 21 to 23 of cycle
F. Wet mounts, vaginal cultures
G. Prolactin level, follicle-stimulating hormone (FSH), luteinizing hormone (LH), thyroid-stimulating hormone (TSH), Rh factor, blood type (preferably day 3–5 of cycle)
H. Hormonal assay (serum) such as FSH, LH, prolactin, estrogen dehydroepiandrosterone sulfate (DHEAS), testosterone, urinary LH 4 to 5 days at midcycle

VII. TREATMENT AND INTERVENTION

A. Infertility workup for the woman
   1. Procedures
      a. Basal body temperature charts, may use test for LH surge instead
      b. Commercially available ovulation tests or devices and fertility monitoring devices[1]
      c. Postcoital test—serial if antispermatozoa antibodies
      d. Cervical mucus test; sperm antibody level; sperm agglutination test; sperm immobilization test; endometrial biopsy 2 to 3 days before menstruation
      e. Hysterosalpingogram after menses, before ovulation
      f. Endometrial biopsy during luteal phase
      g. Tuboscopy
      h. Ultrasound
      i. Laparoscopy with chromotubation, hydrotubation; hysteroscopy; salpingogoscopy
   2. Laboratory
      a. Workup of partner involving tests done by specialist
      b. For complete workup, referral may be in order

VIII. COMPLICATIONS

A. Risks associated with certain tests; costs of testing
B. Persistent infertility, discovery of sterility
C. Effects on couple's relationship

IX. CONSULTATION/REFERRAL

To gynecologist or infertility specialist; reproductive technology centers; genetic counseling.

X. FOLLOW-UP

Long-term process for workup that is staged, so patient would be asked to return for next phase of testing if conception not achieved.

See PCOS, Chapter 19.
See Bibliographies.
Website: http://www.4woman.gov

NOTE

1. Basal body temperature monitoring; saliva microscopes; ovulation predictor tests, such as Ova-Cue Fertility Monitor.

Loss of Integrity of Pelvic Floor Structures

14

I. DEFINITION

Loss of tone of pelvic floor soft tissues can be attributed to various causes, including childbirth, increased body mass index (BMI), exercise, chronic constipation, and/or the general effects of aging and may result in cystocele, rectocele, urethrocele, incontinence, and/or uterine prolapse. It can also result from sexual assault or abuse including incest.

Urinary incontinence is one of the most common results, categorized as stress or urge incontinence, as well as leaking of urine.

II. ETIOLOGY

A. Childbirth trauma resulting in nerve or muscle damage: precipitous delivery, especially of a very large baby, grand multigravida, inadequate repair of episiotomy or of lacerations

B. Aging: loss of muscle tone, relaxation of muscles, ligaments; atrophic vaginitis

C. Trauma caused by sexual assault, incest, abuse

D. Secondary to surgery; infection, especially sexually transmitted diseases (STDs) with scarring

E. Medication side effects; bladder irritants—smoking, caffeine, artificial sweeteners, alcohol

F. Obesity; increase in BMI

G. Diseases: multiple sclerosis, diabetic neuropathy, chronic cough, dementia, stroke, impaired mobility, Parkinson's disease, tumor, congestive heart failure

H. Behavioral: excessive caffeine and alcohol intake, psychological conditions, poor bowel/toilet habits

III. HISTORY

A. What the patient may present with
1. Stress incontinence; urge incontinence; mixed incontinence; leaking of urine
2. Feeling of pressure in pelvic area—heaviness, fullness
3. Pain on defecation, fecal incontinence, chronic constipation
4. Inability to empty bladder completely; frequency, urgency; overactive bladder characterized by sudden urge to urinate with/without urine loss, frequency, nocturia
5. Dyspareunia
6. Lower abdominal, groin, or lower back pulling or aching
7. Bulging of organs against vaginal wall, prolapse through vagina; difficulty starting urination because of rectal prolapse

B. Additional information to be considered
1. Menstrual and reproductive history; pregnancies, route of delivery, any laceration, episiotomy, pelvic surgery or repair, reproductive tract cancers
2. Symptoms: type, onset, frequency, severity, conditions under which they occur, relief measures and results; precipitating factors
3. Contraceptive history: methods used, present method
4. History of sexual assault, abuse, incest

5. STDs, especially with tissue destruction and scarring
6. History of ritual circumcision, genital cutting
7. Caffeine intake, diet, alcohol, smoking
8. Medications use and timing: over the counter (OTC) and herbals, vitamins, homeopathics
9. Overweight: BMI 26 to 30 kg/m^2
10. Hemorrhoids; varicose veins (indication of weak connective tissue)
11. Long-term history of lifting greater than 22 lbs

IV. PHYSICAL EXAMINATION

A. Abdominal examination
1. Masses, fullness
2. Tenderness—suprapubic
B. External examination
1. Urethra
2. Perineum
3. Vulva
a. Cystocele; cystourethrocele
b. Rectocele, enterocele
c. Urethrocele
d. Prolapsed uterus
e. Ritual circumcision, genital cutting
f. Atrophy
g. Skin excoriation
h. Evidence of urine leakage
C. Vaginal examination
1. Speculum
a. Condition of vagina: lax, good tone, any lesions, rugae
b. Presence of cervix
c. Integrity of vaginal walls
d. Visible cystocele, urethrocele, and/or rectocele; uterine prolapse
2. Digital
a. Palpate cystocele, urethrocele
b. Palpate rectocele both vaginally and rectally with patient lying down and standing
D. Biannual examination
1. Uterus
a. Position
b. Tenderness
c. Masses
2. Adnexa
a. Masses
b. Tenderness
3. Palpable cystocele, urethrocele, scars; palpate bladder and urethra for tenderness, assess strength and duration of levator muscle contraction—with fingers in vagina, ask patient to try to squeeze as if stopping urine stream

4. Rectal exam: rectocele; occult blood; masses, anal tone, have patient squeeze Standing evaluation: cough stress test to confirm urine loss from urethra

V. LABORATORY EXAMINATION
A. Urinalysis with culture for stress or urge incontinence, to rule out infection
B. Postvoid residual volume test: catheterization or pelvic ultrasound

VI. DIFFERENTIAL DIAGNOSIS
A. Urinary tract infection (UTI)
B. Genital tract mass/carcinoma
C. Undiagnosed underlying disease (*see Etiology, II.G*)

VII. TREATMENT
A. Medication
1. Prescription for UTI if indicated (*see UTI guideline in Appendix I*)
2. Consider hormone therapy—oral, patch, vaginal ring, or topical
3. Treat any vaginitis, vaginosis, STD
4. Nonhormonal vaginal moisturizers such as Replens
5. Detrol (tolterodine tartrate) 2 mg twice a day or Detrol LA 4 mg/day can reduce to 2 mg/day for overactive bladder, urinary frequency, urgency, or urge incontinence
6. Ditropan XL (oxybutynin chloride) 5 mg/day; or Ditropan 5 mg twice or 3 times a day; Oxytrol (oxybutynin transdermal system) 3.9 mg/day applied twice a week
B. General measures
1. Teach Kegel (pelvic floor muscle training) exercises for stress incontinence (if there is no prolapse, cystocele, or urethrocele). (A commercial product of graduated weighted cones is available to assist in Kegel exercises; a cone is inserted in the vagina and Kegels are performed using the cone's feedback; when weight of cone can be maintained 15 minutes when walking or standing, move to next cone.) Biofeedback devices are available, or electrical stimulation for passive exercise; intravaginal device (sphere) Colpexin to strengthen pelvic organ support.
Phoenix Core Solutions offers a series of pelvic exercises strengthening pelvic bowl muscles
2. Urodynamic testing that may include cystometry or cystography
3. Keep diary of occurrence of incontinence
4. Suggestions for hygiene measures
5. Identify and eliminate bladder irritants, including milk products, sugar, chocolate, many cough medications, caffeine, nicotine, alcohol, artificial sweeteners, spicy and acidic foods Improve hydration.
6. Relaxation training

7. Pessary for uterine prolapse (continence ring, Mar-Land, Evacare, Milex pessaries)
8. Stress incontinence devices: bladder neck support prosthesis (Introl), the Reliance urethral insert, FemAssist, Impress Softpatch, FemSoft insert, Viva plug

VIII. CONSULTATION/REFERRAL
A. To physician or incontinence specialty practice for:
   1. Possible surgical repair, hysterectomy
   2. Possible reconstruction secondary to prior surgery, scarring

See Bibliographies.
Websites: *http://www.kidney.niddk.nih.gov/kudiseases/pubs/bladdercontrol/index.htm; http://www.phoenixcore.com; http://www.medicinenet.com/overactive_bladder/article.htm; http://www.healthcentral.com/incontinence/treatment-000050_12_145.htm*

Medical Abortion

15

I. DEFINITION

To terminate a pregnancy as early as pregnancy can be confirmed, but no later than 63 days from last menstrual period, with the use of misoprostol and mifepristone. The shorter the time a woman has been pregnant, the better the medications work (NAF website).

A. Mifepristone (Mifeprex): a derivative of norenthindrome with a strong affinity for progesterone receptors. The progestin antagonist effect of mifepristone interferes with the maintenance of early pregnancy. Mifepristone acts on the deciduas to break down the capillary epithelial cells, causing the trophoblast to separate from the decidua. This leads to the disruption of the integrity of the pregnancy, bleeding, and a decrease in the maternal human chorionic gonadotropin (hCG).

B. Misoprostol (Cytotec; also known as RU-486): a synthetic prostaglandin analogue. Misoprostol efficiently ripens the cervix and induces uterine contractility. Misoprostol tablets are taken within a few days of taking mifepristone (Mifeprex) and may be taken orally, placed into the vagina, or tucked between the cheek and gum.

II. ETIOLOGY

A. Therapeutic abortion: The patient presents with desire to terminate early pregnancy by nonsurgical means

III. HISTORY

A. Medical guidelines for eligibility
   1. Amenorrhea with positive pregnancy test
   2. Pelvic or transvaginal ultrasound documenting intrauterine pregnancy up to 63 days' gestation
   3. Full medical and surgical, including, but not limited to, the following:
      a. Diabetes
      b. Cardiovascular
      c. Infectious disease (including sexually transmitted infections [STIs], hepatitis, HIV, TB)
      d. Thyroid
      e. Lung
      f. Autoimmune
      g. Metabolic conditions
      h. Psychiatric illness (especially eating disorders if currently active)
      i. Surgeries (especially gynecologic)
      j. Kidney
      k. Epilepsy
      l. Allergies
   4. Full psychosocial history, including, but not limited to, the following:
      a. Drug and alcohol use/abuse/dependence (including prescriptives, nonprescriptives, street drugs, and herbal preparations)
      b. Tobacco use/dependence

c. Domestic violence (with regard to safety of woman)
d. High-risk behaviors
e. Patient's support system, especially with regard to knowledge of her pregnancy and decision to terminate, at home and available support person(s)
f. Cultural beliefs (especially with regard to pregnancy and abortion)
5. Full gynecologic/obstetrical history, including, but not limited to, the following:
a. Menstrual history
b. Gynecologic history
c. Pap smear history (especially with regard to abnormal Pap smears and treatment, including ablations, cryocautery, cone biopsies, etc.)
d. High-risk behaviors (especially STIs and number of sexual partners, prostitution)
e. Pregnancy history, including number of pregnancies, deliveries, miscarriages, previous abortions (medical and surgical), ectopic pregnancies, stillbirths, and other neonatal losses or infant/child deaths (e.g., sudden infant death syndrome [SIDS])
f. Contraceptive history and desire for contraception after abortion is complete
g. Past or current history of attempt to end current pregnancies with prescriptive, nonprescriptive, or herbal preparations or street drugs

IV. CONTRAINDICATIONS AND INELIGIBILITY
A. Greater than 63 days amenorrhea or beyond last menstrual
B. Intrauterine device (IUD) in situ (IUD must be removed prior to taking Mifeprex)
C. Inconclusive pelvic or transvaginal ultrasound for intrauterine pregnancy or documented/suspected extrauterine (ectopic) pregnancy, or documentation of placenta developing abnormally
D. History of severe adrenal failure, severe cardiovascular, liver disease, or diabetes
E. History of current anticoagulant therapy, or blood clotting disorder
F. Taking any medication(s) that interfere with or cannot be combined with either misoprostol or mifepristone
G. Documented allergy to Cytotec or Arthrotec
H. Certain steroidal medication therapies
I. Undiagnosed adnexal mass
J. If breastfeeding, a woman must understand that medications can cross into breast milk and cause diarrhea in the infant

V. ADDITIONAL CONSIDERATIONS
A. Must be certain in decision to terminate pregnancy
B. Must agree to participate her own abortion and take responsibility for her own care

C. Must agree to return for follow-up visit if required by caregiving clinic/facility
D. Must be able to understand and follow instructions for medical abortion, as well as the risks, benefits, and side effects of medications used
E. Must not have comprehension or language barriers
F. Must agree to have a surgical abortion, should the medical abortion fail
G. Must have access to telephone in case of emergency
H. Must have access to transportation to an emergency facility if one is needed
 I. Must agree not to take any herbal medications or supplements or prescription medication without asking the clinician during the medical abortion
J. Must agree not to use any of the following medications/foods/ herbs during the abortion procedure:
1. Ketoconazole
2. Itraconazole
3. Erythromycin
4. Grapefruit juice
5. Klonopin
6. Rifampin
7. Dexamethasone
8. St. John's wort
9. Carbamazepine
10. Corticosteroids

VI. PHYSICAL EXAMINATION
A. Vital signs: blood pressure, pulse, temperature, respirations
B. Pelvic examination: unnecessary unless patient has complaints or need to assess uterine size
C. Pelvic or transvaginal ultrasound (depending upon office protocol)
D. Urine or serum pregnancy test (if ultrasound is inconclusive for intrauterine pregnancy)
E. Laboratory values: hemoglobin and Rh testing
F. Height and weight

VII. COUNSELING AND CONSENT SIGNING
A. Patient should be counseled on options for current pregnancy to include: delivery, adoption, and abortion
B. Patient will be required to read material provided by office on medical abortion
C. Discussion with patient regarding the FDA-approved dosage of misoprostol and mifepristone
D. Patient should be counseled as to instructions for medication use— to include taking mifepristone in the office and when to insert misoprostol at home

E. Patient should be given oral and written instructions to aid her in what to expect and how to identify a complication

F. Patient should be counseled on what she might experience once she takes each medication, including possible bleeding following mifepristone. These include passing tissue (including a grayish sac) and cramping and the possibility of nausea, vomiting, fever, headache, diarrhea, chills, and fatigue. Patient should also be counseled to expect bleeding to last 1 to 2 weeks.

G. Patient should be counseled on what to do if abortion does not occur

H. Patient should be counseled on what to do in case of emergency, including heavy or uncontrolled bleeding, pain that does not respond to medication, or fever greater than 101°F. Patient should be given an information sheet about medical abortion to hand to emergency room personnel in case of emergency.

I. Patient should be counseled on when to begin contraception and that the first period may be heavier than usual

J. Patient will be required to read Mifeprex medication guide and to sign a patient agreement

K. Patient will be given written instructions and information on aftercare that include pain medications, heating pad use, antiemetics and comfort care; discussion about diet, exercise, heavy lifting, return to sexual activity, and other restrictions postabortion

L. Patient will be counseled about the importance of attending follow-up visits if they are scheduled

VIII. MEDICATION REGIMEN (BASED ON INDIVIDUAL CARE FACILITY PROTOCOL)

A. Mifepristone 600 mg orally and 400 µg misoprostol to be used 48 hours after mifepristone dosing orally, vaginally, or bucally

IX. OTHER MEDICATIONS TO CONSIDER

A. Rhogam (D) 1 mL must be given after oral dose of mifepristone to all women who test Rh negative

B. Antiemetic (i.e., Zofran ODT, Compazine, ginger, B_6)

C. Pain medication (i.e., ibuprofen 800 mg every 8 hours; narcotic pain medications per care facility protocol

X. COMPLICATIONS WITH MEDICAL ABORTION

A. Patient to be instructed to seek emergency treatment if:
1. Bleeding (soaking through two thick full-sized sanitary pads per hour for 2 consecutive hours)
2. Pelvic pain uncontrolled with medication regimens recommended
3. Fever greater than 100.4°F or higher that lasts for more than 4 hours
4. Severe abdominal pain
5. Weakness, nausea, vomiting, and/or diarrhea more than 24 hours after taking misoprostol

XI. CONSULTATION/REFERRAL FOR SIGNS OF INCOMPLETE ABORTION OR INFECTION
A. Uncontrolled bleeding
B. Continued pregnancy symptoms (i.e, nausea/vomiting or breast tenderness) 1 week after medical abortion
C. Unexplained fever
D. Failure to return to prepregnancy baseline

XII. FOLLOW-UP
A. Follow-up visit should occur 2 to 3 weeks postabortion and should include:
   1. Vital signs
   2. Pregnancy test
   3. Medical and psychosocial history since medical abortion, including bleeding pattern, pain or cramping, fever, pregnancy symptoms, support network, signs and symptoms of depression, or anxiety caused by the decision to terminate, and signs and symptoms of continued pregnancy
   4. Pelvic exam to assess
      a. Involution of uterus
      b. Vulvovaginal infection postabortion
      c. Resolution of bleeding
      d. Pelvic pain or pelvic inflammatory disease (PID)
   5. Review of birth control management or plan to include
      a. Current method used, evaluate:
         i. effective versus ineffective
         ii. user friendly
         iii. side effect profile
         iv. need for sample, refill, or new prescription
      b. If no current method used, evaluate:
         i. need for method—review options
         ii. review risks, benefits, side effects, and instructions for use
         iii. give sample, new prescription, or referral (as for IUD)

See Bibliographies.
Website: http://www.fwhc.org/abortion/medical-ab.htm

POSTABORTION CARE: MEDICAL AND SURGICAL

Examination After Medical or Surgical Abortion

I. DEFINITION
An examination usually 2 weeks after uncomplicated therapeutic abortion to assess the patient's physical and mental status

II. ETIOLOGY
Therapeutic or elective abortion

III. HISTORY
A. What patient may present with
1. Surgical
a. No unusual complaints
b. Rare complications may include:
i. Excessive blood loss (typical length of light to moderate flow is 9 days)
ii. Pelvic infection
iii. Pelvic perforation
iv. Acute hematometra
2. Medical
a. Nausea
b. Vomiting
c. Headaches
d. Fever
e. Chills
f. Bleeding: Average length of bleeding is 10 to 13 days; however, heavy bleeding may occur
B. Additional information to be considered
1. Date of abortion; type of procedure
2. Date of last menstrual period
3. Are pregnancy symptoms resolved? If not, what symptoms continue?
4. How long after procedure did bleeding continue; any pain associated with bleeding; how much bleeding; any clots, characteristics of bleeding, odor to discharge; fever?
5. Results of pathological examination of products of conception (if available)
6. Any change in relationship with partner?
7. Present emotional status
8. Birth control method
9. Intercourse since procedure
10. Medications taken, including antibiotics, oxytocins, herbals, vitamins, and homeopathics

IV. PHYSICAL EXAMINATION
A. Vital signs: blood pressure, pulse
B. Abdominal examination: suprapubic tenderness, guarding, rigidity
C. Vaginal examination (speculum)
1. Observe for bleeding or other discharge
2. Cervix
a. Os closed
b. Any lesions
c. Any discharge

D. Bimanual exam
  1. Uterus
     a. Size
     b. Consistency
     c. Tenderness
     d. Cervix: positive cervical motion tenderness (CMT); open os (millimeters)
  2. Adnexa
     a. Tenderness
     b. Masses
  3. Rectovaginal: as needed for any abnormal findings on vaginal, uterine, or adnexal exam

V. TREATMENT
A. Birth control
  1. Hormonal contraception: birth control pills, Depo Provera, contraceptive ring, patch, implant
  2. Diaphragm, FemCap
  3. Intrauterine device (IUD) (IUCD): hormonal and nonhormonal
  4. Other methods (over the counter [OTC]): male and female condoms, spermicides, sponge, vaginal contraceptive film
  5. Sterilization (if desired)
B. General measures: review use, potential side effects, and sign informed consent form if necessary (*see Appendix A*)

VI. LABORATORY EXAMINATION
A. Pregnancy test as indicated
B. Wet mount as indicated

VII. DIFFERENTIAL DIAGNOSIS
A. None

VIII. COMPLICATIONS
A. *See Postabortion Complications section*
B. If unresolved issues are apparent, follow-up counseling or referral to medical specialist recommended

IX. CONSULTATION/REFERRAL
A. *See Postabortion Complications section*
B. If unresolved issues are apparent, follow-up counseling will be recommended.

X. FOLLOW-UP
A. Yearly for health examination, Pap smear (per the ASCCP guidelines), reevaluation of family planning needs
B. As per guideline for contraceptive of woman's choice

See Appendix I and Bibliographies.
Website: http://www.nlm.nih.gov/medlineplus/ency/article/001512.htm

POSTABORTION COMPLICATIONS

I. DEFINITION
Any sequelae or unexpected/untoward events or conditions following a therapeutic/elective abortion either medical or surgical

II. ETIOLOGY
Therapeutic/elective abortion: medical or surgical

III. HISTORY
  A. What the patient may present with
    1. Fever, body aches, chills
    2. Pelvic pain, severe cramps
    3. Bleeding; more than one pad per hour
    4. Passing clots larger than a quarter
    5. Abdominal pain: right or left side or bilateral; onset, duration, attempts at relief, and outcomes
    6. Nausea, vomiting, diarrhea
    7. Breast tenderness, discharge
    8. Foul odor to vaginal discharge
    9. Vertigo, headache
  B. Additional information to be considered
    1. Where and when was the procedure done; has the woman spoken to that facility regarding her symptoms or follow-up care; type of procedure (medical or surgical)
    2. How much physical activity since procedure, type of activity
    3. Any intercourse since procedure
    4. Anything used in vagina since procedure: contraceptive device, tampons, sex toy, douching products
    5. Urinary tract symptoms
    6. Bowel symptoms
    7. Any exposure to flu or anyone with similar symptoms
    8. Any medications taken such as analgesics; ergotrate; antibiotics; OTC or prescription drugs, including herbals, vitamins, homeopathics
    9. Still feels pregnant; symptoms of pregnancy

IV. PHYSICAL EXAMINATION
  A. Vital signs
    1. Temperature
    2. Pulse
    3. Blood pressure
    4. Respirations

    B. Breast examination: tender (more or less or same since procedure); discharge from nipples

    C. Abdomen
1. Bowel signs
2. Guarding
3. Rebound tenderness
4. Referred pain (shoulder pain)

    D. Vaginal examination (sterile if within 1 week after procedure):
1. Os dilated or tissue in os
2. Any tissue in vagina
3. Amount of bleeding; character
4. Any discharge present; odor

    E. Bimanual examination
1. Cervical motion tenderness: positive Chandelier's sign
2. Uterine tenderness, enlargement, note consistency
3. Adnexa
    a. Tenderness
    b. Mass
    c. Fullness
4. Rectovaginal examination; if necessary, look for tenderness present

V. LABORATORY EXAMINATION
    A. Serum pregnancy test: quantitative
    B. *Chlamydia* and gonorrhea screening
    C. Cervical culture
    D. Complete blood count with differential and sedimentation rate
    E. Urinalysis and urine culture
    F. Call laboratory of referring facility to get results of pathology report if available

VI. DIFFERENTIAL DIAGNOSIS
    A. Retained secundae, continuation of pregnancy
    B. Uterine infection, endometritis
    C. Delayed involution
    D. Pelvic inflammatory disease
    E. Urinary tract infection
    F. Uterine perforation, bowel perforation
    G. Ectopic pregnancy
    H. *See Acute Pelvic Pain and Abdominal Pain guidelines in Chapter 17*

VII. TREATMENT
As indicated by symptoms and diagnosis; may include appropriate antibiotics, treatment of any urinary infection, ergotrate product to promote involution; re-evacuation or evacuation if failure of medical abortion; referral for evaluation of possible ectopic pregnancy (*see Pelvic Inflammatory Disease, Chapter 17, and Genitourinary Tract Conditions [Urinary Tract Infection], Chapter 12*).

VIII. COMPLICATIONS
A. Sepsis
B. Ruptured ectopic pregnancy
C. Hemorrhage
D. Uterine perforation, bowel perforation
E. Ascherman's syndrome

IX. CONSULTATION/REFERRAL
Call facility or clinician who performed the abortion for a consult and arrangement for return visit and further evaluation or refer to appropriate health provider/specialist

X. FOLLOW-UP
Follow routine postabortion guideline

See Appendix I and Bibliographies.

Menstrual Disorders

16

ABNORMAL VAGINAL BLEEDING

I. DEFINITION
Any variation from a woman's usual menstrual pattern; bleeding post-menopause

II. ETIOLOGY
A. Systemic illnesses: thyroid disease, blood dyscrasias, adrenal imbalance, von Willebrand's disease
B. Submucous leiomyomata in uterus; polyps, liver disease, clotting disorders, kidney disease, leukemia
C. Tumor in vagina, uterus
D. Trauma to vagina, cervix; scar tissue
E. Cervical lesions
    1. Polyps
    2. Carcinoma
F. Abnormal hormone secretion (with anovulatory bleeding)
G. Change in ovarian function (perimenopause)
H. Endometrial polyps or leiomyomata in cervix, uterus
I. Pelvic malignancy—nodes, uterus, bladder, rectum, vagina, ovary
J. Ectopic pregnancy
K. Abortion
L. Placental accidents
M. Hyperplasia
N. Stress
O. Postmenopausal bleed
P. Pharmacotherapeutics
Q. Sexually transmitted diseases (STDs), pelvic inflammatory disease (PID)
R. Structural abnormalities within the endometrium, including synthesis of vasculature vasodilatory proteins
S. Endometriosis/adenomyosis

III. HISTORY
A. The patient may present with
    1. Midcycle bleeding
    2. Spotting
    3. Pain
    4. Sudden onset of heavy bleeding
    5. Perimenopausal bleeding
    6. Postmenopausal bleeding
B. Additional information to be considered
    1. Is bleeding recent or since menarche?
    2. Onset of bleeding
    3. Amount of flow (pads or tampons per hour); clots and size of clots
    4. Normal bleeding pattern: How does this episode differ from normal menstruation?

    5. Current or recent use of medication; complementary therapies (herbals, homeopathics)
    6. Last menstrual period; previous menstrual period
    7. Last sexual contact, if sexually active
    8. Birth control method(s) (including recent insertion of intrauterine device [IUD], intrauterine contraceptive device [IUCD])
    9. Recent trauma to pelvic area or any other part of body (screen for abuse)
    10. Characteristics of present bleeding: clots, tissue
    11. Any related pain
    12. Any fever
    13. Any dizziness; syncope
    14. Symptoms of changing ovarian function (perimenopause)
    15. Recent pelvic surgery, including tubal ligation, uterine ablation

IV. PHYSICAL EXAMINATION
  A. Vital signs
    1. Blood pressure
    2. Pulse
    3. Temperature
  B. Skin: examine for evidence of bleeding disorder (e.g., petechiae or ecchymosis); pallor; fine, thinning hair
  C. Neck—thyroid: examine for enlargement, palpate nodes
  D. Breasts
    1. Development
    2. Masses
    3. Tenderness, appearance of skin, nipples
    4. Discharge
    5. Axillary nodes
  E. Abdomen
    1. Tenderness
    2. Guarding
    3. Bowel sounds
    4. Distension
    5. Hepatosplenomegaly
  F. Genital examination
    1. Observe perineum for trauma
    2. Observe for presence of hemorrhoids
  G. Vaginal examination (speculum)
    1. Observe vaginal walls for lesions or evidence of trauma
    2. Observe cervix for
      a. Polyps
      b. Lesions (evidence of trauma)
      c. Erosion or ectropion
      d. Whether os is closed or dilated; discharge in os
    3. Evaluate amount and type of bleeding

H. Bimanual examination
   1. Uterus: evaluate size, shape, position, any pain
   2. Adnexa: evaluate for possible mass, pain
   3. Recto-vaginal exam
      a. Fullness (fluid)
      b. Pain
      c. Bleeding

V. LABORATORY EXAMINATION (WILL DEPEND ON HISTORY AND ASSESSMENT OF BLEEDING)

A. Complete blood count, differential with hematocrit or hemoglobin; platelet count; bleeding and clotting time if indicated, specific testing for von Willebrand disease, ideally at time of menstruation
B. Serum pregnancy test
C. Gonococcal culture
D. *Chlamydia* smear
E. Thyroid studies
F. Hormone levels—luteinizing hormone (LH), follicle-stimulating hormone (FSH), prolactin, gonadotropin-releasing hormone (GnRH), serum estradiol
G. Urinalysis
H. STD screen, including HIV status
I. Wet mount

VI. DIFFERENTIAL DIAGNOSIS
See Etiology, II

VII. TREATMENT
A. For light flow/regular/irregular bleeding (e.g., midcycle)
   1. Lab work as history demands
   2. May observe 2 to 3 months as indicated by history and physical findings. Woman should be instructed to keep record of days that bleeding occurs.
   3. After 2 to 3 cycles, after normal physical exam and Pap smear as indicated with appropriate lab work, consider:
      a. Progestin preparation
      b. Monophasic oral contraceptive (OC) for 1 to 3 months or 6 to 12 months
      c. Meclofenamate (Meclomen) 100 mg every 8 hours up to 6 days
B. For heavy bleeding
   1. Consult/refer to physician after appropriate workup.
   2. Consider nonhormonal management with tranexamic (Lysteda).
C. For bleeding with IUD in place, *see IUD in Chapter 7*
D. For heavy bleeding with Depo Provera,[1] consider addition of low dose contraceptive for 3 cycles or supplemental estrogen until bleeding stops

E. If bleeding persists with a positive human chorionic gonadotropin (hCG)
   1. Physician consultation
   2. Referral as indicated
F. If bleeding postmenopausal will need an endometrial biopsy (*see Endometrial Biopsy section*)
G. Endometrial biopsy should be considered on a woman of any age if no cause is found

VIII. COMPLICATIONS
   A. Severe hemorrhage
   B. Shock
   C. Of underlying systemic illnesses

IX. CONSULTATION/REFERRAL
   A. After completion of all laboratory work and physical examination, nurse practitioner may:
      1. Consult with physician for possible Mirena insertion
      2. Refer to physician for treatment, that is, endometrial ablation or dilation and curettage (D&C)
      3. Refer to a hematologist if clotting time abnormal
   B. Immediate referral to physician if excessive bleeding after laboratory work and workup by clinician

X. FOLLOW-UP
As indicated by diagnosis and treatment

See Bibliographies.
Website: http://www.womenshealth.about.com/cs/menstrualdisorder/index.htm

AMENORRHEA

I. DEFINITION
   A. Primary amenorrhea: failure of the menses to occur by age 15 years old
   B. Secondary amenorrhea: cessation of the menses for longer than 6 months in a woman who has established menses at least 1 year after menarche

II. ETIOLOGY
   A. Primary amenorrhea
      1. Gonadal failure
      2. Congenital absence of uterus and vagina
      3. Constitutional delay

B. Secondary amenorrhea
1. Pregnancy; breastfeeding
2. Pituitary disease or tumor; disruption of hypothalamic-pituitary axis
3. Menopause
4. Too little body fat (about 22% required for menses)
5. Excessive exercise (e.g., long distance running, ballet dancing, gymnastics, figure skating)
6. Rapid weight loss
7. Cessation of menstruation following use of hormonal contraception
8. Recent change in lifestyle (e.g., increase in stress, travel)
9. Thyroid disease
10. Polycystic ovary syndrome
11. Anorexia nervosa or other eating disorders
12. Premature ovarian failure, ovarian dysgenesis, infection, hemorrhage, necrosis, neoplasm
13. Asherman's syndrome
14. Cervical stenosis—outflow tract anomaly
15. Medications including psychotropics
16. Chronic illness
17. Tuberculosis

III. HISTORY
A. What the patient presents with
1. Absence of menstruation
2. Possible breast discharge
3. Other symptoms secondary to underlying etiology
B. Additional information to be considered
1. Careful menstrual history; pregnancy history
2. Sexual history
3. Contraceptive history
4. Medications—over the counter (OTC), prescription, homeopathic, herbal
5. Sources of emotional stress
6. Symptoms of climacteric
7. Any current acute illness
8. History of chronic illness
9. Present weight, weight 1 year ago
10. Amount of daily exercise
11. Recent D&C or abortion
12. History of tuberculosis
13. Eating disorder—current or history of

IV. PHYSICAL EXAMINATION
A. Weigh patient
B. Neck: thyroid gland (look for nodes: palpable, enlarged)

C. Breast: discharge
1. Breast examination
2. Milky, clear, dark, light, bloody, thick, thin, color
D. Vaginal examination (speculum): vagina may be atrophic and there may be no cervical mucus
E. Bimanual examination
1. Uterus: may be enlarged
2. Cervix—scarring, stenosis
3. Adnexa: ovaries may be enlarged—cystic
4. Recto–vaginal examination
F. Measure ratio of body fat to lean mass; BMI

V. LABORATORY EXAMINATION (MAY INCLUDE)
A. hCG qualitative, quantitative
B. Prolactin level
C. Thyroid stimulating hormone
D. FSH, LH, dehydroepiandrosterone sulfate (DHEAS), and serum testosterone (if patient is hirsute); hemoglobin, erythrocyte sedimentation rate
E. Pap smear
F. Microscopic examination of cervical mucus
G. TB test if no history
H. Consider pituitary function assessment, GnRH stimulation test, ultrasound, CAT scan, MRI, hysterosalpingography, hysteroscopy after consultation with a physician

VI. DIFFERENTIAL DIAGNOSIS
See Etiology, **II**

VII. TREATMENT
A. If breast discharge is present, do not wait: do work up as per breast discharge protocol
B. If hCG and prolactin levels are within normal limits, pregnancy test is negative; may use a progesterone preparation: Prometrium, Provera, Aygestin
1. If no withdrawal bleed in 3 to 7 days after progestin, consider FSH and LH assays 2 weeks after Provera. Try oral estrogen 1.25 mg to 2.5 mg to prime the endometrium (estropipate) daily for 21 to 25 days; if no bleeding, add progestin during last 5 to 10 days of estrogen. If no withdrawal bleed, refer to physician.
2. If woman wishes to start oral or other hormonal contraceptive and has no withdrawal bleed from Provera, repeat hCG if indicated and start OCs or other hormonal method. If no withdrawal bleed after first cycle, consult with physician.
3. If woman wishes to start oral or other hormonal contraceptives and has withdrawal bleed from Provera, start contraceptive after start of bleed; if Provera is not completed by that time, discontinue and discard remainder (some clinicians have woman complete Provera)

4. If withdrawal bleed occurs with Provera, then no menses for 2 months following the bleed, consult with physician, then give Provera 10 mg × 10 days every 2 months. If sexually active, an hCG must be run prior to taking medication each time.
5. If woman has a history of uterine infection or trauma to the uterus through multiple curettages (postpartum or postabortion), or if the workup is negative and there is no response to Provera, referral for further evaluation (hysterosalpingography, hysteroscopy to lyse adhesions, estrogen to restore endometrium)
6. Instruct woman to complete 10 days of Provera even if withdrawal bleed begins, unless starting oral or other hormonal contraceptive as indicated prior in Treatment 3

VIII. COMPLICATIONS
A. Inability to conceive
B. Sequelae of underlying cause

IX. CONSULTATION/REFERRAL
A. As outlined under *Treatment, VII.B.5*
B. After workup for hirsutism is completed (*see Laboratory Examination, V.D*)
C. For all primary amenorrhea cases

X. FOLLOW-UP
A. As deemed necessary with physician consult
B. Yearly
C. PRN if unsatisfactory response to treatment

See Bibliographies.

DYSMENORRHEA

I. DEFINITION
A. Primary dysmenorrhea is the occurrence of painful menses usually beginning within several years of menarche and in the absence of any pelvic pathology but may occur at any time during childbearing years
B. Secondary dysmenorrhea is painful menstruation because of an identifiable pathologic or iatrogenic condition, which may be readily identifiable based on the history and the findings in a physical examination

II. ETIOLOGY
A. Primary dysmenorrhea
1. Caused by prostaglandins produced in the uterine lining and released into the bloodstream as the lining is shed, causing smooth muscle contraction, nausea, and/or diarrhea

B. Secondary dysmenorrhea
   1. Extrauterine causes
      a. Endometriosis
      b. Tumors
         i. Subserosal leiomyomata
         ii. Malignancies
         iii. Pelvic tumors
      c. Ovarian cysts
      d. Pelvic inflammatory disease
   2. Intrauterine causes
      a. Adenomyosis
      b. Endometriosis
      c. Intramural leiomyomata
      d. Polyps
         i. Endometrial
         ii. Cervical
      e. Presence of an intrauterine device
      f. Cervical stenosis
      g. Endometritis

III. HISTORY
   A. What the patient may present with
      1. Regular, recurrent pain may occur monthly, prior to menses, or with menses
         a. Abdominal pain
         b. Pelvic pain
         c. Severe backache
      2. Nausea, diarrhea, or constipation
      3. Weakness
      4. Dizziness
      5. Weight gain
      6. Breast tenderness
      7. Backache
   B. Additional information to be elicited by asking the following questions:
      1. Relationship to menarche
      2. When does pain begin?
      3. How long does it last?
      4. Does anything make it feel better?
      5. Last menstrual period
      6. Birth control method(s) used
      7. Any relationship to intercourse?
      8. Any vaginal discharge?
      9. Any fever related to pain?
      10. What is menstrual flow like?
      11. Is this new? Is this a change in pattern?
      12. Sensitivity to aspirin and nonsteroidal anti-inflammatories
      13. History of chronic illness (kidney disease)

14. Current medications (prescription and OTC)
15. Postcoital bleeding
16. Home remedies and/or folk remedies tried; use of complementary and alternative therapies
17. STD history; vaginitis/vaginosis

IV. PHYSICAL EXAMINATION
A. Vital signs
   1. Blood pressure
   2. Pulse
   3. Temperature, if symptoms are present at time of visit
   4. Weight
B. Vaginal examination (speculum): cervix, cervical pathology
C. Bimanual examination

V. LABORATORY EXAMINATION
A. *Chlamydia* as indicated
B. Gonorrhea culture as indicated
C. Wet mount, as indicated

VI. DIFFERENTIAL DIAGNOSIS
See Etiology, II

VII. TREATMENT
A. Medication
   1. Ibuprofen (Motrin) 400 mg 4 times a day, 200 mg to 400 mg every 4 to 6 hours (max. 1.2 g/day)
   2. Mefenamic acid (Ponstel) 250 mg, two tablets immediately and one every 6 hours
   3. Naproxen (Anaprox) 275 mg, two tablets immediately and one tablet every 6 to 8 hours (no more than 5 tabs [1.375 g] per day); Aleve 200 mg every 8 to 12 hours
   4. Naprosyn 500 mg every 12 hours or 250 mg every 6 to 8 hrs. (max. 1.25 g 1st day then 1.0 g/day)
   5. Anaprox DS 550 mg, one every 12 hours
   6. Aspirin with codeine 1 to 2 tablets every 4 hours as needed
   7. Ibuprofen (Advil) 200 mg, 2 tablets every 4 to 6 hours (max. 1.2 g/day) (OTC)
   8. Flurbiprofen (Ansaid) 100 mg orally twice or 3 times a day
   9. Meclofenamate (Meclomen) 1 tab (100 mg) every 6 hours as needed
   10. Other OTC analogues
   11. Oral or possibly other hormonal contraceptive (to produce anovulatory state)
B. Other measures
   1. Reassurance
   2. Refer to premenstrual syndrome guidelines for diet, complementary therapy, exercise, and vitamin recommendations

3. Heating pad, microwave pad (filled with nonpopping corn or buckwheat)

VIII. COMPLICATIONS
May occur with failure to recognize presence of entity as described in differential diagnosis that results in lack of appropriate treatment

IX. CONSULTATION/REFERRAL
A. Diagnosis of secondary dysmenorrhea
B. Failure to improve after treatment as in *Treatment, VII*

X. FOLLOW-UP
A. Yearly health examination and Pap smear per guidelines
B. Secondary dysmenorrhea follow-up as indicated by physician or with consult

See Bibliographies.

ENDOMETRIAL BIOPSY

I. DEFINITION
Endometrial biopsy is a method of obtaining a sample of the nonpregnant uterine lining for purposes of cytologic and histologic examination. The procedure can be done in an ambulatory setting with or without local anesthesia.

II. ETIOLOGY
A. Reasons for performing this diagnostic procedure may include:
　　1. Unexplained abnormal vaginal bleeding in the premenopausal, perimenopausal, or postmenopausal woman
　　2. Rule out endometrial pathology prior to initiation of hormone therapy (HT), if indicated in the postmenopausal woman, and periodically monitor endometrial status with unopposed estrogen use, if indicated
　　3. Determine response of the endometrium to hormonal intervention in women experiencing infertility
　　4. Evaluate endometrial response during tamoxifen therapy to rule out pathologic response

III. HISTORY
A. What the patient may present with
　　1. Unexplained abnormal vaginal bleeding in a premenopausal, perimenopausal, or postmenopausal woman, with or without hormone therapy
　　2. Unsuccessful attempts at pregnancy
　　3. Current tamoxifen therapy for breast disease

B. Additional information to be considered
  1. Hormone therapy: type, purpose, duration, dosage, side effects, bleeding history; use of hormonal contraception, IUD
  2. Gynecologic and pregnancy
  3. Gynecologic surgery including previous endometrial biopsies and results, tubal ligation, cesarean section
  4. Medical conditions: cardiac, bleeding disorders, hypoglycemia
  5. Current medications including OTC and botanical preparations
  6. Allergies to pharmacologics including local anesthetic agents and povidone-iodine (Betadine, similar products)
  7. Vasovagal episodes especially with pelvic examinations, uterine sounding, IUD insertion, elective abortion
  8. Symptoms of vaginitis, cervicitis, STD, PID
  9. Contraceptive methods including current method and consistency of use; any recent exposure to pregnancy risk and date
  10. Menstrual cycles, peri- and postmenopausal bleeding; LMP, PMP
  11. General status: last meal or snack, fluids (rule out hypoglycemia); offer juice or snack

IV. PHYSICAL EXAMINATION
  A. Prior to exam (20 minutes), consider administering a mild prostaglandin inhibitor
  B. Bimanual examination: uterine position, pain, flexion, size, shape, adnexal or uterine masses, cervical motion tenderness, adnexal exam; any pelvic pain; determine involution if woman is postpartum, postabortion
  C. Speculum exam, presence of vaginal discharge
  D. Cervical inspection, position, presence of polyps, nebothian cysts, IUD string, mucopurulent discharge
  E. Recto–vaginal examination to determine uterine size, position, rule out pregnancy
  F. Vital signs: blood pressure, temperature (rule out fever)
  G. Teach woman about the procedure and possible complications, and obtain her consent to proceed

V. REASONS TO DEFER PROCEDURE
  A. Pregnancy or possible pregnancy
  B. PID, STD with PID as complication, cervicitis
  C. Poor involution of uterus postpartum or postabortion
  D. Fever
  E. Blood dyscrasias, especially bleeding disorders, severe anemia
  F. Extremely anteflexed or retroflexed uterus or cervical stenosis— may need to do biopsy under general anesthesia
  G. Vaginitis—defer procedure until diagnosis and treatment regimen completed

VI. LABORATORY
A. Pregnancy test
B. Hematocrit as indicated
C. Vaginal and cervical cultures as indicated
D. Postprocedure biopsy specimen(s) for histologic screening
E. Other per workup for abnormal uterine bleeding

VII. BIOPSY TECHNIQUE
A. Cleanse cervix and vagina with antiseptic, considering any sensitivities, allergies
B. Administer local anesthetic agent to the cervix (lidocaine gels, other topical gel or spray products, or paracervical block) if necessary/desired depending on sampling technique and equipment to be used
C. Sound the uterus (if using curette for sampling); prior to this, grasping the cervix with a fine tenaculum is necessary (using local anesthetic gel at the site for tenaculum placement reduces pain for the woman). Having the patient cough when applying and removing the tenaculum often reduces discomfort.
D. Insert the sampling device in the os, taking care not to force the device through a resistant os. If the os is stenotic, cervical dilators may be used. Use one of the following techniques:
   1. Pipelle device (flexible sampler with a piston to create suction for sampling): Insert up to fundus. Pull back completely on the piston to create suction, and rotate the pipelle continuously, moving it from the fundus and back again several times to collect the sample completely, filling the plastic tube. Withdraw the pipelle and push in the piston to deposit sample into the preservative. Some devices require cutting off the tip to expel the specimen.
   2. Pipelle device attached to suction pump: Insert as previously mentioned, and collect specimen by connecting the external pump, continuing suction until the device is filled
   3. Suction curette that is steel and reusable or plastic and disposable: Sound the uterus, stabilizing the cervix with a tenaculum, and then insert the curette and gently sample in a manner similar to using the pipelle devices (some are attached to a 10 mL syringe to provide the suction and some to an external pump). Withdraw the curette, deposit the specimen in the preservative.
E. Monitor patient's condition during and after the procedure to assess for vasovagal response, signs, and symptoms of uterine perforation
F. Allow patient to rest briefly with her legs flat before getting off the examination table. Assure that she is not feeling faint and is able to get dressed safely.
G. Instruct patient about post procedure care.
   1. Signs and symptoms of complications: severe cramping or pelvic pain; bright red bleeding with or without clots; fever, chills, foul-smelling vaginal discharge—call provider and/or go to urgent care setting

2. Expect spotting for 1 to 2 days after the biopsy. Define spotting and the difference between spotting and bleeding.
3. Patient may resume vaginal intercourse in 3 days or whenever she desires
4. Prostaglandin inhibitor for mild cramping
5. Resumption of menses if premenopausal and having menstrual cycles

VIII. REFERRAL/CONSULTATION FOR PROCEDURE
A. Patients with severe cervical stenosis to consider procedure under general anesthesia
B. Patients with contraindications for procedure

IX. FOLLOW-UP
A. Arrange for an opportunity to review laboratory findings
B. Care based on reason for endometrial biopsy and laboratory results
C. Treatment of any positive culture results

X. REFERRAL/CONSULTATION FOR RESULTS
A. Endometrial carcinoma—referral for treatment or comanagement
B. Hyperplasia without atypia—usually means atrophic changes
   1. Secretory: follow but no need for treatment unless bleeding persists and consider a progestin
   2. Proliferative may benefit from a progestin
C. Complex hyperplasia without atypia
   1. Desires pregnancy: consider risks and comanage with physician
   2. Does not desire pregnancy: to remove unopposed estrogen, cycle with progestins and repeat endometrial biopsy in 3 to 6 months
D. Complex hyperplasia with atypia—referral for D&C
   1. Comanagement for pregnancy if desired and no malignancy or for surgical high risk
   2. Surgery and/or treatment per staging if malignant
   3. Hysterectomy if nonmalignant and no pregnancy desired

See Bibliographies.
Websites: http://www.mayoclinic.com/health/vaginal-bleeding/HO000159; http://www.medicinenet.com/endometrial_biopsy/article.htm; http://www.webmd.com/hw/healthy-women/hw4583.asp

PREMENSTRUAL SYNDROME

I. DEFINITION
Premenstrual syndrome (PMS) is a cluster of physical, emotional, and behavioral symptoms related to the menstrual cycle, developing or

worsening during the luteal phase and clearing with the onset of the menstrual flow.

Premenstrual dysphoric disorder (PMDD) is a severe form of PMS sharing symptoms but set apart by the exaggeration and severity.

II. ETIOLOGY

No single etiology explains the various symptoms associated with PMS. A multifactorial cause is probable, involving psychosocial, genetic, hormonal, and neurotransmitter components (serotonergic dysfunction).

III. HISTORY

A. What the patient presents with (may include some or all of the following symptoms, in varying degrees)
 1. Headache, backache, migraine, syncope
 2. Edema
 3. Breast tenderness, engorgement, enlargement, heaviness
 4. Hot flashes
 5. Paresthesia of hands and feet, aggravation of epilepsy, joint or muscle pain
 6. Weight gain
 7. Fluid retention
 8. Abdominal bloating
 9. Increase in appetite and/or impulsive eating; craving for sweets and/or salt; food cravings in general
 10. Nausea, vomiting, constipation
 11. Decreased urine output, cystitis, urethritis, enuresis
 12. Exacerbation or recurrence of acne, boils, urticaria, easy bruising, herpes, rhinitis, colds, hoarseness, increased asthma, sore throat, sinusitis
 13. Emotional lability (anxiety, depression, crying, fatigue, persistent and marked anger, aggression, irritability); difficulty in concentrating; decreased interest in usual activities
 14. Changes in libido
 15. Lethargy, fatigue, depression in mood, feeling hopeless
 16. Sleep disturbances—hypersomnia, insomnia
 17. Palpitations
 18. Any symptoms, physical or emotional, that cluster during the same phase of menstrual cycle
B. Additional information to be considered
 1. When did these symptoms first occur in relationship to menarche?
 2. When do they begin and end in relationship to menses?
 3. Has there been a recent change in symptoms?
 4. Do you have cramps with your period?
 5. Has there been any change in your lifestyle (work, personal, family)?
 6. What is your diet like?
 7. How much exercise do you get?

    8. Are you or have you ever been in counseling?
    9. What medications are you taking?
   10. Do you have a history of chronic illness; if so, which, including depression?
   11. When was your last menstrual period?
   12. What birth control method do you use, if any?
   13. Have you had tubal ligation and if so, when?
   14. Have you ever thought about suicide or harm to others?
   15. Have you experienced depression or agitation at other times in your life?

IV. PHYSICAL EXAMINATION
  A. Vital signs
  B. Complete physical and gynecologic exam within past year examination
  C. Mental status examination

V. LABORATORY EXAMINATION
  A. Only as indicated medically

VI. TREATMENT
  A. Treatment is multifaceted and diverse, aimed at symptoms that patient finds most debilitating. To aid in diagnosis and treatment, 2 months of retrospective daily logs or symptom calendars help to confirm diagnosis and guide selection of appropriate treatment.
    1. Vitamin B^6 (pyridoxine). Begin with 50 mg to 100 mg total daily dose. Do not exceed recommended dosage. This vitamin has been shown to be toxic in large doses.
    2. Vitamin E 400 mg daily or twice a day
    3. Evening primrose oil. Begin with two capsules twice a day. May increase to four capsules twice a day. Improvement will occur slowly more than 3 to 9 months. Contains vitamin E, so patient should not take both.
    4. Prostaglandin inhibitors may provide relief taken during the second half of the menstrual cycle
    5. May consider
      a. Diuretics
      b. Antidepressants
      c. Antianxiety drugs
      d. Birth control pills (Yaz has been approved for PMDD), contraceptive patch, ring, Depo Provera
    6. Calcium 1,000 to 1,200 mg daily; magnesium 300 to 400 mg daily
  B. General measures
    1. Lifestyle changes, including stress reduction (i.e., meditation, yoga, or other relaxation techniques)

2. Diet recommendations (These dietary changes should be ongoing. It is not enough to modify one's diet only on the days prior to menstruation.)
   a. Limit consumption of refined sugar (e.g., cookies, cakes, jelly, honey) to 5 tablespoons/day
   b. Limit salt intake to 3 g or less per day (e.g., avoid using saltshaker)
   c. Limit intake of alcohol and nicotine
   d. Avoid caffeine (e.g., coffee, tea, chocolate, soft drinks)
   e. Increase intake of complex carbohydrates (e.g., fresh fruits, vegetables, whole grains, pasta, rice, potatoes)
   f. Consume moderate amounts of protein and fat (decrease animal fats and increase vegetable oils)
   g. Limit red meat consumption to twice weekly or less
3. Exercise plan recommendations: exercise 3 times per week for 30 to 40 minutes (brisk walking, jogging, aerobic dancing, swimming)
4. Consider other complementary therapies, including botanicals, aroma and music therapy, acupuncture, and energy healing
5. Keep a diary of daily symptoms, diet, and body temperature

VII. DIFFERENTIAL DIAGNOSIS
A. Sexual dysfunction
B. Chronic pelvic pain
C. Endometriosis
D. Primary dysmenorrhea
E. Post-tubal ligation syndrome
F. Prolactin-producing tumors
G. Perimenopausal symptoms
H. Fibrocystic breast disease
I. Depression
J. Psychopathology
K. Somatization of stress
L. Life stressors
M. Systemic lupus erythematosus
N. Hypertension
O. Meningioma
P. Attention-deficit disorder (residual type)
Q. Thyroid disorders

VIII. COMPLICATIONS
A. Serious psychological problem misdiagnosed as PMS
B. Systemic disease misdiagnosed as premenstrual syndrome

IX. CONSULTATION/REFERRAL
A. Referral at discretion of the nurse practitioner, after review of history and physical examination

 B. Mental health referral if appropriate
 C. Referral to nutritionist if needed/desired by patient
 D. Support group referral if desired

X. FOLLOW-UP
 A. Check up once a month for each of 3 months
 B. Yearly if improvement in relief of symptoms
 C. If symptoms increase or change

*See Appendix F, Complementary and Alternative Medicine and Bibliographies.
Website: http://womenshealth.gov*

NOTE

1. Approach this regime with caution remembering that menstrual changes are recognized as an early phenomenon with progestin-only contraception, decreasing with prolonged use. If patient is a longtime user, the onset of new bleeding may indicate underlying pathology.

Miscellaneous Gynecologic Conditions

17

ABDOMINAL PAIN

I. DEFINITION
Pain (mild to severe) in any region of the abdomen as differentiated from the pelvic area, including the area from the costal margins to the beginning of the mons pubis, including, but not limited to, the abdominal organs and anatomical structure. Usually refers to pain originating from the organs within the abdomen.

II. ETIOLOGY
  A. Inflammation, ulceration, infection, irritation, referred pain
  B. Space occupying lesion
  C. Response to injury: intra-abdominal or extra-abdominal
  D. Sequelae of surgery: adhesions, presence of foreign body, unrepaired perforation
  E. Systemic, hematologic, metabolic/endocrine, infectious, inflammatory, toxic, functional
  F. Tension pain
  G. May occur with stretching or distention of an organ

III. HISTORY
  A. What the patient may present with
    1. Pain that interrupts sleep, pain with sitting, dull aching, sharp pain, or cramping
    2. Pressure or heaviness deep in the pelvic area
    3. Dyspareunia
    4. Anorexia
    5. Vomiting
    6. Nausea
    7. Change in bowel habits, constipation; pain with bowel movement
    8. Urinary symptoms; dark urine
    9. Gynecologic symptoms and history (*see sections on Acute Pelvic Pain and Chronic Pelvic Pain*); menstrual, contraceptive history
    10. Diaphoresis
    11. Fainting, malaise, confusion, fatigue, joint pain
    12. Distension of the abdomen
    13. Dyspnea, tachycardia, bradycardia
    14. Fever
    15. Chills
  B. Additional information to be considered (patient will generally complain only of abdominal pain; history must be very thorough). Specific questioning is needed to elicit information about and sequence of symptoms.
    1. Onset (sudden, gradual, chronic, and so on)
    2. Character (e.g., throbbing, aching, burning, knife-like)
    3. Intensity: difficult to define, but can be likened to other pain such as toothache, cramps, or labor pain

4. Location: where did pain originate, quadrant, generalized, epigastric
5. Radiation: does it travel elsewhere
6. Pain relief measures: what helps, what makes it worse
7. Any weight gain or loss
8. Pregnancy history; infertility diagnostics or treatments
9. Psychosocial history including life stressors, major life changes, and timing in relation to onset of symptoms
10. History of incest, other sexual assault or abuse, violence or battering in relationships
11. History of bowel obstruction, polyps, hernias
12. History of abdominal tumors, benign or malignant
13. Use of gastrointestinal (GI) irritants including spicy foods, lactose, infectious agents; nonfood substances
14. Possible contaminated drinking water source in home country and/or abroad; food allergies, food poisoning
15. History of pelvic and/or abdominal surgery including organ transplant
16. History of extrauterine pregnancy
17. History of ovarian cysts, rupture of cysts
18. History of chronic bowel syndrome, any bowel disease
19. History of gallbladder disease
20. History of hepatitis, jaundice, liver disease, mononucleosis, abnormal liver function
21. History of trauma to the abdomen; accident, battering
22. History of travel abroad; recent immigrant and from where
23. History of exposure to industrial toxins, pesticides
24. History of kidney anomaly or disease; other genitourinary (GU) problems
25. History of appendicitis, chronic or acute
26. History of ulcers; gastric surgery
27. History of cardiovascular, respiratory problems
28. Previous care for abdominal pain; type of pain, origin, any treatments

IV. PHYSICAL EXAMINATION
A. Vital signs as appropriate
B. Cardiovascular, respiratory examinations; general appearance
C. Abdominal examination
   1. Bowel sounds; normal, hypoactive or hyperactive, sluggish, absent, adventitious sounds, bruits
   2. Abdominal tenderness; sites of acute, dull pain elicited on superficial and/or deep palpation
   3. Any guarding
   4. Any rebound tenderness
   5. Scars
   6. Distension, symmetry or asymmetry
   7. Patient's perception of pain location

8. On percussion, liver or spleen is enlarged, and other abdominal organs are enlarged as well
9. Organomegaly, masses, blood in the stool
10. Abdominal bruits

D. Vaginal and bimanual examination
   1. Examine cervix for presence of intrauterine device (IUD) string
   2. Examine vagina for masses, lesions, discharge, unusual odor, color
   3. Examine cervix for cervical motion tenderness, mucopurulent discharge
   4. Examine uterus for tenderness, masses, shape, size, consistency
   5. Examine adnexa for ovarian shape, size, tenderness, masses; other adnexal masses or tenderness

E. Rectal examination
   1. Pain, tenderness
   2. Masses
   3. Melena
   4. Rectovaginal masses, fistulas, adhesions
   5. Rectocele

F. Psoas sign, obturator sign

V. LABORATORY EXAMINATION

A. Cultures as indicated by history, physical findings
B. Complete blood count (CBC)/differential, serum electrolytes
C. Liver function studies, enzymes; pancreatic enzymes, *H. pylori* culture, stool cultures
D. Urinary tract infection screen; hepatitis panel
E. Pregnancy test; cervical, vaginal smears, cultures
F. Ultrasound evaluation based on examination
G. X-ray if indicated; abdomen, chest, posterior, anterior and lateral, KUB films
H. May consider consultation for CT scan and/or MRI if abdominal or pelvic examination is abnormal
I. Sickle-cell prep if indicated
J. Erythrocyte sedimentation rate; tuberculosis skin test, blood, sputum cultures, stool cultures, stool for ova and parasites
K. Thyroid-stimulating hormone (TSH) test
L. Toxicology screen
M. Barium X-rays

VI. DIFFERENTIAL DIAGNOSIS

A. Consider possible causes under acute and chronic pelvic pain and rule out the following:
   1. GI and GU pathology, including appendicitis, pancreatitis, bowel obstruction, ulcers, cholecystitis, cholelithiasis, renal colic, biliary colic, rupture of spleen, diverticulitis, ileitis, carcinoma, irritable bowel syndrome, ulcerative colitis, pyelonephritis, hepatitis, hernias, urinary calculus, mesenteric thrombosis, urethral

syndrome, perforation, strangulation, abscess, urinary tract infections, interstitial cystitis
2. Acute or chronic constipation
3. Dissecting aneurysm; embolism
4. Ectopic pregnancy or other gynecologic findings
5. Acute gastritis
6. Drug or toxin reaction; toxic systemic causes
7. Injury secondary to accident, violence including organ rupture
8. Abdominal pain, undetermined etiology
9. Referred pain from thoracic pathology: coronary thrombosis, pleural pneumonia, pleurisy, herpes zoster
10. Gastritis, coronitis, ileitis secondary to parasitic infection, cholera, waterborne diseases
11. Systemic diseases: hematologic, metabolic/endocrine, infectious, inflammatory, functional

VII. CONSULTATION/REFERRAL
A. For laparoscopic diagnostic examination
B. For medical evaluation of suspected GI, GU conditions as indicated by history and physical examination
C. To confirm a suspected diagnosis and initiate treatment as comanagers of care
D. For surgical consultation as indicated by history and findings
E. For CT scan, MRI

VIII. TREATMENT
A. As indicated by findings and history
B. Etiology undetermined, pain persists
   1. Follow-up to any diagnostic workup
   2. Multidisciplinary approach to pain or symptom management

IX. FOLLOW-UP
A. As appropriate for diagnosis and treatment
B. As desired by patient if no definitive cause is found, and palliative treatments are suggested

See Bibliographies.
Websites: http://www.mayoclinic.com/health/abdominal-pain/DG00013; http://www.familydoctor.org/x2593.xml; http://www.medicinenet.com/abdominal_pain/article.htm

ACUTE PELVIC PAIN

I. DEFINITION
Acute pelvic pain can be defined as sudden onset of severe lower abdominal pain assessed to be gynecologic in nature.

II. ETIOLOGY
A. Physiologic causes
1. Infection from several organisms, resulting in pelvic inflammatory disease (PID)
2. Extrauterine pregnancy
3. Ovarian pathology
4. Uterine perforation
5. Ruptured pelvic abscess in several sites
6. Aberrant uterine leiomyomata
7. Bladder pathology; bowel pathology
8. Urethral pathology
9. Proliferate endometrium beyond the uterine corpus
10. Postsurgical sequelae, adhesions from previous pelvic surgeries
11. Mittelschmerz
12. Trauma, abuse, sexual assault
13. Age-related physiologic change
14. Acute cholecystitis
15. Pancreatitis
16. Appendicitis
17. Vascular
B. Psychological causes
1. Secondary to pelvic surgery
2. Secondary to pregnancy whatever the outcome
3. Secondary to resolved pelvic pathology
4. Primary or secondary as a focal site for stress; posttraumatic stress disorder secondary to sexual abuse, assault

III. HISTORY
A. What the patient may present with
1. Sudden onset of symptoms
2. Chills, fever, body aches
3. May have nausea, vomiting, and/or diarrhea
4. May have constipation
5. Increased vaginal discharge
6. Acute, continuous, or intermittent cramping
7. Urinary symptoms including frequency, urgency, and pain
8. Missed menses
9. Menses at time of onset
10. History of pelvic surgery
11. History of ovarian cysts
12. History of extrauterine pregnancy
13. History of PID
14. History of urinary tract infection
15. History of endometriosis
16. History of gonorrhea or *Chlamydia* infection
17. History of rape, sexual assault, incest
18. History of bowel disease
19. Symptoms of depression or anxiety

B. Additional information to be considered
   1. Location of pain: whether it stays in any one place or is variable; whether the patient has ever had this pain before
   2. Description of pain: sharp, dull, throbbing; have patient rate her pain
   3. When does pain occur; does it wake patient up
   4. Does anything induce the pain such as eating, defecating, urinating, sexual intercourse, sexual stimulation; beliefs about cause of pain
   5. What, if anything, relieves the pain
   6. Any weight gain or loss
   7. Associated symptoms such as diarrhea, blood in stool or urine, increase in vaginal discharge, or vaginal bleeding
   8. Timing in relation to menses, if any association
   9. Duration of symptoms: days, weeks, months; regularity of symptoms
   10. Sexual history: exposure to sexually transmitted disease (STD), unprotected intercourse, new partner, change in contraception, methods used in recent past and currently, use of sex toys
   11. Psychosocial history: unusual stressors at time of onset when pain occurs; life changes such as moving, new job, new relationship, end of relationship
   12. Pelvic surgery in the past 12 to 24 months such as hysterectomy, laparotomy, tubal ligation, or occlusion
   13. Diagnostic pelvic workup such as laparoscopy, endometrial biopsy, colonoscopy, infertility workup
   14. Change in character of menses: heavier, lighter, more or less frequent

IV. PHYSICAL EXAMINATION
   A. Vital signs as appropriate
      1. Temperature
      2. Blood pressure
      3. Pulse
      4. Respirations
   B. Abdominal examination
      1. Bowel sounds: normal, hyperactive, sluggish, absent, any adventitious sounds, any bruits
      2. Generalized or localized lower abdominal tenderness
      3. Any guarding, pulsations observed
      4. Any rebound tenderness
      5. Any old scars
      6. Any distention
      7. Patient's perception of location of pain
      8. On percussion, are liver or spleen enlarged or is bladder distended
      9. Any pain elicited with light touch, with deep palpation
      10. Any organomegaly or masses

   C. Vaginal examination
      1. Examine cervix for discharge
      2. Examine vagina for lesions, discharge, and any unusual odor
   D. Bimanual examination
      1. Examine cervix for cervical motion tenderness
      2. Examine uterus for tenderness
      3. Examine adnexa for ovarian tenderness, masses, or tenderness
         in rest of adnexa
   E. Rectal examination
      1. Pain or tenderness
      2. Masses
   F. Elicit psoas sign; perform obturator maneuver

V. LABORATORY EXAMINATION
   A. Cultures as indicated might include gonococcus culture, *Chlamydia*
      smear; wet mount; pH of vaginal fluids; vaginal and cervical cul-
      tures; HIV testing
   B. CBC/differential—normal white blood cell (WBC) count may oc-
      cur in 56% of patients with PID
   C. Sedimentation rate; C-reactive protein
   D. Urinary tract infection screen; urinalysis with microscopic
      examination
   E. Pregnancy test—urine, ultrasound cardiography (UCG) quantita-
      tive; do serial if positive
   F. Ultrasound transvaginal, pelvic, abdominal
   G. Flat plate of abdomen; renal ultrasonography; MRI in pregnant
      women with acute pain
   H. Other tests as symptoms and/or history indicate
   I. Consider CA-125 if age, history, family history, and/or physical
      findings indicate
   J. Diagnostic laparoscope with a diagnosis that is not clear

VI. DIFFERENTIAL DIAGNOSIS
   A. Septic abortion
   B. Ectopic pregnancy
   C. Threatened or incomplete abortion
   D. Uterine leiomyomas with hemorrhage or infarction
   E. Ovarian cyst with rupture extruding blood, cyst fluid, and der-
      moid contents into pelvic cavity; torsion of ovary (sudden onset of
      pain, often after recent activity, nausea, vomiting, and sometimes,
      prior pain reported)
   F. Uterine perforation
   G. Ruptured abscess from ovary, uterus, bowel; tubo-ovarian abscess
   H. Urinary tract infection: cystitis or pyelonephritis; kidney stones;
      interstitial cystitis
   I. Appendicitis
   J. Adhesions
   K. Solid ovarian tumor

  L. Irritable bowel syndrome; diverticulitis, acute bowel

  M. Primary dysmenorrhea, especially in women older than 35 years old

  N. PID

  O. Mittelschmerz, especially in women younger than 35 years old

  P. Endometriosis

  Q. Adenomatosis

  R. Complications of IUD—migration out of the uterus

  S. Posttubal ligation syndrome; pelvic pain syndrome

  T. Constipation

  U. Lower bowel tumor; inflammatory bowel disease

  V. Uterovaginal prolapse

  W. Sexual/physical abuse

  X. Vascular etiology— deep vein thrombosis in pelvis

  Y. Pelvic pain associated with infertility treatment; ovarian hyper-stimulation syndrome: tachycardia, hypotension, abdominal pain, tense ascites; may have multisystem failure

VII. TREATMENT

  A. Medication as indicated for diagnosis

  B. Physician consult for suspected ectopic pregnancy, appendicitis, ovarian pathology, abscess, complications of uterine leiomyomas or infertility treatment, suspected pelvic adhesions, irritable bowel syndrome, suspected bowel or other tumors

  C. Treatment for primary dysmenorrhea per guideline

  D. Removal of IUD; consult as needed for complications

  E. Teaching and comfort measures for Mittelschmerz

VIII. COMPLICATIONS

  A. Generalized sepsis

  B. Hemorrhage

  C. Perforation of bowel

  D. Rupture of abscess

  E. Rupture of site of extrauterine pregnancy

  F. Shock

  G. Bowel obstruction

  H. Torsion of ovary with rupture and loss of ovarian function

  I. Development of chronic pelvic pain

  J. Scarring from salpingotomy, infertility

IX. CONSULTATION/REFERRAL

  A. Unable to find cause

  B. Physician consult for medical or surgical intervention

  C. For hospitalization if no admitting privileges

  D. If symptoms worsen or recur after treatment

  E. No response to treatment

  F. Unable to remove or find IUD (intrauterine contraceptive device [IUCD]) or differentiate cause of problem with method

X. FOLLOW-UP
  A. Consider reevaluation in 48 hours as warranted by clinical findings
  B. Consider repeating bimanual and/or abdominal examination in 1 week, and review status
  C. Seek immediate clinical consultation if symptoms worsen
  D. Follow up as appropriate for specific conditions such as PID

See Bibliographies.
  Websites: http://womenshealth.about.com/cs/pelvicpain/a/pelvicpainpt2.htm; http://www.familydoctor.org/x2593.xml; http://www.medicinenet.com/abdominal_pain/article.htm; http://www.mayoclinic.com/health/abdominal-pain/DG00013

BARTHOLIN'S CYST, BARTHOLINITIS

I. DEFINITION
Bartholin's duct cyst is a postinflammatory pseudocyst that forms proximally to the obstructed duct of a Bartholin's gland. The obstruction leads to dilatation of the duct. Bartholinitis is inflammation of one or both of the Bartholin's glands.

II. ETIOLOGY
  A. Responsible organisms include:
    1. *Staphylococcus aureus*
    2. *Streptococcus faecalis*
    3. *Escherichia coli*
    4. *Pseudomonas* may also be cultured from abscess
    5. *Gonococcus*
    6. *Chlamydia trachomatis*
    7. *Trichomonas vaginalis*
    8. *Bacteroides*

III. HISTORY
  A. What the patient may present with
    1. Deep, diffuse, painful, swollen lump and/or swelling in posterior vaginal (vestibular) area—can be unilateral, bilateral, or asymptomatic
    2. Can become large
    3. Difficulty sitting and walking because of severe pain and swelling as a result of trauma or infection
  B. Additional information to be considered
    1. Previous infection of a Bartholin's gland or duct; if yes, how was it treated
    2. History of STD

IV. PHYSICAL EXAMINATION
A. Vital signs
   1. Temperature
   2. Blood pressure
B. Visual examination of external genitalia
   1. Cyst is characteristically located in the lower half of the labia, with its inner wall immediately adjacent to the lower vaginal canal
   2. Lesions may vary in size from 1 to 10 cm
   3. The involved area may be painfully tender
   4. There may be no subjective symptoms
   5. Diagnosis is usually made by clinical appearance at the vulva
   6. Histology examination of the lesion presents atypically

V. LABORATORY EXAMINATION
A. Culture lesion at time of incision and drainage
B. Consider cervical cultures for *Chlamydia* and gonorrhea

VI. DIFFERENTIAL DIAGNOSIS
A. Lipoma
B. Fibroma
C. Hydrocele
D. Carcinoma of Bartholin's gland (extremely rare); suspicion arises if the cyst is firm or irregular to palpation
E. Inclusion cysts, sebaceous cysts
F. Congenital anomaly
G. Secondary metastatic malignancy
H. Hernia

VII. TREATMENT
A. May not be necessary unless it is quite large, symptomatic, or infected
B. Sitz bath 4 times a day for 2 to 3 days, then reexamine. If size has increased or there is no change, perform incision and drainage, or refer to physician for possible marsupialization (surgical excision and unroofing of lesion). If cyst or gland is extremely painful or large, immediately refer to a physician.
C. Antibiotics as appropriate to organism; most common is ampicillin, 500 mg 4 times a day for 7 days; ceftriaxone 125 mg IM single dose; cefixime 400 mg orally in single dose; azithromycin 1 g orally in a single dose; or doxycycline 100 mg orally twice a day for 7 days

VIII. COMPLICATIONS
Recurrence

IX. CONSULTATION/REFERRAL (*see Treatment, VII.A and B*)

X. FOLLOW-UP
At the clinician's discretion after incision and drainage or marsupialization

See Bibliography.
Website: http://www.mayoclinic.com/health/bartholin-cyst/DS00667

CHRONIC PELVIC PAIN

I. DEFINITION
Pain in any region of the pelvis that is long term and unresponsive to treatment of symptoms and/or undiagnosed

II. ETIOLOGY
    A. 50% enigmatic
    B. 25% endometriosis
    C. 25% other pathology including subacute and chronic salpingitis

III. HISTORY
    A. What the patient may present with
        1. Chronic pelvic pain with or without menstrual exacerbation
        2. Dysmenorrhea
        3. Dyspareunia
        4. Dyschezia
        5. Chronicity of symptoms
        6. Absence of chills, fever associated with pain
        7. Nausea, vomiting, and/or diarrhea associated with pain
        8. Chronic constipation
        9. Chronic intermittent cramping

IV. ADDITIONAL INFORMATION TO BE CONSIDERED
    A. Any symptoms of chronic bowel disease, any previous assessments for such, and results
    B. Any symptoms of chronic urinary tract infection, urinary tract anomaly, kidney disease
    C. Location of pain, duration, exacerbation, and what precedes increased symptoms
    D. Description of pain: sharp, dull, aching, cramping, intermittent, continuous
    E. Pain relief measures; what helps; use of over-the-counter (OTC) analgesics
    F. Any weight gain or loss
    G. Symptoms that accompany pain
    H. Sexual history including sexual responsiveness; STDs, PID; contraceptive history including IUD (IUCD)
    I. Surgical history including hernia repair

    J. Medical history

    K. Pelvic surgery including laparoscopy, laparotomy, tubal ligation, hysterectomy, repair of cystocele, rectocele, urethrocele, appendectomy, myomectomy, cervical cone biopsy, loop electrosurgical excision procedure (LEEP), also called LOOP excision (surgical excision with a small wire loop)

    L. Menstrual history

    M. Pregnancy history including extrauterine pregnancy(ies), infertility assessments, and/or treatments

    N. Psychosocial history including life stressors, major life changes, and timing in relation to onset of symptoms; depression, anxiety disorder, personality disorder

    O. History of incest, other sexual assault, or abuse

V. PHYSICAL EXAMINATION

    A. Vital signs as appropriate

    B. Abdominal examination

        1. Bowel sounds: normal, hypoactive or hyperactive, sluggish, absent, adventitious sounds, bruits

        2. Lower abdominal tenderness; sites of acute, dull pain elicited on superficial and/or deep palpation

        3. Guarding

        4. Rebound tenderness

        5. Scars

        6. Distention, asymmetry

        7. Patient's perception of pain location

        8. On percussion, liver, spleen enlarged, bladder distended

        9. Organomegaly, masses, hernias

    C. Vaginal examination

        1. Examine cervix for discharge

        2. Examine vagina for masses, lesions, discharge, unusual odor, color

    D. Bimanual examination

        1. Examine cervix for cervical motion tenderness

        2. Examine uterus for tenderness, masses, shape, size, consistency

        3. Examine adnexa for ovarian shape, size, tenderness, masses, other adnexal masses or tenderness

    E. Rectal examination

        1. Pain, tenderness

        2. Masses

        3. Melena

        4. Rectovaginal masses, fistulas, adhesions

        5. Rectocele

    F. Elicit psoas sign; perform obturator maneuver

VI. LABORATORY EXAMINATION

    A. Cultures as indicated by history, physical findings

    B. CBC/differential

    C. Sedimentation rate, C-reactive protein

    D. Urinary tract infection screen
    E. Pregnancy test
    F. Ultrasound evaluation based on pelvic examination
    G. Consider consultation for CT scan and/or MRI if pelvic examination is abnormal
    H. Consider psychological testing
    I. Hormone testing including TSH
    J. Hysterosalpingography (HSG)
    K. Barium enema, upper GI
    L. Colonoscopy
    M. CA-125

VII. DIFFERENTIAL DIAGNOSIS

    A. Uterine
        1. Dysmenorrhea (primary or secondary)
        2. Adenomyosis
        3. Leiomyomata
        4. Positional (prolapse)
        5. Pelvic congestion
    B. Adnexal
        1. Adhesive disease (infection, postsurgical)
        2. Neoplasm
        3. Functional ovarian cysts (Mittelschmerz)
        4. Endometriosis
    C. Peritoneal
        1. Endometriosis
        2. Adhesive disease
        3. Adenomyosis—cells that normally line the uterus invade the myometrium
    D. GI
        1. Irritable bowel syndrome
        2. Other bowel disease (e.g., Crohn's disease, inflammatory)
    E. Urinary
    F. Musculoskeletal
    G. Psychogenic (e.g., sexual abuse, rape)
    H. Congenital, anatomical
    I. Neurologic (neuroma)
    J. Infections

VIII. CONSULTATION/REFERRAL

    A. For laparoscopic diagnostic examination
    B. For medical evaluation of suspected GI, GU conditions as indicated by history and physical examination
    C. For pelvic venography
    D. To confirm a suspected diagnosis and initiate treatment as comanagers of care
    E. For psychological evaluation
    F. For ultrasound, MRI

IX. TREATMENT
A. Endometriosis: pain-only treatment; lowers estrogen
  1. Create a pseudomenopause with Danocrine 200 to 800 mg orally twice a day for 6 months; or GnRH analogues for 3 to 6 months or leuprolide acetate (Lupron depot) as per protocol
  2. Continuous monophasic oral contraceptives—no pregnancy plans—oral contraceptive pill (OCP), patch, ring, nonsteroidal anti-inflammatory drugs (NSAIDs)
B. Other pathologic causes
  1. Diagnose and treat cause according to established guidelines (such as salpingitis, trauma from sexual assault, incest or rape, childbirth)
C. Enigmatic pelvic pain
  1. Follow-up to diagnostic laparoscopy as appropriate to any findings
  2. Multidisciplinary approach to pain management
D. Consideration of empiric therapy
  1. Antidepressant
  2. GnRH agonist
  3. Musculoskeletal relaxant

X. FOLLOW-UP
A. As appropriate for diagnosis and treatment
B. As desired by patient if no definitive cause is found and palliative treatments are suggested
C. If symptoms continue, introduce the team approach.
  1. Mental health care specialist
  2. Physical therapist
  3. Nutritionist
  4. Urogynecologist
  5. Gastroenterologist

See Bibliographies.
Websites: http://www.mayoclinic.com/health/chronic-pelvic-pain/DS00571; http://women.webmd.com/endometriosis/endometriosis-treatment-overview

DYSESTHETIC VULVODYNIA

I. DEFINITION
Chronic mild-to-severe vulvar pain that is described as burning, stinging, irritating, and/or rawness that occurs alone or in conjunction with other vulvar pain syndromes or dermatoses and may occur with or without an identifiable provocation. The name is derived from the Greek word *odynia*, which means *pain*. The vulvar discomfort may involve the urethra, perianal area, and the thighs, as well as the generalized vulvar area. Accounts for 15% of gynecology visits and includes women of all ages. Current thinking is that vulvar pain is a symptom and not a diagnosis.

II. ETIOLOGY

A. May not be one single etiology, but rather a mixed etiology

B. Chronic infection could be the precipitating factor, careful diagnosis of *Candida* by positive wet mount or fungal culture, whereby the vulva becomes permanently sensitized from infection

C. Cutaneous perception or sensory nerve damage—neuropathic pain

  1. The vulva is rich with nerve fibers that may be disrupted or altered by inflammation and cause a sustained prolonged firing along the nerve even after the initial causative agent is removed or treated (i.e., infection)

    a. C fibers in the vestibule that are unmyelinated and are mechanosensitive and thermosensitive nociceptors. Inflammatory cytokines wrap around C fibers (nociceptors) and fire repeatedly.

    b. The remainder of the vulva is rich with A delta fibers that are mechanosensitive and myelinated and sensitive to light touch and thermosensitive nociceptors + C fibers. A delta fibers are hypersensitive.

  2. Sensitization occurs with chronic stimulation or irritation, resulting in allodynia (pain from a nonnoxious stimulus)

  3. Pain or hypersensitivity in radiating areas, such as the thighs and perianal area, may be suggestive of pudendal neuralgia

  4. Hyperpathia—stimulus causes greater pain than would be expected

  5. Central sensitization—related to lower parts of the brain and the cortex as well as centers of the spine. This sensitization is caused by a persistent signal to the nerve center that causes sensitization. Neurotransmitters activate these pain centers as well, and are the same chemicals that are increased in stress and anxiety. Lower peripheral pain thresholds in other sites such as the thumb and shin have been noted in women with vulvodynia that help to support this theory. Brain interpretation of pain results in motor and sensory abnormalities in body located outside of vulva. Lowered pain thresholds may precede genital pain (e.g., migraines).

  6. Dysesthetic vulvodynia is associated with cutaneous pain perception unrelated to touch

  7. Neuroimmunologic mechanisms involved in the allodynia/hyperpathia process in vulvodynia. These proposed mechanisms are under study.

D. Embryogenic correlation with interstitial cystitis—tissue from two anatomic sites that have a common embryonic origin, the urogenital sinus; because of this common origin, this may have a similar pathology response when provoked

E. Inflammatory dermatosis—related to prolonged topical steroid use, where temporary relief rebounded with more severe discomfort upon discontinuing the topical, or associated with benzylkonium chloride in pads and tampons or meds such as benzocaine and lidocaine or lotrisone

F. Genetic relationship—check whether other female family members have had problems with tampon use or dyspareunia

G. Pelvic floor dysfunction—the muscles involved in the pelvic floor are both tight and weak; the increase in muscle tone decreases blood flow to the vulvar tissue, with decreases in nutrients and buildup of lactic acid, causing tightness and pain. The resting tone of the muscle is most associated with the pain, and second, the variability of the contractile signal.

III. HISTORY
A. What the patient may present with
   1. High incidence of anxiety and emotional distress as a result of the vulvar pain
   2. Experiencing the pain for years
   3. In a stable relationship
   4. Having been examined by several clinicians
   5. History of one or more chronic pain conditions
      a. Migraines
      b. Fibromyalgia
      c. Irritable bowel syndrome
      d. Low back pain
      e. Interstitial cystitis
      f. Chronic fatigue syndrome
      g. Other
B. Begin with a thorough history
   1. Use open-ended questions about the pain and associated factors
      a. Location and duration of pain
      b. Any initiating factors
      c. Medications used and their effects on the pain
      d. Family history of similar pain
      e. Use of soaps, detergents, feminine products
      f. Contraceptive use
      g. History of trauma—vulvar surgery, episiotomy
      h. Discomfort with intercourse or pelvic exams
      i. Impact on daily living
      j. Any associated symptoms—urinary, bowel
      k. Pain or discomfort for hours or days following a pelvic exam or intercourse
      l. Constant or intermittent discomfort not related to touch or pressure
      m. History of seeing many clinicians without successful therapy

IV. PHYSICAL EXAMINATION
A. As appropriate to the history
B. Pelvic exam
   1. Inspect for erythema, erosions, ulcers, vesicles, whitened epithelium, any vulvar lesions, or alterations in the vulvar architecture

2. Cotton Q-tip test, light pressure, indent 5 mm to labia, ure-thra, hymenal remnants, and thighs, especially the posterior introitus and posterior hymenal remnants, and note areas of tenderness—patients with vulvodynia will have more gen-eralized pain, not necessarily made worse by touch or any pressure
3. Signs and symptoms of infection/potassium hydroxide (KOH) for fungal infection
4. Maybe no objective findings or some mild erythema are noted
5. Pelvic exam—note any associated pelvic pain and vaginal mus-cle tone
6. Check for vaginismus
7. Check for dermographia, because antihistamine may be helpful if the test is positive

V. LABORATORY EXAMINATION AS INDICATED BY HISTORY AND PHYSICAL EXAMINATION
A. Bacterial cultures and wet mount (KOH, saline)
B. If wet mount is negative for *Candida*, do a fungal culture
C. Herpes simplex virus (HSV) culture if erosions, fissures, or vesicles are present
D. Vulvar biopsy if there is a suspicious vulvar lesion, ulcers, vesicles, papules

VI. DIFFERENTIAL DIAGNOSIS
A. Infection: *Candida* or other fungal, herpes or other viral, bacterial
B. Inflammatory dermatoses: contact dermatitis, immunobullous dis-orders, lichen planus, lichen sclerosus, erosive lichen planus
C. Neoplastic: squamous cell carcinoma, Paget's disease, vulvar intra-epithelial neoplasia (VIN) neoplasm
D. Neurologic: HSV neuralgia, spinal nerve compression, pudendal nerve compression

VII. TREATMENT
A. Chronic pain model emphasizing ameliorating pain rather than cure
B. Patient education: good vulvar care—avoid tight clothes, 100% cot-ton underwear, as well as tampons or pads. Use of hypoallergenic detergents and stress-reduction methods; avoid chemical irritants—soaps, feminine sprays.
C. Multidisciplinary team approach; consider gynecologist, derma-tologist, urologist, gastroenterologist, physical therapist, and pain specialist per individual situation and accompanying symptoms. Acupuncture may be helpful.
D. Establish a sound, communicative, and trusting relationship
E. Establish one clinician as coordinator for the multidiscipline team (nurse practitioner [NP] ideal)

F. Treat any identified infections first, vaginal atrophy, or HSV with appropriate medication, including topical estrogen if indicated

G. Begin with local topical anesthetics, such as Lidocaine 5% ointment, applied to a cotton ball and placed at the vestibule overnight

H. Medications for neuropathic pain include:
1. Tricyclics: Use initially amitriptyline or nortriptyline, with gradual dose increases to numb the nerves by decreasing the electrical signals. Improvement may be sporadic at first and takes weeks—allow 3 months of use initially. Educate patient about tricyclic side effects.
2. Neurontin (gabapentin) antiseizure medication that is used for neuropathic pain
3. Selective serotonin and norepinephrine reuptake inhibitors such as Cymbalta, Effexor
4. None of these medications are U.S. Food and Drug Administration (FDA) approved for use in neuropathic pain
a. Refer to an appropriate clinician with experience with these drugs, or
b. Work with an appropriate clinician in treating the patients
c. Doses and effectiveness will vary, as will adverse events
d. Closely monitor
5. Alpha interferon injections intralesionally to the vestibule in vestibulodynia only

I. Advise a low oxalate diet with calcium citrate—eliminates irritants so may be beneficial, but as yet no scientific data to support its effectiveness

J. Refer to physical therapy (PT) for biofeedback to train the muscles to relax and teach the patients some control of these muscles
1. Specific surface electromyography (sEMG) to identify pelvic floor muscle abnormality and treatment to those muscles (craniosacral, myofascial)
2. Trigger point muscle massage—work with a physical therapist or massage therapist trained in women's health
3. Muscle stabilizing program, based on each woman's individual needs (6–8 months of PT)

K. Suggest acupuncture and/or hypnosis

L. Suggest personal counseling to decrease the woman's personal distress related to vulvar pain when necessary

M. Suggest marital counseling and sexual counseling when appropriate for issues related to intimacy discomforts that may arise with vulvodynia. As a woman's pain decreases, so may her sexual discomforts, distress, and anxiety, because these are correlated.

VIII. COMPLICATIONS
A. Development of additional symptoms following institution of treatment

    B. Side effects of any medications
    C. Coexistence of life-threatening condition

IX. CONSULTATION/REFERRAL
    A. Specialist in vulvodynia, dermatologist
    B. Psychotherapy, marital, sexual counseling
    C. PT, massage therapy, other complementary and alternative therapies
    D. Nutritional therapy
    E. Gastroenterologist
    F. Pain specialist or pain clinic
    G. If treating vulvar pain, consider taking a postgraduate course, seek to further educate yourself about this complex condition

X. FOLLOW-UP
    A. Return for recheck after treatment is initiated
    B. Team review as warranted by patient's response to interventions
    C. As indicated by therapy or for further diagnostic work and consultation

Website: http://www.mayoclinic.com/health/vulvodynia/DS00159

PEDICULOSIS

I. DEFINITION
Pediculosis is the state of being infested with lice that may be found on the skin, particularly the hairy areas such as the scalp and pubis, and may cause intense itching

II. ETIOLOGY
    A. Two species that look like each other but have different feeding habits are the following:
        1. *Pediculus humanus* var. *capitis* inhabits the skin of the head or body; transmitted by shared clothing, towels, brushes, combs, batting helmets, stuffed animals, car seats, bedding, headphones, hats; *P. humanus* var. *corporis* body louse lives in clothes
        2. *Phthirus pubis* ("crab louse," pubic louse) inhabits the genital area, but may colonize other areas including axillae, eyelashes, head hair; transmitted by close personal contact, bedding
    B. Nits hatch in 5 to 10 days incubation; adult pubic lice probably survive no more than 24 hours off their host; nits can survive in hot and humid climates up to 10 days. Symptoms may manifest in 2 to 3 weeks to develop pruritus.

III. HISTORY
  A. What the patient may present with
1. Pruritus
2. Visual identification of the parasite or its feces on bed pillow
3. Known exposure to household member or intimate partner with head, body, or pubic lice
4. Rarely, lymphadenopathy at back of neck; an allergic reaction to saliva and feces of lice
  B. Additional information to be considered
1. Lifestyle: shared clothing, towels, beds, pillows; shag rugs or carpets, upholstered furniture

IV. PHYSICAL EXAMINATION
  A. *Pediculosis capitis* (infestation with head lice); examine for:
1. Parasite
2. Greenish-white oval attachments to hair shaft (nits)
3. Secondary impetigo and furunculosis
4. Cervical lymphadenopathy
  B. *Pediculosis corporis* (infestation with body lice); examine for:
1. Parallel linear scratch marks on back, shoulders, trunk, buttocks (areas easily reached for scratching)
2. Impetigo lesions and furuncles associated with scratch marks secondary to scratching
3. Lice on clothing, especially the seams, as lice are rarely found on the body
  C. *Pediculosis pubis* (infestation with pubic [crab] lice); examine for:
1. Parasite (rarely found)
2. Oval attachments on pubic hair (nits)
3. Black dots (representing excreta) on surrounding skin and underclothing
4. Nits in eyebrows, eyelashes, scalp hair, axillary hair, and other body hair
5. Crusts or scabs in pubic area

V. LABORATORY EXAMINATION
May be able to see parasite on microscope slide after removal from hairy area.

VI. DIFFERENTIAL DIAGNOSIS (*see Etiology, II*)

VII. TREATMENT
  A. General measures
1. Wash with hot water, dry-clean, or run through a dryer on heat cycle all contaminated clothing, hats, towels, bedclothes, and so on to destroy nits and lice; wash combs and hairbrushes in hot soapy water, letting them soak for at least 15 minutes

2. Spray couches, chairs, car seats, and items that cannot be washed or dry-cleaned with OTC product (A-200 Pyrinate [pyrethrin]), Triplex, or RID (permethrin); alternative is to vacuum carefully to pick up living lice and nits

B. Specific treatment
1. *P. capitis* (infestation with head lice)
   a. Thoroughly wet hair with permethrin 1% cream rinse applied to affected areas and washed off after 10 minutes or Triplex Kit (pyrethrins + piperonyl butoxide); Pronto (piperonyl butoxide), RID (permethrin) shampoo or R&C shampoo (pyrethrins and piperonyl butoxide), or End Lice (pyrethrins and piperonyl); work up lather, adding water as necessary; shampoo thoroughly, leaving shampoo on head for 5 minutes; rinse, or use Pronto shampoo/conditioner (piperonyl butoxide); or Clear lice-killing shampoo (pyrethrin-based) and lice egg remover (permethrin-based) per directions on product or Klout (nonpesticide ingredients include isopropanol, methylparaben, propylparaben) per directions on product
   b. Rinse thoroughly, towel dry
   c. Remove remaining nits with fine-tooth metal comb or tweezers (use of vinegar solution and hair conditioner or olive oil make combing easier)
   d. Use LiceMeister comb to remove nits and check hair preventatively
2. *P. corporis* (infestation with body lice)
   a. Bathe with soap and water if no lice are found
   b. Wash with hot water and dry in dryer all clothing, bedclothes, towels, and so on
   c. Dry-clean items that cannot be washed; for items that cannot be washed or dry-cleaned, seal in a plastic bag for 1 week— lice will suffocate (in cold climates, put bags outside for 10 days; temperature change kills lice)
   d. If evidence of lice is found or patient is not relieved by a. and b., malathion 0.5% lotion applied for 8 to 12 hours, and thoroughly rinsed off
3. *P. pubis* (infestation with pubic lice)
   a. Permethrin 1% cream (NIX) rinse applied to affected area and washed off after 10 minutes; OR
   b. Pyrethrins with piperonyl butoxide (RID, Clear, A-200, Pronto, generics) applied to affected area and washed off after 10 minutes; OR
   c. Malathion 0.5% lotion applied for 8 to 12 hours, and thoroughly rinsed off; OR
   d. Ivermectin 200 µg/kg in a single dose. Adult minimum/maximum dose is 0.15 mg/kg or 0.2 mg/kg.
   e. Pregnancy, lactation: use permethrin or pyrethrins with piperonyl butoxide, not lindane

     f. Lindane is not recommended as first-line therapy because of toxicity; it should only be used as an alternative when other therapies fail, and only in adults; not in pregnancy or lactation

     g. Treat sexual partners within past month

     h. Wash in hot water and thoroughly dry on heat cycle or dry-clean all clothing, bed linen, towels, and so on, or remove from body contact for at least 72 hours

C. Stress the importance of careful checking of family and household members and close contacts; no treatment is needed unless there is evidence of contamination

D. Put nonwashable items in hot dryer; or spray with permethrin (RID, NIX)—check safety with children and pets

E. Screen patients with *P. pubis* for other STDs

VIII. COMPLICATIONS
A. Secondary infection
B. Sensitivity reactions to treatment
C. Excoriations
D. Resistance of lice to pediculicides

IX. CONSULTATION/REFERRAL
A. Lice found in eyelashes: because shampoo cannot be used, occlusive ophthalmic ointment is applied to the eyelid margins
B. Treatment failures
C. Coexisting dermatologic conditions

X. FOLLOW-UP
A. Evaluate in 1 week if symptoms persist
B. Instruct patient to return for repeat treatment if symptoms or parasites recur
C. Treat with alternative regimen if patient's infestation is nonresponsive

See Appendix I and Bibliographies.
Websites: http://www.health.state.ny.us/diseases/communicable/pediculosis/ fact_sheet.htm; http://www.headlice.org

PELVIC INFLAMMATORY DISEASE

I. DEFINITION
PID comprises a spectrum of inflammatory disorders of the upper genital tract. This may include any combination of endometritis, salpingitis, tubo-ovarian abscess, and pelvic peritonitis.

II. ETIOLOGY
  A. Causative organisms include:
    1. *Neisseria gonorrhoeae*
    2. *Streptococcus agalactiae*
    3. *Peptostreptococcus, Peptococcus*
    4. *Bacteroides*
    5. *C. trachomatis*
    6. *E. coli*
    7. *Mycoplasma hominis*
    8. RNA virus of the family *Orthomyxoviridae*
    9. *Urealyticum*
    10. *Gardnerella vaginalis*
    11. Trichomonads
    12. *Staphylococcus*
    13. *Pseudomonas*
    14. Diphtheroids
    15. Cytomegalovirus
    16. *Haemophilus agalactiae*
    17. *Mycoplasma hominis*

III. HISTORY
  A. What the patient may present with (wide variation in symptomatology, making diagnosis difficult)
    1. Lower abdominal pain, usually bilateral
    2. Chills, fever
    3. May have anorexia
    4. May have nausea
    5. May have vomiting
    6. Increased vaginal discharge
    7. Heavier than usual period; abnormal bleeding
    8. Urinary symptoms: frequency, pain
    9. May complain of right upper quadrant pain; also Fitz-Hugh-Curtis syndrome
    10. Dyspareunia
    11. Back pain
  B. Additional information to be considered
    1. Known exposure to STD
    2. Previous STD
    3. Previous diagnosis of PID
    4. Previously diagnosed endometriosis
    5. History of abdominal surgery
    6. Chronic illness
    7. Sexual activity (present and recent past)
    8. Last menstrual period (LMP); birth control method; presence of an IUD or recent insertion; recent pregnancy, childbirth, or abortion
    9. Medication allergy
    10. Currently taking any medication

11. Recent pelvic surgery (i.e., therapeutic abortion or dilatation and curettage)
12. Smoker or nonsmoker (smoking cigarettes has recently been implicated as a risk factor for PID)
13. History of douching

IV. PHYSICAL EXAMINATION
A. Vital signs
   1. Temperature
   2. Blood pressure
   3. Pulse
   4. Respiration
B. Abdominal examination
   1. Bowel sounds: normal, hyperactive, sluggish, absent
   2. Generalized lower abdominal tenderness
   3. Guarding
   4. Rebound tenderness
C. External genitalia
   1. Lesions
   2. Observe and palpate Skene's and Bartholin's glands
D. Vaginal examination (speculum)
   1. Profuse vaginal discharge (may be purulent)
   2. Examine cervix for
      a. Erosion, ectropion
      b. Friability
      c. Discharge in os
E. Bimanual examination
   1. Examine cervix for cervical motion tenderness
   2. Examine uterus for tenderness
   3. Examine adnexa for
      a. Tenderness
      b. Mass
   4. Rectovaginal examination for tenderness; if present, describe location (e.g., cervix, uterus, adnexa)

V. LABORATORY EXAMINATION
A. Gonococcal culture
B. *Chlamydia* smear
C. CBC/differential, C-reactive protein
D. Sedimentation rate
E. Urinary tract infection screen
F. Serology test for syphilis; HIV
G. Human chorionic gonadotropin (hCG) if history indicates: urine, serum
H. Transvaginal ultrasound
I. MRI—severe symptoms
J. Endometrial biopsy with histologic evidence of endometritis

    K. Laparoscopic abnormalities consistent with PID
    L. Culdocentesis (refer to a physician)

VI. CRITERIA FOR CLINICAL DIAGNOSIS
    A. Criteria for ambulatory treatment
        1. The three minimum criteria for diagnosis of PID
           a. History of uterine tenderness
           b. Cervical motion tenderness
           c. Adnexal tenderness (may be unilateral)
        2. Additional criteria that will increase the specificity of diagnosis
           a. Temperature of 101°F (38.3°C) or higher
           b. WBCs on saline microscopy of vaginal secretions
           c. Abnormal cervical or vaginal mucopurulent discharge
           d. Elevated C-reactive protein
           e. Culdocentesis yielding peritoneal fluid, which contains bacteria; WBCs
           f. Presence of adnexal mass noted on bimanual examination; tubo-ovarian abscess on sonography
           g. Elevated sedimentation rate greater than 15 mm/hour
           h. Positive gonococcal culture from cervix
           i. Positive *Chlamydia* smear from cervix
    B. Criteria for hospitalization
        1. Surgical emergencies such as appendicitis cannot be excluded
        2. The patient is pregnant
        3. The patient does not respond clinically to oral antimicrobial therapy
        4. The patient is unable to follow or tolerate an outpatient oral regimen
        5. The patient has severe illness, nausea, and vomiting or high fever
        6. The patient has a tubo-ovarian abscess
        7. The patient is immunodeficient (i.e., has HIV infection with low counts; is taking immunosuppressant therapy), or has another disease

VII. DIFFERENTIAL DIAGNOSIS
    A. Septic abortion
    B. Ectopic gestation
    C. Ovarian cyst
    D. Ruptured ovarian cyst
    E. Cystitis
    F. Pyelonephritis
    G. Peptic ulcer disease
    H. Hepatitis
    I. Appendicitis
    J. Adhesions
    K. Endometriosis/endometritis

L. Diverticular disease
M. Pelvic neoplasms
N. Irritable bowel syndrome
O. Ovarian torsion
P. Inflammatory bowel disease

VIII. TREATMENT (CENTERS FOR DISEASE CONTROL AND PREVENTION [CDC] RECOMMENDATIONS 2010) FOR UNCOMPLICATED PELVIC INFLAMMATORY DISEASE (MILD TO MODERATELY SEVERE ACUTE PID)

A. Medication
   1. Ceftriaxone 250 mg IM in a single dose *plus* doxycycline 100 mg orally twice a day for 14 days *with* or *without* metronidazole 500 mg orally twice a day for 14 days OR
   Cefoxitin 2 g IM and probenecid 1 g orally concurrently in a single dose *plus* doxycycline 100 mg orally twice a day for 14 days *with* or *without* metronidazole 500 mg orally twice a day for 14 days OR
   2. Other parenteral third-generation cephalosporin (e.g., ceftizoxime or cefotaxime *plus* doxycycline 100 mg orally twice a day for 14 days *with* or *without* metronidazole 500 mg orally twice a day for 14 days)
   3. Pregnant women: Hospitalize and treat with parenteral antibiotics per CDC guidelines for hospitalization
   4. Refer to CDC guidelines (2010) if patient meets hospitalization criteria
B. General measures
   1. Bed rest
   2. Increased fluid intake
   3. General diet
   4. Stress the importance of partner being examined and treated
   5. Stress the use of condoms to prevent reinfection or future infections
   6. No douching
C. Management of sex partners
   1. Examine and treat if sexual contact with patient during 60 days prior to onset of symptoms

IX. COMPLICATIONS

A. Sterility
B. Generalized sepsis
C. Chronic pelvic pain
D. Tubal pregnancy
E. Surgical interventions
F. Dyspareunia
G. Tubo-ovarian abscess
H. Fitz-Hugh-Curtis syndrome: perihepatitis

X. CONSULTATION/REFERRAL
A. If failure to improve within 3 days (48–72 hours) after starting the aforementioned treatment
B. For hospitalization
C. For culdocentesis or diagnostic laparoscopy if indicated

XI. FOLLOW-UP
A. Reevaluate within 72 hours or sooner if symptoms worsen or do not improve. Patients should demonstrate substantial clinical improvement within 3 days.
B. After completion of medication course (no sooner than 7 days)
   1. Bimanual
   2. Cultures if indicated (i.e., positive lab results prior to treatment); some specialists recommend rescreening for gonorrhea and *C. trachomatis* regardless of prior culture results 4 to 6 weeks after completion of therapy
C. Male sex partners of women with PID should be examined and treated if sexual contact was 60 days or less preceding symptom onset

See Bibliographies.
Websites: http://www.cdc.gov/node.do/id/0900f3ec800e9b48;
www.cdc.gov/mmwr for December 17, 2010, STD Treatment Guidelines, 2010

PELVIC MASS

I. DEFINITION
Mass found in adnexa, cul-de-sac, or uterus during bimanual examination

II. ETIOLOGY
A pelvic mass may be caused by any number of factors. This guideline is meant to assist the clinician in the screening and referral process.

III. HISTORY
A. What the patient may present with
   1. May be asymptomatic
   2. Bloating
   3. Abdominal pain: generalized or localized/duration/onset
   4. Flatulence
   5. Dysfunctional bleeding—can be heavy
   6. Amenorrhea; number of weeks
   7. Vaginal discharge
   8. Low back pain and/or pressure
   9. Dyspareunia
   10. Bowel or bladder dysfunction; chronic bowel disease
   11. Prior abdominal surgery

12. Prior pelvic surgery
13. Endometriosis
14. Pregnancy history; assisted reproduction
B. Additional information to be obtained
1. LMP
2. Contraception used
3. Menstruation, pregnancy, and infertility history
4. Any change in bowel habits; last bowel movement
5. History of ovarian cysts
6. History of uterine fibroids
7. History of PID
8. History of *Chlamydia* or gonorrhea
9. History of IUD use
10. History of ectopic pregnancy
11. Family history
12. Results of recent Papanicolaou smear; any follow-up if abnormal
13. Diagnostic tests including colonoscopy, laparoscopy, flexible sigmoidoscopy

IV. PHYSICAL EXAMINATION
A. Abdominal exam
1. Bowel sounds
2. Pain
3. Organomegaly
B. Vaginal examination
1. Examine cervix for discharge and presence of IUD string
2. Examine vagina for masses, lesions, discharge
C. Bimanual examination
1. Examine cervix for cervical motion tenderness
2. Examine uterus for tenderness, masses, shape, size, and consistency; prolapse
3. Examine adnexa for masses, attempting to differentiate between ovaries and bowel
4. Evaluate mass for shape, consistency, size, mobility, and tenderness
5. Examine bladder; check for cystocele
6. Cul-de-sac for mass
7. Thickening or tenderness at or near uterosacral ligaments
D. Rectal examination
1. Pain, tenderness
2. Masses
3. Melena
4. Rectovaginal masses, fistulas
5. Rectocele/occult blood

V. LABORATORY EXAMINATION
A. Cultures as indicated
B. Wet prep as indicated
C. Serum pregnancy test as indicated

D. CBC with sedimentation rate; C-reactive protein
E. Ultrasound; transvaginal and transabdominal, or with Doppler as indicated
F. CA-125, ovarian cancer tumor marker as indicated
G. Consider carcinoembryonic antigen
H. Endometrial biopsy as indicated

VI. TREATMENT
A. Adnexal masses
1. If thought to be retained stool or intestinal gas, patient should have bowel prep and be reexamined
2. If thought to be ovarian in origin, the following differentiation may be made
   a. Age of patient (ovulation or using ovulation inhibitor, perimenopausal or menopausal)
   b. Menstrual history
   c. Indication of infection
   d. Positive result of the pregnancy test
3. If ovulation is presumed, assess size of mass with ultrasound
   a. If greater than 5 to 6 cm, physician referral is indicated
   b. If less than 5 cm and asymptomatic, reexamine after next menses; if unchanged, may
      i. Recommend ovulatory inhibitor for 3 months and reexamine. If remaining after 3 months, refer to a physician.
      ii. Consider ultrasound as baseline. If functional cyst is confirmed, wait 2 months and repeat ultrasound.
4. If on ovulatory inhibitor, do appropriate workup (i.e., ultrasound) and refer, or refer immediately depending on setting
5. If perimenopausal/menopausal
   a. Do appropriate workup (i.e., ultrasound); refer for a physician evaluation as indicated
B. Uterine mass
1. Do ultrasound; small, nonsymptomatic fibroids may be followed and assessed on a 6- to 12-month basis as appropriate to setting. Large fibroids or other finding, refer to a physician.
C. Ectopic pregnancy
1. Do ultrasound; if confirmed to be ectopic, consult or refer to a physician for treatment. Current treatment includes
   a. Serial serum human gonadotropin levels (hCG level <2,000 mIU, and <50% rise in 48 hours) followed by consultation with a physician
   b. Medical management (per guidelines of clinical site) consultation with or prescription by a physician
      i. Methotrexate in single dose IM 50 mg/m^2 of body surface calculated on body weight
      ii. Monitor hCG per guidelines of clinical site and possible ultrasound monitoring
   c. Consult and referral for surgical management

VII. DIFFERENTIAL DIAGNOSIS
A. Inflammatory
  1. Tubo-ovarian abscess
  2. Appendiceal abscess
  3. Diverticular abscess
B. Functional
  1. Ovarian cysts
    a. Follicular
    b. Luteal
    c. Polycystic ovaries
C. Neoplastic
  1. Benign
  2. Malignant
D. Anatomic anomalies
  1. Pelvic kidney
  2. Bicornuate uterus
E. Other
  1. Ectopic pregnancy
  2. Endometrioma
  3. Paratubal/ovarian cyst
  4. Hydrosalpinx

VIII. COMPLICATIONS
Complication of individual entity as listed in differential diagnosis

IX. CONSULTATION AND REFERRAL
As indicated by laboratory workup and physical findings indicated in *Treatment, VI*

X. FOLLOW-UP
As indicated by diagnosis

See Bibliographies.
  Websites: http://www.mamc.amedd.army.mil/referral/guidelines/obgyn_pelvic mass.htm; http://www.merck.com/mmpr/sec18/ch242/ch242c.html

SCABIES

I. DEFINITION
A highly contagious papulofollicular skin rash whose chief symptom is pruritus. Infestation of the human itch mite that burrows into upper layer of the skin. Rash and itching are thought to be hypersensitivity reactions to the mites, and are not confined to the locations of mite burrows. With first exposure, sensitization can take several weeks. After reinfestation, pruritus can occur within 24 hours. Transmitted by skin-to-skin

contact with an individual who has scabies. Scabies among adults may be sexually transmitted.

II. ETIOLOGY

Sarcoptes scabiei mite. The mite burrows into skin and deposits eggs along a tunnel. Larvae hatch in 3 to 5 days and gather around hair follicles. Newly hatched female burrows into the skin, maturing in 10 to 19 days, then mates and starts a new cycle. Crusted scabies (Norwegian scabies) is an aggressive infestation.

III. HISTORY

    A. What the patient may present with
        1. Pruritus—worse at night or at times when body temperature is raised (i.e., after exercise). Pruritus exists prior to physical manifestations.
        2. Lesions are usually on interdigital webs of hands, flexor aspects of wrists, extensor surfaces of the elbows, areas surrounding the nipples, anterior axillary folds, umbilicus, belt line, lower abdomen, genitalia and gluteal cleft; male genitals; can be all over body especially with immunosuppression
    B. Additional information to be considered
        1. Known contact with scabies. Incubation period in persons without previous exposure is usually 4 to 6 weeks (mean 3 weeks). Persons who were previously infected develop symptoms 1 to 3 days after repeat exposure to the mite. These reinfections are usually milder.
        2. Lifestyle. Persons in crowded living conditions and living in proximity with others, such as in nursing homes, dormitories, and shelters, and those who share clothing are at increased risk for nonsexual exposures.
        3. History of atopic dermatitis, HIV+, or other immunosuppressed condition; hematologic malignancies
        4. At high risk for crusted scabies

IV. PHYSICAL EXAMINATION

    A. Skin: thorough examination of lesions and of those areas most frequently involved
        1. Linear burrows about 1.5 to 2 cm in length, terminating in a papule or vesicle
        2. Lesions: papules or vesicles
        3. Scaling, crustation lesions, furuncles, or excoriations may be present with secondary infection
    B. Lymph nodes exhibit generalized lymphadenopathy

V. LABORATORY

    A. Mineral oil to skin, and then a scraping from several of the excoriated lesions onto a slide, examined under low power. It may be difficult to find mites. Application of water, alcohol, or mineral oil

to the skin facilitates collection of the scraping. Scraping is done at the edge of a burrow.
B. Diagnosis is usually made based on clinical presentation

VI. DIFFERENTIAL DIAGNOSIS
A. Atopic dermatitis
B. Impetigo
C. Urticaria
D. Psoriasis
E. Drug-induced eruption
F. Insect bites

VII. TREATMENT
A. Medication
 1. 5% permethrin cream (Elimite), applied to all areas of the body from neck down, and washed off after 8 to 14 hours, and then repeat treatment 1 week later; OR
 2. Ivermectin 200 μg/kg single oral dose, repeated in 2 weeks (safety in children <15 years of age not determined)
 3. In pregnancy and lactation and for children younger than 2 years old, use only permethrin. Do not use ivermectin or lindane.
 4. Lindane is not recommended as first-line therapy because of toxicity. Use only as alternative in patients who cannot tolerate other therapies or when other therapies have failed. Lindane 1% lotion or 30 mg of cream applied in a thin layer to all areas of the body from the neck down and thoroughly washed off after 8 hours. It should not be used immediately after a bath or shower, or by persons with extensive dermatitis.
B. Symptomatic treatment
 1. Antihistamines may be given to relieve pruritus
 2. Patient should be informed that pruritus may persist for several weeks. If the patient does not respond to therapy and itching is still persistent after 1 week, he or she should be instructed to contact the health care provider to decide whether further therapy is necessary. The patient may need mild-to-moderate potency topical steroids for pruritus.
C. General measures
 1. Clothing, towels, and bed linens should be laundered at 60°C (hot cycle) or dry-cleaned on the day of treatment
 2. If clothing items cannot be washed or dry-cleaned, these should be separated from washed clothes and not worn for at least 72 hours. Mites cannot exist for more than 2 to 3 days away from the body.
 3. Sexual partners and close personal or household contacts within the past month should be informed, examined, and treated if necessary

4. Patient should be instructed to follow treatment regimen carefully
5. Although fumigation of living areas is not necessary, some patients may wish to decontaminate mattresses, sofas, and other inanimate objects that cannot be washed. OTC sprays and powders are available for this purpose. This is usually discouraged because it is generally unnecessary.

VIII. COMPLICATIONS
A. Secondary infection (may require systemic antibiotics)
B. Reaction to lindane (Kwell, Scabene)
   1. Dermatitis
   2. Central nervous system toxicity

IX. CONSULTATION AND REFERRAL
A. Secondary infection
B. Generalized widespread inflammatory response
C. Failure to respond to therapy
D. Reaction to lindane (Kwell, Scabene)
E. Patients with coexisting dermatitis or other dermatologic condition
F. Patients with coexisting HIV infection or who are otherwise immunosuppressed; those with crusted scabies

X. FOLLOW-UP
A. Failure to respond to therapy. Some experts recommend retreatment after 1 to 2 weeks for patients who are still symptomatic; others recommend retreatment only if live mites can be observed. Retreatment should be with an alternative regimen.
B. Recurrence

Appendix I may be copied or adapted for your patients.
Website: www.cdc.gov/NCIDOD/DPD/parasites/scabies/factsht_scabies.htm

UTERINE LEIOMYOMATA

I. DEFINITION
Often referred to as uterine fibroids, fibromyomas, myomas, or fibromas, leiomyomas are benign uterine tumors arising from the smooth muscle and having some connective tissue elements as well. They are nonmalignant growths that do not pose any increased risk for uterine cancer.

II. ETIOLOGY
A. Physiology
   1. Appear to arise from single (monoclonal) neoplastic smooth muscle cells (fourth and fifth decades) within the myometrium
   2. May be single or multiple

3. May range in size from microscopic to more than 20 cm (filling the abdomen)
4. May occur within the uterine wall (intramural) or extend externally from the serosal surface (subserosal) internally into endometrial cavity (submucous); have both estrogen and progesterone receptors
5. Can also be in broad ligament, ovary, or cervix
6. Occur most commonly during a woman's fertile years (35–50), usually asymptomatic
7. Usually undergo regression with menopause; rare before menarche
8. Sometimes increase in size with hormonal contraceptives or pregnancy

III. HISTORY
A. What the patient may present with
   1. May be asymptomatic
   2. Pelvic pain (acute or chronic) 1:3 women
   3. Abnormal vaginal bleeding (30%), menorrhagia
   4. Urinary frequency, retention, incontinence, urgency
   5. Constipation
   6. Pelvic pressure
   7. Dyspareunia
   8. Backache or leg aches
   9. Occasionally acute pain
B. Additional information to be considered
   1. Menstrual history, menorrhagia, dysmenorrhea
   2. History of infertility
   3. Habitual spontaneous abortions—may need surgical removal of fibroids
   4. Menopausal symptoms
   5. LMP, methods of birth control, IUD in place, or history of IUD use
   6. Any pelvic surgery
   7. Pregnancy history; parity—may have a protective effect
   8. Use of hormones: oral contraceptives, hormone therapy, infertility drugs
   9. Family history; ethnic background; genetic alterations, may run in families—Black women more likely to have fibroids
   10. Obesity (elevated body mass index [BMI])
   11. OCP use—usually lowers risk for fibroids to develop

IV. PHYSICAL EXAMINATION
A. Vital signs as indicated
B. Abdominal examination
   1. Any abdominal guarding or tenderness
   2. Location of any pain
   3. Bladder (palpable or distended)

   C. Vaginal examination
     1. Examine cervix for any extraneous tissue, distortion of configuration
     2. Palpate vagina for any masses
     3. Examine any bleeding or discharge
   D. Bimanual examination
     1. Examine uterus for tenderness, masses
     2. Examine adnexa for masses, tenderness
     3. Locate any pain if possible
   E. Rectovaginal examination for tenderness, masses

V. LABORATORY EXAMINATION
   A. Ultrasound—more detail with transvaginal
   B. Pregnancy test if premenopausal or perimenopausal
   C. CBC
   D. MRI
   E. Endoscopic visualization
   F. HSG
   G. Sonohysterography

VI. DIFFERENTIAL DIAGNOSIS
   A. Uterine pregnancy
   B. Malignant uterine tumor
   C. Ovarian cyst or tumor
   D. Extrauterine pelvic mass
   E. Bowel tumor
   F. Bladder tumor
   G. Tumor of ureter, kidney
   H. Pelvic abscess
   I. Extrauterine pregnancy
   J. Bicornuate uterus

VII. TREATMENT
   A. As indicated by ultrasound
     1. Note the size of leiomyomata with bimanual examination and repeat ultrasound and monitor with exams and/or ultrasounds
     2. Consultation for medical management: progestins, gonadotropin-releasing hormone (GnRH) agonists cause estrogen and progesterone levels to decrease, thus fibroids shrink
     3. Consultation for surgical management: hysterectomy, myomectomy, hysteroscope, resectoscope, laser ablation; myolysis or myoma coagulation; cryomyolysis; fibroid embolization
     4. Progesterone IUD may provide relief from symptoms of fibroids
     5. Androgens such as Danazol can relieve symptoms; no menstruation thus decrease in fibroid size and uterine size

VIII. COMPLICATIONS
A. Torsion of pedunculated leiomyomata resulting in necrosis
B. Uterine abscess
C. Infarction
D. Hemorrhage
E. Degeneration: hyalinization, cystic, calcification, fatty
F. May affect fertility, increase risk of miscarriage; may also create malposition of fetus, premature labor and delivery

IX. CONSULTATION/REFERRAL
A. Rapid change in size
B. Signs of complications
C. Menorrhagia
D. Compromise of adjacent organs
E. Intractable pelvic pressure or pain

X. FOLLOW-UP
A. Reevaluate every 6 to 12 months or as indicated
B. As indicated under medical management with medication
   1. Long-term GnRH agonists >6 months add estrogen for osteoporosis, menopausal symptom relief

See Bibliographies.
Website: http://www.mayoclinic.com/health/uterine-fibroids/DS00078/DSECTION=symptoms

VULVAR CONDITIONS

I. DEFINITION
Primary vulvar conditions are those that arise from abnormal epithelial growth, which can be inflammatory, dermatologic, or congenital in origin, or from neoplastic alterations. Because the vulva includes the labia majora and minora, the mons veneris, fourchette, and vestibule, and encompasses the urethral and vaginal orifices and the ducts of the Skene's and Bartholin's glands, vulvar conditions are varied both in origin and in clinical manifestations. Please refer to separate guidelines for STDs that can cause clinical signs and symptoms on the vulva, and guidelines for Bartholin's cyst, molluscum contagiosum, herpes, and condyloma.

II. ETIOLOGY
A. Nonneoplastic epithelial disorders
   1. Squamous cell hyperplasia
   2. Lichen simplex chronicus

    3. Lichen sclerosis
    4. Lichen planus
    5. Pigmented lesions
    6. Systemic diseases (inflammatory bowel disease, Behcet's syndrome)
    7. Psoriasis
  B. Neoplastic disorder (VIN)
    1. Vulvar intraepithelial neoplasia
      a. Low-grade squamous intraepithelial lesion (SIL) mild dysplasia
      b. High-grade SIL moderate to severe dysplasia
      c. Squamous cell carcinoma in situ—Bowen's disease, bowenoid papulosis
      d. Basal cell carcinoma
      e. VIN 2 to 3
      f. Invasive VIN
    2. Other neoplastic disorders
      a. Extramammary Paget versus vulvar vaginal *Candidiasis*
      b. Melanoma (5% is vulvar)

III. HISTORY

  A. What the patient may present with
    1. Pruritus, rash
    2. Hypopigmentation or hyperpigmentation
    3. Bullae
    4. Weeping, scaling, crusting
    5. Excoriation
    6. Maceration
    7. Thickening
    8. Hyperkeratosis
    9. Fissures
    10. Abscesses
    11. Lesions: macules, papules, vesicles, warty, pedunculated, domed, flat, plaques
    12. Lichenification
    13. Change in color of vulva
    14. Dyspareunia
    15. Burning
    16. Genital erosions
    17. Vaginal/vulvar discharge
  B. Additional information to be considered
    1. Type of clothing commonly worn
    2. Type of underwear: cotton, synthetic
    3. Use of feminine deodorant products
    4. Use of scented, deodorant tampons, pads, panty liners
    5. Douching; shaving of perineum
    6. Detergents, bathing soap, fabric softeners
    7. Bubble bath or oils, body washes, lotions, creams

8. Family or personal history of diabetes
9. Sexual partners, activity; contraception; STD history
10. Fungal infection of hands and feet, self or partner; oral *Candidiasis*
11. LMP
12. Perimenopausal symptoms
13. History of dermatologic conditions: human papillomavirus (HPV), psoriasis, eczema, seborrheic dermatitis
14. Fever, malaise, flu-like symptoms, recent streptococcal infection
15. Character and changes in lesions
16. Partner with symptoms
17. History of Crohn's disease; other systemic disease
18. Genital HPV history, history of Pap smear with HPV, any abnormal Pap history
19. Any other possible allergens: plant, make-up, nail polish, depilatories, piercings, and jewelry

IV. PHYSICAL EXAMINATION
A. Vulva
1. Skin appearance: inflammation, edema, dry or moist, thickening hyperkeratosis, erythema with a demarcation between normal and abnormal tissue (strawberries and cream appearance)
2. Lesions present
3. Weeping, scaling, crusting
4. Fissuring
5. Lichenification
6. Excoriation
7. Hypopigmentation
8. Hyperpigmentation
9. Ulcers
B. Adenopathy
C. Groin, inner thighs, buttocks
1. Lesions
D. Other systems as indicated by history and drugs

V. LABORATORY EXAMINATION AS INDICATED BY HISTORY AND APPEARANCE OF LESIONS
A. Bacterial cultures and sensitivities
B. Wood's lamp examination
C. Gram-stained scraping from lesions
D. Scrapings for KOH
E. Punch biopsy of lesions
F. Colposcopic examination
G. Staining with 1% toluidine blue
H. Fasting blood sugar
I. HPV testing

VI. DIFFERENTIAL DIAGNOSIS
   A. Allergic vulvitis, cellulitis
   B. Inflammatory conditions and reactions
   C. Bacterial, viral, fungal infections
   D. Lichen sclerosis
   E. Necrotizing fasciitis
   F. Lichen planus
   G. Pigmentation disorders
      1. Hyperpigmentation
      2. Congenital hypopigmentation
   H. Benign epithelial changes
   I. Neoplasms: vulvar intraepithelial neoplasia, Paget's disease, melanoma
   J. Lesions from Crohn's disease
   K. Trauma
   L. Infestation
   M. Zinc deficiency
   N. Fixed drug reaction
   O. HSV infection

VII. TREATMENT
   A. Medication
      1. Contact dermatitis: cool, tepid, warm compresses or sitz baths; midpotent corticosteroid ointment, triamcinolone oil 1% twice a day; identify and remove irritant. Apply petrolatum to open areas.
      2. Bacterial infections: Erythromycin 250 mg 4 times a day for 14 days; tetracycline 250 mg 4 times a day for 10 to 14 days or until resolved/culture and sensitivity for medication coverage
      3. Tinea: topical antifungals such as Gyne-Lotrimin, Mycelex, Monistat Derm, Loprox
      4. Analgesics for pain: no topical Lanacane creams—high degree of sensitivity; Xylocaine 5% ointment 1/8 teaspoon 3 times daily and cotton ball in the vestibule at bedtime. If burning continues, have it buffered by compounding pharmacy.
      5. Topical antibiotics Bactroban 2% ointment may be considered
      6. Fixed drug reaction—check on any new medication; must go off medication for 2 months to see resolution; contact primary care provider to change medication
   B. Lifestyle changes and self-care measures
      1. Wear loose, cotton underwear; do not wear underwear in bed
      2. Keep area dry and clean
      3. Discontinue use of irritant or allergen
      4. Sitz baths
   C. Teaching and reassurance

VIII. COMPLICATIONS
   A. Secondary infection
   B. Progressive disease
   C. Masking more serious disease

IX. CONSULTATION/REFERRAL
   A. Unable to identify lesion or condition
   B. No response to treatment
   C. Progression of disease or persistence of condition
   D. For biopsy, diagnostic workup
   E. For surgical excision or other surgical intervention
   F. To specialist for systemic disease or dermatoses beyond the vulva
   G. To specialist for vulvar vestibulitis and vulvodynia

X. FOLLOW-UP
   A. See patient again in 1 to 2 weeks to assess therapy/treatment
   B. As indicated by therapy or for further diagnostic work

See Bibliographies.
Website: http://www.cancer.about.com/od/vulvarcancer/a/vulvarexam.htm

18

Perimenopause and Postmenopause

GENERAL CARE MEASURES

I. DEFINITION
The menopause is the landmark event of the climacteric, the 10- to 15-year period, beginning at about age 35 to 40 years old, when women's bodies are changing and preparing for cessation of menses. A woman cannot say that she has gone through menopause until at least one year has passed without any menstrual period (uterine bleeding). The postmenopausal time begins when menopause is complete and menses no longer occur. For women today, the postmenopausal years may comprise as much as three-eighths of their lives or more, the age for menopause being about 50 years old in the United States (mean 50.4 years). A woman who has had a hysterectomy (removal of uterus only) is not considered menopausal with cessation of menses.

II. ETIOLOGY
    A. Physiologic: The gradual diminution of estrogens, resulting in cessation of ovulation and thus of menstruation
    B. Anatomic: Surgical removal of the uterus and ovaries resulting in surgical menopause, an abrupt end to ovulation and menstruation

III. HISTORY
    A. What the patient presents with
        1. Changes in character of the menstrual cycle
            a. Menstrual periods that are more frequent, less frequent, of longer duration or shorter duration
            b. Scanty flow
            c. Flooding at onset of flow
            d. Gradual or abrupt cessation of menses for 1 or more months
            e. Irregular periods over a period or abrupt cessation of menstruation
        2. Changes related to menopause and/or the aging process
            a. Hot flashes, hot flushes
            b. Vaginal dryness, atrophy of vaginal tissues
            c. Night sweats
            d. Dry skin and hair; skeletal pain or stiffness
            e. Graying of hair
            f. Loss of skin elasticity
            g. Alterations in sleep patterns
            h. Alterations in sexual response: longer time needed for arousal, lessened vaginal lubrication
            i. Mons and vulva flatten, less fatty tissue padding, thinning of pubic hair
        3. Recent history of gynecologic surgery: hysterectomy, oophorectomy, salpingectomy, dilatation, and curettage

B. Additional information to be considered
   1. Menstrual history, past year
   2. Contraceptive use to present
   3. Obstetrical history: pregnancies, abortions, stillbirths
   4. Gynecologic history: surgery, endometriosis, infertility, anomalies, last Pap smear, any breast problems, last mammogram, sexually transmitted disease (STD), infections; any stress or urge incontinence
   5. Sexual history: dysfunction, unresponsiveness, recent changes, use of sex toys (*see Sexual Dysfunction, Chapter 20*); high-risk sexual behaviors
   6. Life event changes: resumption of career, retirement, caring for older family members, adult children in or out of home, divorce, separation, marriage, new sexual relationship, caring for grandchildren, loss of a child
   7. Lifestyle: exercise, diet, smoking, recreation, stressors, recreational drugs
   8. Medical history: chronic disease, medications (over the counter [OTC], prescription); depression, anxiety
   9. Family medical history
   10. Use of complementary therapies (botanicals, homeopathics, massage, Tai Chi, acupuncture, Chinese medicine, aromatherapy, etc.)
   11. Beliefs about menopause and expectations
   12. Domestic violence, elder abuse

IV. PHYSICAL EXAMINATION
   A. Vital signs
      1. Blood pressure
      2. Pulse
      3. Height
      4. Weight, body mass index (BMI)
   B. General health examination
      1. Head
      2. Neck
      3. Heart
      4. Lungs
      5. Abdomen
      6. Extremities, joints, spine
   C. External examination for lesions, infection, atrophy, anomaly
      1. Urethral os
      2. Clitoris
      3. Labia
      4. Perineum
   D. Vaginal examination (speculum)
      1. Walls
      2. Discharge
      3. Lesions in the vaginal vault, noting if posthysterectomy

    4. Cervix
    5. Careful inspection of entire vagina
  E. Bimanual examination
    1. Adnexa
      a. Tenderness
      b. Masses
      c. Palpable ovaries, if present
    2. Uterus
      a. Size
      b. Mobility
      c. Tenderness
      d. Masses
    3. Cystocele, rectocele, urethrocele
  F. Rectal examination: fecal occult blood

V. LABORATORY EXAMINATION
  A. Appropriate cultures, smears if suspicion of infection
  B. Pap smear per the ASCCP guidelines
  C. Mammogram per American Cancer Society guidelines: (annually at 40 and after); may be altered with family history or personal risk factors for breast cancer and new recommendations from ACS or NCI
  D. Consider serum follicle-stimulating hormone (FSH) level to assess for menopause if no menses for 12 months or on hormonal contraception age 50 years or older and/or desire to consider hormone therapy (HT; FSH equal to or >2–40 mIU/ml); discontinue hormones for the 2 weeks prior to serum assay of FSH
  E. Blood glucose and lipid levels, TSH, 25-hydroxyvitamin D

VI. DIFFERENTIAL DIAGNOSIS
  A. Carcinoma of genital tract
  B. Pregnancy
  C. Endocrine disorders
  D. Decreased nutritional state; obesity
  E. Marked increase in exercise regimen

VII. TREATMENT
  A. Medication
    1. Perimenopausal: consider low dose oral contraceptive or other hormonal contraception after assessment for risks, desire for contraceptive protection; consider cycling with a progestin if intermenstrual time decreases and/or heavy bleeding/flooding characterize menses
    2. Postmenopausal: consider nonhormonal or hormone (*see Hormone Therapy section*) interventions per clinical picture and patient's wishes

B. General measures
1. Teaching about normal menopausal symptoms, changes with aging, need for more time for arousal, use of supplemental lubrication (saliva, water soluble lubricants—these come as creams, jellies, and as vaginal inserts); nonhormonal agents to restore/maintain vaginal mucosa and vaginal moisture such as Replens, Comfrey ointment, vitamin E supplement + 100 to 600 mg/day, or evening primrose oil 2 to 4 capsules/day 1 (also helpful for hot flashes); *Calendula*, black cohosh (20–40 mg twice a day), changes in sexual response that accompany the removal of the uterus/ovaries
2. Teaching about self-care: diet, exercise—aerobic, weight bearing, and strengthening—prevention of osteoporosis (calcium intake 1,200–1,500 g/day and vitamin in foods or supplement (dosage will vary according to individual need); breast self-examination, need for Pap smear as indicated by history and past Pap tests and pelvic examination yearly; regular mammograms; contraception until 1 year without menses (some say 2 years); signs and symptoms of problems: postmenopausal bleeding; prevention of vaginal infections
3. Teaching about urinary health: 6 to 8 glasses of water a day, decrease caffeine, Kegel exercises; quit smoking
4. Teaching about triggers for hot flashes—electric blanket, alcohol, spicy foods, overheating, constrictive clothing; symptom management with evening primrose oil, licorice root, phytoestrogens, sage or sarsaparilla, black cohosh (*see Complementary and Alternative Therapies, Chapter 3*)
5. Consider nonhormonal synthetic medication and bioflavonoid alternatives for symptom management; other botanicals, homeopathic medicines (e.g., for sleep disorders: hops, valerian tea or tincture, melatonin, exercise, relaxation techniques; for memory: ginkgo biloba [120–240 mg/day]; for irritability: anise, chasteberry, dong quai, flaxseed, ginseng, kava kava [60–120 mg], red raspberry leaf) (*see Complementary and Alternative Therapies, Chapter 3)*
6. Diet: low fat, avoid or decrease caffeine, zinc 15 mg/day in foods and/or in supplements; vitamin B and C complex vitamins, fiber; phytoestrogens (soy protein isoflavone 40–160 mg/day; lignans such as flaxseed, cereal bran; other isoflavones: chick peas, legumes, bluegrass, clover)

VIII. COMPLICATIONS/RISKS
A. Pregnancy
B. Carcinoma of reproductive tract
C. Breast cancer (risk is higher after menopausal years)
D. Incapacitating menopausal symptoms: hot flashes that disrupt normal life, night sweats, sleep disturbances

    E. Osteoporosis
    F. Possible increased risk for heart attacks, coronary heart disease (*see Appendix E*)
    G. Interactions, adverse effects of herbals, vitamins; negative interactions with prescription medications

IX. CONSULTATION/REFERRAL
    A. To physician or other clinician, as appropriate for complications previously listed
    B. Sex therapist for prolonged or severe disruption in sexual relationship
    C. Counseling: stresses of the middle years, depression
    D. Mammogram, sigmoidoscopy, or colonoscopy per protocol and risk
    E. Bone mineral density
    F. Consider consultation with homeopath, herbalist, naturopath, Ayurvedic practitioner

X. FOLLOW-UP
    A. Annual examination, Pap smear as recommended, pelvic examination
    B. Mammograms and bone mineral density testing as recommended
    C. As needed if problems continue or become exacerbated

See Bibliographies.
    Websites: http://www.menopause.org; http://www.herbalgram.org; http://womenshealth.med.ucla.edu/community/newsletter

HORMONE THERAPY[1]

I. DEFINITION
HT is the use of exogenous natural or synthetic estrogen or estrogen and progestin in combination by the postmenopausal woman (whether natural or surgical menopause has occurred) to alleviate the symptoms of lower amounts of natural estrogen

II. ETIOLOGY
    A. The theca interna and granulosa cells of the ovarian follicles and the corpus luteum produce three naturally occurring estrogens: estradiol, estrone, and estriol together with precursors luteinizing hormone (LH) and FSH from the anterior pituitary and androstenedione from the adrenals. The corpus luteum and ovarian follicle produce progesterone. The stromal tissues of the ovaries produce insignificant amounts of androgens; the major sources of androgens in women are the adrenals. During the perimenopausal years, there is a gradual decrease of the production of these hormones.

III. HISTORY
A. What the patient may present with
   1. Irregular menstrual cycles: longer than 35 days, shorter than 21 days
   2. Changes in character of cycles: scanty, brief duration, begin with flooding, clots, dysmenorrhea
   3. Sleep disturbances, night sweats
   4. Experiencing hot flashes and hot flushes
   5. Dyspareunia
   6. Changes in vaginal tissue: dryness, itching, burning of vulva
   7. Urinary urgency or frequency; urethral pain; irritation at meatus
   8. No vaginal bleeding for prior 12 months or more
   9. Surgical menopause: hysterectomy with bilateral oophorectomy and salpingectomy
B. Additional information to be considered
   1. Age of patient and of her biological mother at menopause
   2. Last Pap smear, breast self-examination, mammogram, bone density testing
   3. Medical, surgical, and gynecologic/obstetric history; history of pelvic surgery
   4. Family medical history, especially osteoporosis, heart disease, carcinoma, Alzheimer's disease
   5. Signs, symptoms of possible vaginitis, vaginosis, STD, cystitis
   6. Lifestyle: diet, exercise, smoking, alcohol
   7. Change in mood or sense of well-being
   8. All medications, including OTC, herbals, homeopathics

IV. PHYSICAL EXAMINATION
A. Vital signs
B. Complete physical examination
C. Pelvic examination
   1. Vulva and perineum, noting any signs of infection, atrophy, irritation; hair distribution and signs of thinning; loss of adipose tissue
   2. Vagina: color, rugae, signs of atrophy, infection or irritation, length
   3. Cervix: color, any lesions, ectropion
   4. Urethral os: signs of irritation, atrophy, urethrocele
   5. Pelvic floor integrity: cystocele, rectocele, uterine prolapse
   6. Uterus: size, shape, position, contour, mobility, presence of masses, tenderness
   7. Adnexa: masses, tenderness
   8. Rectal examination: masses, rectocele, uterine anomalies, occult blood

V. LABORATORY
A. Pap smear with maturation index
B. Mammogram
C. May consider endometrial biopsy with intact uterus

    D. Vaginal and/or urine cultures: HIV, STD screen as appropriate
    E. Serum FSH or testosterone assay as indicated
    F. Lipid profiles, thyroid function test, serum glucose
    G. Hematocrit or hemoglobin as indicated
    H. Bone density assays if indicated
    I. Pelvic/transvaginal ultrasound if pelvic examination is positive for masses
    J. Per findings of physical examination and from history

VI. CONSIDERING HT[2]
    A. Contraindications[3]
      1. Undiagnosed vaginal bleeding
      2. Known or suspected pregnancy
      3. History of nontraumatic pulmonary embolism (PE) or deep vein thrombosis (DVT), or PE or DVT in the past 6 months
      4. Known or suspected cancer of the breast or reproductive tract (estrogen-dependent carcinomas); malignant melanoma at any stage
      5. Currently on anticoagulants or tamoxifen
    B. Precautions: consider clinical data, risk, and benefits
      1. Active gallbladder disease
      2. Family history of breast cancer
      3. Migraine headaches
      4. Elevated triglycerides, high low-density lipoprotein (LDL), low high-density lipoprotein (HDL)
      5. Leiomyomata
    C. Weighing risks and benefits
      1. Osteoporosis in family or personal history; risk factors for osteoporosis (*see osteoporosis handout in Appendix I*)
      2. Personal and family medical history, including heart and Alzheimegr's disease, breast cancer, ovarian, endometrial, colon cancer
      3. Presence of indicators for benefits in absence of absolute contraindications and weighing of relative risks
      4. Consideration of risks with smoking, hypertension, epilepsy, migraines, benign breast or uterine disease, endometriosis
      5. Consideration of benefits to genitourinary tract, feelings of well-being
      6. The use of HT remains a highly individualized decision, and controversial issues remain
      7. Access to health care for follow-up: endometrial biopsy, mammography, monitoring for side effects, danger signs
      8. Alternatives to HT: diet, exercise, calcium from exogenous source in addition to foods, botanicals, vitamins, nonhormonal vaginal lubricants (such as Astroglide), naturalistic interventions, homeopathic preparations (*see General Care Measures section, this chapter and Complementary and Alternative Therapies, Chapter 3*)
      9. Recommendation currently is for lowest effective dose for shortest amount of time

VII. HORMONE REGIMENS
  A. Absence of uterus: estrogen only or estrogen and androgen
    1. May be synthetic or compounded bioidentical
    2. Types of preparations
      a. Oral
      b. Transdermal
        i. Patch
        ii. Gel/spray/cream
      c. Vaginal
        i. Ring
        ii. Tablet
        iii. Cream
  B. Presence of uterus: add progestin
    1. Types of preparation
      a. Oral
      b. Transdermal (compounded cream)
      c. Progesterone intrauterine device (IUD)
    2. Regimes
      a. Sequential
      b. Continuous
  C. Other
    1. Raloxifene hydrochloride (Evista) synthetic selective estrogen receptor modulator 60 mg orally daily. Use daily for osteoporosis protection.
    2. Custom compounded HT, oral, topical, and pellet implant (estrogen, progesterone, and testosterone) may be compounded by many pharmacists and mail order pharmacies specializing in natural hormones
      a. Referral to compounding pharmacists at http://www.iacprx. org (International Academy of Compounding Pharmacists)
  D. Withdrawal bleeding
    1. Will occur with sequential use of progestin
    2. No bleeding should occur with continuous use

VIII. CLINICAL MANAGEMENT
  A. Side effects
    1. Bleeding with hormone use
      a. With sequential use
      b. With continuous use
        i. Consider change in dosage or medication
        ii. If not effective, do endometrial biopsy
      c. Unopposed estrogen use (still prescribed by some providers)
        i. Encourage combination therapy; prior to changing therapy, consider using a progestin. If no bleeding, begin new regimen. If bleeding does occur, do endometrial biopsy or do an ultrasound to measure lining.
    2. Breast tenderness
    3. Fluid retention

    4. Weight gain (increased appetite)
    5. Dysmenorrhea with withdrawal bleeding
    6. Depression
    7. Irritability or emotional lability
    8. Possible increase in size of uterine leiomyomata
    9. Allergic response to patch
    10. Virilization with androgens (rare)
 B. Other clinical management strategies
    1. Topical estrogen for vaginal dryness
    2. Alternative nonhormonal vaginal lubricants such as Astroglide or Replens
    3. Complementary/alternative modalities to be considered, including many botanicals as well as acupuncture, massage, and relaxation; can increase a woman's feeling of well-being
    4. Careful teaching about modalities used
 C. Follow-up and lifestyle on HT
    1. Reinforce need for calcium intake both from food and supplementary sources; will also need a consistent source of vitamin D + magnesium in appropriate dose for adequate absorption
    2. Regular program of exercise, strength training
    3. Reinforce knowledge of risks and benefits
    4. Preventive health care: annual examination, Pap smear as indicated, mammography, breast, and vulvar self-examination
    5. Consider periodic monitoring for bone density, lipid profile
    6. Vaginal lubricants, signs of vaginal infection or cystitis versus dryness, Kegel exercises, sexuality
    7. Careful use of herbals, vitamins, and isoflavones with HT

See Appendix I and Bibliographies.

OSTEOPOROSIS

I. DEFINITION
Osteoporosis, a largely preventable skeletal disease, is characterized by low bone mass and microarchitectural deterioration of bone tissue, leading to enhanced bone fragility and a consequent increase in fracture risk

II. ETIOLOGY
 A. Two main factors are responsible for the fragility of bone:
    1. Reduced bone mass
    2. Impaired repair of microdamage caused by normal wear and tear of bone, with disruption in continuity of the plates in cancellous (trabecular) bone

III. CLINICAL TYPES
A. Primary or idiopathic osteoporosis
1. Type I bone loss occurs primarily in the trabecular compartment and is closely related to postmenopausal loss of ovarian function
2. Type II bone loss involves cortical bone and is thought to be an exaggeration of the physiologic aging process
B. Secondary osteoporosis
1. Medical conditions
a. Chronic renal failure
b. Gastrectomy and intestinal bypass
c. Malabsorption syndrome
d. Metastatic cancer
e. Fractures
f. Alcoholism
g. Celiac disease
h. Vitamin B_{12} deficiency
i. Vitamin D deficiency
j. Rheumatoid arthritis
2. Endocrinopathies
a. Hyperprolactinemia
b. Hyperthyroidism
c. Hyperparathyroidism
d. Adrenocortical
e. Diabetes
f. Turner's syndrome
g. Premature ovarian failure
h. Hypogonadism overactivity
i. Hypercalciuria
3. Connective tissue disorder
a. Osteogenesis imperfecta
b. Ehlers-Danlos syndrome
c. Homocystinuria
d. Rheumatoid arthritis
4. Medications
a. Anticonvulsants
b. Antacids (with aluminum)
c. Thyroid HT
d. Glucocorticoids: oral, inhaled
e. Luteinizing hormone-releasing hormone
f. Lithium
g. Long-term Depo Provera use
h. Aromatase inhibitors
i. Immunosuppressants
j. Insulin
k. Phenothiazines
l. Butyrophenones
m. Methotrexate

      n. Heparin
      o. Sodium fluoride

IV. HISTORY
  A. Woman's medical history, including but not limited to: refer to *Clinical Types, III.B*
  B. Medication history
    1. Current prescription medication
    2. Current OTC medication
    3. Current vitamin and botanical use
  C. OB-GYN history
    1. Age at menarche
    2. Age at menopause
    3. Months (years) of oral or other hormonal contraceptive, Depo Provera use
    4. Parity
    5. Estrogen use
    6. History of menstrual dysfunction
      a. Late menarche
      b. Oligohypomenorrhea
      c. Exercise-induced amenorrhea
      d. Previous hysterectomy with oophorectomy
    7. History of extended breastfeeding
  D. Nutritional status
    1. Height and weight
    2. Eating habits
    3. Excessive consumption of caffeine and alcoholic beverages
    4. History of an eating disorder
  E. Lifestyle
    1. Excessive use of alcohol
    2. Smoking
    3. High caffeine intake
    4. Current and past exercise habits
  F. Family history
    1. Maternal history of osteoporosis or fractures

V. PHYSICAL EXAMINATION
  A. Height (compare to previous measurement), (loss of 1.5 in.)
  B. Weight; BMI
  C. Observe back for dorsal kyphosis and cervical lordosis
  D. Assess for physical abnormalities that interfere with mobility
  E. Assess for bone pain
  F. Assess for change of stature

VI. LABORATORY
  A. Consider one of the following screening tests:
    1. X-ray densitometry (DEXA) gold standard
    2. Bone ultrasound

3. Genotyping
4. Bone turnover markers (urinary N-telopeptide; NTX)
5. Single energy X-ray absorptiometry (measures the bones of the wrist or heel)
6. Quantitative computed tomography (measures the bone density of the spine); this test is expensive and exposes the woman to a higher dose of radiation than other screening tests
7. Consider calcium and albumin (hyperparathyroidism)
8. Consider 25-hydroxyvitamin D (vitamin D deficiency)
9. Consider thyroid-stimulating hormone (TSH; hyperthyroidism)
10. Consider complete blood count (CBC) with sedimentation rate
11. Consider liver function test
12. Immunoglobulin A (IgA)
13. Antitissue transglutaminase (+TGA)
14. IgA antiendomysial antibodies (AEA)
15. Serum protein electrophoresis

VII. TREATMENT RECOMMENDATIONS

A. Initiate treatment in postmenopausal women over 50 years of age with:
1. T-score <2.5 (excluding 2 causes)
2. Hip or vertebral fracture
3. Low bone mass and 10-year probability of hip fracture ≥3% or 10-year probability of any major osteoporosis-related fracture
4. Clinician's judgment and/or patient preferences may indicate treatment for people with 10-year fracture probabilities above or below these levels
B. Medication
1. Estrogen (*see Hormone Therapy section*)
2. Bisphosphonates regime should include Fosamax, Actonel, and Boniva; an alendronate regimen should include:
   a. 5 mg/10 mg a day or 35 to 70 mg once a week with 6 to 8 oz of water on arising, at least half an hour before breakfast; or 150 mg monthly with 6 to 8 oz of water on arising, at least 1 hour before breakfast
   b. Calcium supplements and antacids interfere with absorption of alendronate; these should be taken at least half an hour later
   c. To prevent gastrointestinal complications, the woman must remain in an upright position for 1.5 hours after taking medication
3. Calcitonin-Salmon—Fortical
   a. Injection treatment: 100 IU subcutaneously or intramuscularly every other day
   b. Nasal spray treatment: 200 IU intranasally once a day (Miacalcin or Fortical)
4. Selective estrogen receptor modulators: raloxifene (Evista) 60 mg daily

5. Calcium, 1,200 mg with vitamin D, 800 to 1,000 IU daily (20 mg), and a multivitamin with magnesium 320 mg daily per CDC 2011
6. Forteo (parathyroid hormone) 20 μg subcutaneously daily (may treat up to 2 years)
7. Denosumab (Prolia) 60 mg, subcutaneous injected into deltoid, quadriceps, or abdomen every 6 months (persons with latex allergy should not handle grey cap on syringe)
8. Zoledronic acid (Reclast) 5 mg IV infusion every year
9. Phytoestrogens
10. Medical Food, Fosteum (Genistein, Chelazome, Cholecaliferol), 1 capsule, twice daily
11. Promising new selective estrogen receptor medication is in the pipe line

B. General measures
   1. Increase exercise
      a. Muscle strengthening exercises concentrating on large muscle groups
      b. Aerobic exercise: walking, walking on a treadmill, climbing a Stairmaster, riding a bicycle, using a cross-country ski-type apparatus
   2. Increase dietary intake of calcium, vitamin D, magnesium
   3. Decrease dietary intake of alcohol and red meat
   4. Decrease or stop smoking (*see Smoking Cessation, Chapter 4*)

VIII. DIFFERENTIAL DIAGNOSIS
A. Osteopenia—reduced bone mass caused by inadequate osteoid synthesis
B. Arthritis
C. Paget's disease
D. Fracture

IX. COMPLICATIONS
A. Fracture with associated complications
B. Physical deformity
C. The benefits of long-term oral bisphosphonate use are unknown because most clinical trials have not exceeded 5 years. Indeed, some experts recommend "drug holidays" for patients who have taken oral bisphosphonates for extended periods.

X. REFERRAL/CONSULTATION
A. Lack of response to treatment
B. Fractures
C. Nutritional guidance
D. Exercise program (organizations providing moderate to low cost for physical fitness)
E. Smoking cessation

See Appendix I and Bibliographies.

Websites: for menopause: http://www.menopauseonline.com; http://www.mayoclinic.com/health/menopause/DS00119; for hormone therapy: http://www.nlm.nih.gov/medlineplus/hormonereplacementtherapy.html; http://www.osteo.org; http://www.womenshealth.gov/; http://www.womenshealth.gov/minority/africanamerican/osteoporosis.cfm

NOTES

1. *See Complementary and Alternative Therapies, Chapter 3.*
2. The use of HT continues to be controversial. The decision about the use of HT requires evaluation of the risks and benefits for each individual woman. Clinicians should keep up to date with ACOG guidelines to assist them with decision making.
3. The decision about the use of HT requires evaluation of the risks and benefits for each individual woman. For women currently using HT, it is important to assess their reasons for use and to evaluate potential risks, benefits, and alternatives (see ACOG website: *http://www.acog.org*).

19

Polycystic Ovary Syndrome

I. DEFINITION
Polycystic ovary syndrome (PCOS), formerly known as Stein-Leventhal syndrome, is an endocrinologic condition with complex pathophysiology and various clinical presentations. It is one of the most common problems in women of reproductive age. Typical clinical and biochemical manifestations are anovulatory cycles, infertility, and hyperandrogenicity, but many women do not exhibit these characteristic signs. Some women with PCOS have ovaries with a thickened capsule and multiple follicular cysts (polycystic ovaries [PCO]). Women with PCO do not necessarily have PCOS, and those with PCOS do not always have PCO.

II. ETIOLOGY (UNKNOWN BUT POSITED)
A. Genetic factors
B. Possible autosomal transmission of responsible genetic sequences
C. A gene or gene series may render the ovary susceptible to insulin stimulation of androgen secretion and block follicular maturation

III. HISTORY
A. What the patient may present with (only 20%–30% symptomatic)
  1. Anovulatory cycles
  2. History or infertility
  3. Oligomenorrhea
  4. Amenorrhea
  5. Prolonged erratic menstrual bleeding
  6. Signs of hyperandrogenism, including hirsutism, acne, and alopecia (especially crown pattern baldness)
  7. Galactorrhea
  8. Increased waist to hip ratio: >0.85
  9. Hyperpigmentation: nape of neck, axillae, and inguinal areas (acanthosis nigricans)
B. Additional information to be considered
  1. Menstrual cycle history or patterns (onset, length, duration, amount of bleeding)
  2. Pregnancy history
  3. Contraceptive history
  4. History of weight gain, hirsutism
  5. Voice changes, frontal balding, increased muscle mass, acromegaly
  6. Any chronic diseases, especially diabetes
  7. Family history of PCOS, infertility, or diabetes
  8. Medication history

IV. PHYSICAL EXAMINATION
A. Complete physical examination, including height, weight, and blood pressure
B. Pelvic examination—speculum and bimanual to check for enlarged PCO
C. Breast examination to rule out galactorrhea

   D. Full body scan for hirsutism, acanthosis nigricans, body shape, waist-to-hip ratio, and hair growth patterns

V. LABORATORY AND OTHER DIAGNOSTICS
   A. Follicle-stimulating hormone (FSH)
   B. Luteinizing hormone (LH)
   C. LH/FSH ratio
   D. Prolactin
   E. Androstenedione
   F. Glucose (fasting)
   G. Testosterone (total and free)
   H. 17-ketosteroids
   I. Dehydroepiandrosterone sulfate (DHEAS)
   J. Sex hormone binding globulin
   K. Comprehensive metabolic panel
   L. Transvaginal ultrasound preferably on cycle days 3, 4, or 5
   M. Thyroid-stimulating hormone (TSH)
   N. Lipid profile
   O. Insulin (fasting)
   P. Human chorionic gonadotropin (hCG)

VI. DIFFERENTIAL DIAGNOSIS
   A. Late manifestation of congenital adrenal hyperplasia
   B. Adrenal adenoma
   C. Adrenal carcinoma
   D. Hyperthecosis
   E. Ovarian carcinoma
   F. Cushing's syndrome
   G. Acromegaly
   H. Idiopathic hirsutism
   I. Hyperprolactinemias
   J. Thyroid disorders
   K. Disorders of adrenal and pituitary glands

VII. TREATMENT
   A. Weight loss and exercise program
   B. Low dose, low androgenic combination of oral contraceptives to restore cyclic menses
   C. Possibly use antiandrogens for hirsutism and acne
   D. Insulin-sensitizing agents: metformin and troglitazone (not generally recommended as first-line, single therapy for infertility)
   E. Electrolysis, depilatories
   F. Ovulation induction

VIII. COMPLICATIONS
   A. Insulin resistance and development of Type 2 diabetes, metabolic syndrome
   B. Miscarriage

    C. Infertility
    D. Hysterectomy
    E. Endometrial cancer
    F. Ovarian cancer
    G. Cardiovascular disease (atherosclerosis, hypertension, increased triglycerides)

IX. CONSULTATION AND REFERRAL
    A. For infertility treatment
    B. For nonpharmacologic treatment of hirsutism

X. FOLLOW-UP
    A. Education about PCOS and lifestyle alterations
    B. Education about pharmacologic interventions
    C. Education about fertility

See Bibliographies.
Websites: http://www.pcosupport.org; http://www.obgyn.net/pcos/pcos.asp

Sexual Dysfunction

20

I. DEFINITION
Diminished libido or lack of libido, diminished sexual response, or lack of response to sexual stimulation; vaginismus, involuntary spasm, or constriction of the distal third of the vaginal musculature around the introitus on one or more occasions

II. ETIOLOGY
A. Organic and physiologic disorders
   1. Hormonal imbalance
   2. Injuries or anomalies of the genital tract
   3. Infection of the genitalia
   4. Lesions
   5. Nerve impairment
   6. Substance abuse: alcohol, recreational drugs
   7. Recent pregnancy
   8. Effects of medications—prescription or over the counter
   9. Chronic illness
B. Relationship disorders
   1. Partner's and/or patient's lack of desire for sex
   2. Medical conditions
   3. Lack of privacy
   4. Fear of failure in the sexual act; lack of knowledge about sexual response(s)
   5. Shame, guilt
   6. Expectations different from those of partner; miscommunication
   7. Rape trauma; sexual assault or abuse at any age; domestic violence
   8. Improper use of barrier or chemical contraceptives
   9. Recent gynecologic event affecting sexuality, such as sterilization, pregnancy, tubal ligation or occlusion, abortion, hysterectomy, and mastectomy
   10. Difficulties in sexual orientation; confusion over gender identity
   11. Clinical depression of patient and/or partner

III. HISTORY
A. What the patient may present with
   1. Lack of sexual desire
   2. Lack of response to stimulation
   3. Inability to have an orgasm
   4. Vaginal or vulvar irritation, bleeding, soreness
   5. Lack of vaginal lubrication
   6. Inability to have vaginal intercourse
   7. Dyspareunia may be associated with vaginal dryness
B. Other signs and symptoms
   1. Rectal or perineal pain
   2. Perineal lesions

3. Abdominal pain, pelvic pain
4. Fever
5. Bladder, urethral pain
C. Additional information to be considered
1. Sexual history: ever had intercourse; ever experienced orgasm; partners—men, women, both
2. Contraceptive history and method presently using
3. Any gynecologic/obstetrical history, diethylstilbestrol exposure, perimenopausal problems, pelvic surgery, tubal ligation, carcinomas
4. Any recent contributing events: change of partner or new relationship, marriage, divorce, separation, sterilization, pregnancy, infection, surgery, sexual assault, incest, domestic violence
5. Any cultural or religious beliefs that relate to sexual activity
6. Alcohol, drug use; any changes
7. Expectations of self and partner, health of sexual partner
8. Any problems with privacy, time together, living arrangements
9. Use of sex toys
10. Pattern of sexual expression; availability of sexual partner
11. You might ask, "What do you do?" "How do you do it?" and "How does it make you feel?"
12. Sexual fantasies, preoccupations
13. Difficulties focusing on tactile or other sensations previously erotic

IV. PHYSICAL EXAMINATION
A. Vital signs
1. Blood pressure
2. Weight
B. General physical examination, including thyroid, breasts, costovertebral angle (CVA) tenderness, and neurologic
C. Abdominal examination with special attention to:
1. Guarding
2. Pain
3. Masses
D. External examination
1. Anomalies
2. Skene's glands
3. Clitoris
4. Status of hymen
5. Perineum
6. Bartholin's glands
7. Urethra
8. Lesions, signs of infection, injury
E. Vaginal examination (speculum)
1. Vaginal walls: infection, anomalies, atrophy, injuries
2. Discharge, lesions

3. Cervix: lesions, signs of infection, anomalies, scarring
    4. Tolerance of speculum and size accommodated, length of vagina
  F. Bimanual examination
    1. Pain on cervical manipulation
    2. Uterus: tenderness, position
    3. Adnexa: mass, tenderness
    4. Vaginal lesions

V. LABORATORY EXAMINATION
  A. Appropriate cultures when evidence of infection; wet mount; urinalysis
  B. Consider thyroid panel, fasting blood sugar (FBS), liver, renal function tests, serum corticosteroids if history and/or clinical findings warrant
  C. Hormone assays as indicated

VI. DIFFERENTIAL DIAGNOSIS
  A. Hormonal imbalance: estrogen, androgens
  B. Anomaly, injury
  C. Infection
  D. Substance abuse: drugs, alcohol, smoking
  E. Nerve impairment: spinal cord injury, neurologic diseases
  F. Changes caused by aging: slower responses
  G. Adrenal, thyroid, liver, kidney problems
  H. Diabetes, diabetic neuropathy
  I. Medication side effects
  J. Depression
  K. Psychosocial problems, eating disorders
  L. Posttraumatic stress disorder (PTSD) secondary to incest, rape, sexual assault, and domestic violence
  M. Vestibulitis, vulvodynia
  N. Physical and/or intellectual disabilities

VII. TREATMENT
  A. Medications
    1. Treat any infection present (*see Genitourinary Tract Conditions, Chapter 12, Miscellaneous Gynecologic Conditions, Chapter 17, and Vaginal Conditions, Chapter 21*)
    2. Consider hormones especially if perimenopausal or postmenopausal; new drugs for women—analogues to sildenafil citrate (Viagra) when available. Nonprescription dietary supplement Avlimil (salvia rubus).
    3. At present, no U.S. Food and Drug Administration (FDA)-approved testosterone preparation for women is available. The use of bioidentical preparations or off-label use might be considered.
    4. Nonprescription dietary supplement (i.e., Avlimil)

     5. Vaginal estrogen

     6. *See Complementary and Alternative Therapies, Chapter 3*

  B. General measures

     1. Education about changes in sexual response that accompany aging; need for privacy; making time for intimacy

     2. Education about a woman's sexual response and how it differs from that of a man; teach Kegel (pelvic floor) exercises; positions

     3. Explore partner relationship: changes, previous responsiveness, sexual preference, communication, expectations, guilt; screen for abuse

     4. Education on techniques for stretching hymen, vagina

     5. Education and techniques for learning about sexual response and excitation, self and partner

     6. Emphasize role of self-care: diet, exercise, vitamins, hygiene, stress reduction

     7. Education about lubricants, nonhormonal agents to restore/maintain vaginal mucosa and moisture, other sexual aids

VIII. COMPLICATIONS

  A. Long-term disruption of relationships

  B. Exploitation in relationships: abuse, violence, infidelity

IX. CONSULTATION/REFERRAL

  A. Physician for possible hormonal imbalance, genital anomaly, nerve impairment, medical conditions underlying problem

  B. Counselor for rape trauma, PTSD, exploitative relationships, abuse, depression, gender identity, sexual preferences

  C. Sex therapist—single or couples

  D. Support group

X. FOLLOW-UP

  A. Check if infection is present; reevaluate for further treatment

  B. Arrange repeat visit as appropriate for discussion of relationship problems

  C. Assess the success of vaginal, hymenal stretching; stimulation techniques

  D. For medical/medication problems, laboratory results as appropriate

See Bibliographies.
Websites: http://familydoctor.org/612.xml; https://www.avlimil.com

Vaginal Conditions

21

CHECKLIST FOR VAGINAL DISCHARGE WORKUP

I. SUBJECTIVE DATA
  A. Social history
   1. Age
   2. Occupation
   3. Partner status
     a. Frequency of sexual contact
     b. Last sexual act and type
     c. Age of first intercourse
   4. Pregnancy history including elective or spontaneous abortion
   5. Sexual preference
   6. Number of sexual partners over lifetime, known partner history, history of new partner(s) within past month
   7. Documented sexually transmitted disease (STD) history including HIV status
   8. Recent weight change
  B. Previous gynecologic surgery including surgical abortion, tubal ligation, dilation and curettage (D&C), cesarean section, cone biopsy, loop electrosurgical excision procedure (LEEP)
  C. Past or current medical illness; chronic diseases
  D. Family history of diabetes, personal history of Type 1 or Type 2
  E. Diet, alcohol, cigarettes, recent change in habits; use of street drugs including injectables, inhalants; use of sex toys, stimulants, genital jewelry
  F. Medications (past and present); recent antibiotics; use of vaginal medications (over the counter [OTC] and prescription)
  G. Past history of similar problems
   1. Dates
   2. Treatment
   3. Follow-up
  H. Vaginal discharge
   1. Onset
   2. Color
   3. Odor
   4. Consistency
   5. Amount
   6. Constant versus intermittent
   7. Related to sexual contact
   8. Relationship to menses
   9. Relation to other life events
   10. Wear pads, tampons
  I. Papanicolaou history: last Pap smear, any history of abnormal Pap smears, and any interventions
  J. Sores anywhere on the body; rashes
  K. Genital itching, swelling, or burning; genital sores or tears
  L. Abdominal and/or pelvic pain

M. Fever, chills
N. Achy joints
O. Nausea and vomiting; diarrhea
P. Dyspareunia
Q. Known contact with STD; AIDS risk (*see Appendix D for AIDS risk assessment tool*)
R. Birth control (including recent changes in method or products used previously and currently)
  1. Hormonal contraception, vaginal ring, patch, implant, intrauterine device (IUD), pills; type and length of use
  2. IUD: type, how long in place
  3. Diaphragm; cervical cap; Lea's Shield; FemCap
  4. Depo-Provera
  5. Implant
  6. Condom (male or female); foam, jelly, gel, cream, vaginal film, tablets, suppositories, gels, sponge
S. History of douching; use of soaps, chemicals
T. Personal hygiene
  1. Use of feminine hygiene sprays or deodorant tampons, panty liners, or pads
  2. Poor personal hygiene
U. Clothing: consistent wearing of tight-crotched pants; type of underwear; panty hose; panty hose under slacks or jeans
V. Last menstrual period (LMP); last normal menstrual period
W. Urinary problems
  1. Frequency
  2. Dysuria
  3. Urgency
  4. Hematuria: other debris in urine
  5. Odor
  6. Dark or cloudy urine; color
X. Allergies to drugs: reactions
Y. Partner(s) problems, symptoms

II. OBJECTIVE DATA
A. Vital signs: blood pressure, pulse, respiration, temperature
B. Inguinal lymph nodes
C. Abdominal examination: rebound, bowel sounds, suprapubic tenderness, masses, organomegaly, enlarged bladder, costovertebral angle (CVA) tenderness
D. External genitalia: Bartholin's glands, Skene's glands, sores, rash, genital warts, swollen reddened urethra, urethral discharge; lesions on labia, between labial folds; signs of scratching
E. Vaginal examination (speculum)
  1. Inspection of vaginal walls, vaginal lesions, tears, discharge
  2. Inspection of cervix: friability, ectropion, cervical erosion, discharge from os, cervical tenderness; color

3. Discharge: if present, characteristically is thick, mucus at cervical os, difficult to remove
F. Bimanual examination: pain on cervical motion, fullness or pain in adnexa, tenderness of uterus, size and shape of uterus

III. ASSESSMENT AND PLAN

A. Normal discharge: usually clear or white, nonirritating or nonpruritic, pH is 3.8 to 4.2, does not pool, has body, can write initials in it
B. Diagnosis
1. Wet prep will be negative
2. Gram stain will be negative
3. pH within normal range
4. Card test for elevated pH and trimethylamine, and for proline amino-peptidase (e.g., FemExam pH and Amines TestCard, FemExam *Gardnerella vaginalis* Proline Imino-Peptidase (PIP) Activity TestCard)
C. Treatment: none required
D. Patient education
1. Reassurance
2. If clinical and/or laboratory findings are not within normal limits, refer to protocol for suspected organism(s) for further workup

IV. HINTS ON PREPARATION OF A WET SMEAR[1]

A. Collect a copious amount of vaginal discharge from the lateral walls with a wooden Pap spatula (some say a cotton swab moistened with saline); repeat so you have two samples to work with
B. Place a drop of the specimen mixture at each end of a clean glass slide, or on two separate slides, when you are ready to read the slides; or place a drop of saline on one slide and a drop of potassium hydroxide (KOH) on the second slide before collecting specimens; place in cardboard slide holders if available.
C. Add a drop of KOH[2] (10%) to one specimen or stir one specimen into the KOH on the slide and sniff immediately for the characteristic "fishy" odor of bacterial vaginosis (BV; positive whiff test).
D. Cover both specimens with cover slips once you reach the microscope. Plan to view the plain saline specimen first to allow time for the KOH to lyse cells prior to looking for *Candida*, noting that *Candida torulopsis* does not have the same characteristics as *Candida albicans*, so KOH will be negative. If you suspect *Trichomonas*, you may want to examine the slide without a cover slip because the slip can sometimes immobilize the organism. Warming the slide will also increase the possibility of seeing trichomonads.
E. With the 10× objective in place on the microscope, the light on low power, and the condenser in the lowest position, place the slide on

the stage and lower the objective until it is as close to the slide as possible.

F. Adjust the eyepieces until a single, round field is seen. Turn the coarse focus knob until the specimen is focused. Use the fine focus knob to bring the specimen into sharp focus.

G. Be sure to use subdued light and a lowered condenser for a wet specimen. Try increasing the light and raising the condenser while viewing the specimen to see how the cells and bacteria disappear from view.

H. Move the slide until you have a general impression of the number of squamous cells. Switch to high power (40×); it may be necessary to increase the amount of light slightly.

I. Evaluate the slide for bacteria, white blood cells (WBCs), clue cells, trichomonads, hyphae, and yeast buds. Even if one organism is identified, continue to scan the slide systematically to fully evaluate the specimen. Vaginitis/vaginosis may have multiple causes.

J. Move the KOH slide into position; switch back to low power to scan the slide for *Candida*. If hyphae are noted, switch to high power to confirm the impression.

K. Be sure to wipe spilled fluid from the stage. If the objective becomes contaminated, clean it only with special lens paper.

L. To perform Gram staining:

1. Spread a *thin* smear of the specimen on a glass slide. Air dry the slide completely, or dry it carefully high above a flame.

2. After the specimen is dry, fix it by passing it through a flame several times (with the specimen side away from the flame). Allow it to cool completely; otherwise, the reagents used in the staining process may precipitate on the slide.

3. Flood the slide with Gram crystal violet. Wait 10 seconds, and then rinse with tap water.

4. Flood the slide with Gram iodine. Wait 10 seconds, and then rinse with tap water.

5. Wash the slide with decolorizer just until the fluid dripping from the slide changes from blue to colorless, and then immediately rinse the slide with tap water. This step is crucial to ensure correct decolorizing.

6. Flood the slide with Gram sufranin. Wait 10 seconds, and then rinse the slide with tap water.

7. Allow the slide to air dry, or blot dry. Place the slide on the microscope stage and put a small drop of oil on the stained specimen. With the oil power objective in place, the condenser tip and the diaphragm open (for bright-field illumination), focus and examine several fields on the slide.

8. When finished, remove the oil from the lens with lens paper.

Appendix I contains information on vaginal discharge to copy or adapt for your patients. See Bibliographies.

CHECKLIST FOR VAGINAL DISCHARGE WITH ODOR WORKUP

I. DEFINITION
Vaginal discharge with or without a distinctive odor may result from vaginitis or vaginosis. Discharge may also be caused by cervicitis (*see Cervical Aberrations, Chapter 10*).

Vaginitis: Inflammation of the vagina, characterized by an increased vaginal discharge containing many WBCs

Vaginosis: Characterized by increased discharge without inflammatory cells (WBCs)

II. ETIOLOGY
A. Foreign body (e.g., forgotten tampon, retained cap, condom, or diaphragm)
B. Allergy to soap or feminine hygiene spray
C. Deodorants
D. Scented toilet tissue; scented or deodorant menstrual products
E. Vaginal contamination through oral or rectal intercourse
F. Poor personal hygiene
G. Sensitivity to contraceptive spermicides or lubricants
H. Condom allergy (Hint: If the woman is allergic to latex, then use latex condom with animal skin or polyurethane condom over; if the man is allergic to latex, use animal skin condom or polyurethane with a latex condom over.)
I. Presence of a pathogen

III. HISTORY
A. What patient may present with
1. Vaginal discharge, may be chronic
2. Vaginal odor
3. Vulvar/vaginal irritation, pruritus, and/or burning made worse by urination, intercourse
4. Postcoital bleeding
5. Difficulty urinating or pain with urination
B. Additional information to be considered
1. Relationship of discharge to birth control method; any recently discontinued method
2. Relationship of discharge to sexual contact: recency, partner affected, recent change in partners
3. Relationship of discharge to personal hygiene: any recent change in hygiene products or toiletries, douching
4. Any history of vaginal infection associated with STD or pelvic inflammatory disease (PID)
5. History of
a. Previous infection or STD
b. Chronic cervicitis
c. Cervical surgery

  d. Abnormal Pap smear
  e. Diethylstilbestrol (DES) exposure
6. Description of discharge
  a. Color
  b. Onset
  c. Odor
  d. Consistency
  e. Constant versus intermittent
  f. Color of discharge on underwear; changes

IV. PHYSICAL EXAMINATION
  A. External examination: external genitalia
   1. Erythema
   2. Excoriations
   3. Lesions
   4. Edema
  B. Vaginal examination (speculum)
   1. Presence of foreign body
   2. Erythema and edema of the vaginal vault
   3. Inspection of cervix
    a. Erythema
    b. Erosion
    c. Severe physiologic ectropion
    d. Friability
    e. Serous sanguineous discharge
    f. Lesions
  C. Bimanual examination if indicated

V. LABORATORY EXAMINATION
  A. As indicated by findings
   1. Wet saline prep; KOH slide
   2. Gram stain
   3. Gonorrhea culture if indicated
   4. *Chlamydia* test if indicated
   5. Urinalysis if indicated
   6. Herpes culture if indicated
   7. Cervical culture
   8. pH with nitrazine paper, Affirm VPIII, QuickVue Advance pH and Amines Test, QuickVue Advance *G. vaginalis* Test
   9. HIV testing

VI. DIFFERENTIAL DIAGNOSIS
  A. Normal physiologic discharge
  B. DES exposure
  C. *Chlamydia*
  D. *Neisseria gonorrhoeae*
  E. *C. albicans* or other *Candida* infection; BV
  F. Urinary tract infection

G. Condylomata
H. Herpes simplex
I. Contact dermatitis
J. Tinea or other fungus
K. Cervicitis symptomatic for *Chlamydia* infection, gonorrhea, trichomoniasis, genital herpes

VII. TREATMENT
A. General measures
1. Removal of causative factor
2. Education about
a. Personal hygiene
b. Avoidance through the use of alternatives to causative factors
B. Medications
1. No treatment, depending on evaluation of clinical data
2. If a pathogen is identified, treat through appropriate protocol
3. If after 1 week of no treatment, try Aci-Jel to restore and maintain normal vaginal acidity, one applicatorful intravaginally at bedtime for 7 to 14 days or until tube is used up

VIII. COMPLICATIONS
Abnormal Pap smear resulting from continuing irritation; reparative process

IX. CONSULTATION/REFERRAL
In case of unresolved symptomatology

X. FOLLOW-UP
A. One week if indicated, then as needed
B. If no improvement at 1 week after treatment of Aci-Jel, refer to a physician

See Appendix I and Bibliographies.

CANDIDIASIS

I. DEFINITION
Candidiasis, or monilia, is a microscopic, yeastlike fungal infection of the vagina usually caused by *C. albicans* (+90%). *Candida tropicalis, Torulopsis glabrata, Candida krusei, Candida parapsilosis,* and other lesser known *Candida* species are also clinically implicated.

II. ETIOLOGY
A. A fungus of the genus *Candida,* species *C. albicans, C. tropicalis,* or *T. glabrata;* part of the normal flora of the mouth, gastrointestinal (GI) tract, and vagina; may become pathogenic under variable conditions, such as change in the vaginal pH, which encourage an overgrowth of the organism
B. Incubation period: about 96 hours

III. HISTORY
A. What patient may present with
1. Vulvar pruritus
2. Vulvar and vaginal swelling
3. Vulvar excoriation
4. Vulvar burning and external dysuria with urination
5. Dyspareunia or burning during and/or after intercourse
B. Additional information to be considered
1. Previous vaginal infections or vaginosis; diagnosis, treatment, and compliance with treatment
2. Chronic illness (diabetes); immunocompromised patients
3. Sexual activity including oral and anal sex
4. History of STD or PID
5. Last intercourse, changes in frequency, new partner
6. LMP
7. Method(s) of birth control
8. Other medications
   a. Antibiotics
   b. Steroids
   c. Estrogens
9. Description of discharge
   a. Color
   b. Onset
   c. Odor
   d. Consistency
10. Constant versus intermittent
    a. Relationship to sexual contact
    b. Relationship to menses
    c. Use of vaginal deodorant sprays, deodorant or scented tampons, panty liners, or pads, douches, perfumed toilet tissue
    d. Change in laundry soaps, fabric softener, body soap (amount of soap used and application inside labia)
    e. Clothing: consistent wearing of tight-crotched pants, wearing nylon underwear, panty hose under slacks, wearing underwear to bed
11. "Jock" itch (partner); athlete's foot (self or partner); itchy rash on thighs, buttocks, under breasts; oral candidiasis (thrush)
12. Diet high in refined sugar

IV. PHYSICAL EXAMINATION
A. External examination
   Observe perineum for excoriation, erythema, edema, ulcerations, lesions
B. Vaginal examination (speculum)
1. Inspection of vaginal mucosa: may be erythematous, irritated, with white patches along side walls
2. Cervix

3. Discharge: characteristically thick, odorless, white, curdlike, resembling cottage cheese, with pH remaining in the normal range of 3.8 to 4.2 (nitrazine paper)
C. Bimanual examination

V. LABORATORY EXAMINATION

A. Wet prep microscopic examination to visualize hyphae, pseudohyphae, spores, or buds
B. Affirm VPIII Microbial Identification Test
C. Consider vaginal or cervical culture
D. Consider fasting blood sugar and 2-hour postprandial blood sugar on women with chronic yeast infections
E. Further laboratory work as indicated by history including HIV testing

VI. DIFFERENTIAL DIAGNOSIS

A. Herpes genitalis
B. Chemical vaginitis
C. Contact dermatitis
D. Normal physiologic discharge
E. Candidiasis secondary to diabetes, pregnancy, positive HIV status
F. *T. glabrata* or *C. tropicalis* or lesser known species (*C. krusei*, *C. parapsilosis*, other *Candida* species)
G. *Trichomonas*, BV, *Chlamydia*, or gonococcal infection

VII. TREATMENT

A. Medications (some of these are now over the counter)
    1. Butoconazole 2% cream 5 g intravaginally for 3 days (Femstat3) OR
    2. Clotrimazole (Gyne-Lotrimin, Lotrimin, Mycelex, Mycelex 7, Mycelex-G) 1% cream 5 g (1 applicatorful) intravaginally at bedtime for 7 to 14 days
    3. Clotrimazole (Femcare, Gyne-Lotrimin, Lotrimin, Mycelex, Mycelex-G) 2% cream 5 g (1 applicatorful) intravaginally at bedtime for 3 days OR
    4. Miconazole 2% cream 5 g intravaginally for 7 days OR
    5. Miconazole 4% cream 5 g intravaginally for 3 days OR
    6. Miconazole 100 mg vaginal suppository, one suppository daily intravaginally for 7 days OR
    7. Miconazole 200 mg vaginal suppository, one suppository daily intravaginally for 3 days OR
    8. Miconazole 1,200 mg vaginal suppository, one suppository intravaginally for 1 day OR
    9. Tioconazole (Vagistat-1) 6.5% ointment 5 g intravaginally in a single application *or* prescription intravaginal agents
    10. Nystatin 100,000 unit vaginal tablet, one tablet once a day for 14 days OR

11. Terconazole (Terazol) 0.4% cream 5 g (1 applicatorful) intravaginally for 7 days OR
12. Terconazole 0.8% cream 5 g (1 applicatorful) intravaginally for 3 days OR
13. Terconazole 80 mg vaginal suppository, one suppository for 3 days
14. Oral agent: Fluconazole (Diflucan) 150 mg oral tablet, one tablet in a single dose (pregnancy category C)
15. In pregnancy: use only topical azole therapies; most effective in pregnancy are butoconazole, clotrimazole, miconazole, and terconazole; Centers for Disease Control and Prevention (CDC) STD Guidelines 2010 recommend 7-day therapy
16. Miconazole cream (Monistat-Derm) or clotrimazole cream (Mycelex) can be used for external irritation
17. If treatment is unsuccessful, may refill script once; if still unsuccessful, consider treating partner and/or fasting blood sugar and 2-hour postprandial blood sugar; review history carefully with the woman
18. If fasting blood sugar and 2-hour postprandial blood sugar are within normal limits, several options may be considered:
    a. Clotrimazole 1 applicatorful intravaginally every other week for 2 months. If patient remains symptom free, reduce treatment to every month, the week prior to menses.
    b. If the first option is not successful, consider non-*C. albicans* species: *T. glabrata* or *C. tropicalis*. If laboratory result confirms diagnosis, treat with gentian violet one tampon at bedtime for 12 days; triazole compounds have also been found to be effective (Terazol, terconazole; Noxafil, posaconazole; ravuconazole; voriconazole; itraconazole).
    c. Boric acid capsules: 600 mg 1 capsule twice a week intravaginally for recurrent *C. vaginitis* (four or more episodes per year) as organism may be *T. glabrata* (less sensitive to fluconazole or imidazoles)
    d. Clove of garlic in gauze placed in vagina for 10 to 12 hours; other complementary therapies (*see Complementary and Alternative Therapies, Chapter 3 and Bibliographies*)
B. General measures
    1. No intercourse until symptoms subside; then use condoms until end of treatment
    2. No douching
    3. Stress the importance of continuing medication even if menses begin
    4. Do not use tampons during treatment
    5. Stress hygiene, cotton underwear, loose clothing, no underpants while sleeping, wipe front first and then back
    6. Do not use feminine hygiene sprays, deodorants, and so forth
    7. Treat athlete's foot, "jock" itch, or rash with OTC antifungals (such as Lotrimin, Tinactin) or prescription dual-action Lotrisone

8. Consider the use of vitamin C 500 mg twice to 4 times a day to increase acidity of vaginal secretions, or oral acidophilus tablets 40 million to 1 billion units daily (1 tablet); eat live culture yogurt several times a week

VIII. COMPLICATIONS
A. Drug interactions; adverse reactions to treatment
B. Need for maintenance regimens: oral fluconazole 100 mg, 150 mg, or 200 mg dose weekly for 6 months
C. Severe vulvovaginitis: extensive vulvar erythema, edema, excoriation, fissure formation: 7 to 14 days of topical azole or 150 mg of fluconazole in two sequential doses: initial does and second dose 72 hours after initial dose

IX. CONSULTATION/REFERRAL
A. No response to treatment as outlined previously
B. Elevated fasting blood sugar or 2-hour postprandial blood sugar
C. Presence of concurrent systemic disease

X. FOLLOW-UP
A. None necessary unless
   1. Symptoms persist after treatment
   2. Symptoms recur or exacerbate

Appendix I has information on candidiasis that you may wish to photocopy or adapt for your patients. See Bibliographies.

BACTERIAL VAGINOSIS

I. DEFINITION
A polymicrobial clinical syndrome characterized by replacement of the normal hydrogen peroxide-producing *Lactobacillus* species with an overgrowth of anaerobic bacteria (e.g., *Prevotella* and *Mobiluncus* species), *G. vaginalis*, *Ureaplasma*, and numerous fastidious or uncultivated anaerobes (per CDC STD Guidelines 2010)

II. ETIOLOGY
A. Bacterial vaginosis (BV) is a vaginosis rather than vaginitis. As such, there is usually little or no inflammation of the epithelium associated with the syndrome (relative absence of polymorphonuclear leukocytes). It is not caused by a single pathogen, but is **probably** a disturbance of the vaginal microbial ecology, with a displacement of normal lactobacillary flora by anaerobic microorganisms.

B. It is a sexually associated rather than a sexually transmitted syndrome (BV is found more often in sexually active women). A male version of BV has not been identified.

III. HISTORY
A. What the patient may present with
   1. History of having multiple sex partners—male and female, a new sex partner, douching, no use of condoms; but also negative history of sexual activity
   2. Vaginal odor (fishy)
   3. Increased vaginal discharge—milky white, thin adherent discharge, or dark or dull gray discharge
   4. Vaginal burning after intercourse; vulvar pruritis (15% of women)
   5. No symptoms in many patients
B. Additional information to be considered
   1. Previous vaginal infections; diagnosis, treatment; compliance with treatment
   2. Chronic illness; careful history of seizure disorders
   3. Sexual activity; partner preference; multiple partners, new sex partner
   4. History of STD or PID
   5. Last intercourse
   6. LMP, pregnancy
   7. Method of birth control, other medications
   8. Description of discharge
      a. Onset
      b. Color
      c. Odor stronger during intercourse
      d. Consistency
      e. Constant versus intermittent
      f. Relationship of symptoms to sexual contact
      g. Relationship of symptoms to menses
      h. Amount
   9. Use of vaginal deodorant sprays, deodorant tampons, panty liners or pads, douches, or perfumed toilet tissue
   10. Change in laundry soaps, fabric softener, body soap
   11. Clothing: consistent wearing of tight-crotched pants; nylon underwear, underwear to bed
   12. Personal hygiene
   13. Recent change in lifestyle (stress, personal crisis)
   14. Partner symptoms

IV. PHYSICAL EXAMINATION
A. External examination
   Perineum usually has a normal appearance; occasional irritation
B. Vaginal examination (speculum)
   1. Inspection of vaginal walls—check if smoothly covered with white discharge

  2. Inspection of cervix
  3. Discharge: characteristically adherent, homogenous, whitish in color, and of a fishy, musty odor with a pH of >4.5. Take smear from lateral walls of vagina, not cervix, for accurate pH (use nitrazine paper for test).
C. Bimanual examination if indicated

V. LABORATORY EXAMINATION
  A. Diagnosis (3 of 4 Amsel criteria)
   1. White, thin adherent discharge
   2. pH >4.5
   3. Positive whiff test (fishy amine odor from vaginal fluid mixed with 10% KOH)
   4. Clue cells on wet mount: epithelial cells dotted with large numbers of bacteria that obscure cell borders, should see >20% of clue cells
   5. Gram stain
  B. Office lab tests: FemExam, proline amino-peptidase test card (PIP Activity TestCard); Affirm VPIII DNA probe-based test OSOM BVBlue test—vaginal swab in test tube with reagent—positive for BV if it turns blue or green (performance of these tests comparable to Gram stain)
  C. Few WBCs seen on wet mount; decreased *Lactobacilli*
  D. Further laboratory work as indicated by history or wet prep/card, BVBlue test results

VI. DIFFERENTIAL DIAGNOSIS
  A. Trichomoniasis
  B. Presence of foreign body

VII. TREATMENT: ACUTE BACTERIAL VAGINOSIS— RECOMMENDED REGIMENS
  A. Medications
   1. Metronidazole 500 mg orally twice a day for 7 days OR
   2. Metronidazole gel 0.75% one applicatorful (5 g) once a day for 5 days *or*
   3. Clindamycin phosphate cream (Cleocin vaginal cream 2% one applicatorful, 5 g) intravaginally at bedtime for 7 nights. Clindamycin is contraindicated with colitis and other chronic bowel disease. Use cautiously in patients with asthma or impaired renal or hepatic function. (*Note:* The mineral oil in Cleocin vaginal cream may weaken latex or rubber products such as condoms or vaginal diaphragms for 5 days after use.)
  B. Alternative regimens
   1. Tinidazole 2 g orally once daily for 3 days OR
   2. Tinidazole 1 g orally once daily for 5 days OR
   3. Clindamycin 300 mg orally twice daily for 7 days *or*
   4. Clindamycin (Cleocin) vaginal ovules 100 mg intravaginally once at bedtime for 3 days

5. In pregnancy: symptomatic women require treatment with:
   a. Metronidazole 500 mg orally twice a day for 7 days OR
   b. Metronidazole 250 mg orally 3 times a day for 7 days OR
   c. Clindamycin 300 mg orally twice a day for 7 days
6. In pregnancy: asymptomatic women at low risk for preterm delivery
   a. Controversial whether to treat or not to treat. Conclusion: Use of clindamycin cream in the second half of pregnancy might be associated with adverse outcomes.
   b. Increase in adverse events. Conclusion: Use clindamycin only in the first half of pregnancy per CDC 2010 recommendations.
7. Treatment for partner not recommended by CDC (no decrease in recurrences with partner treatment and no effect on cure rates)
8. *Note:* If BV coexists with candidiasis:
   a. Treat a predominant organism first. If symptoms persist, recheck and treat as indicated.
   b. Consider local treatment for candidiasis concurrently with oral treatment for BV as previously mentioned
   c. Clindamycin also kills *Lactobacilli*, so candidiasis is common after treatment. Consider sequential treatment.
   d. If BV coexists with Group B Streptococcus, treat concurrently
C. General measures
   1. Stress avoidance of intercourse until symptoms subside, then use condoms until end of treatment; condom therapy for 4 to 6 weeks (without antibiotic treatment) often results in resolution of BV
   2. Stress no douching during treatment or after
   3. Stress necessity of completing course of medication
   4. Nausea, vomiting, and cramps can occur (if patient is on metronidazole). Stress no alcohol intake during treatment and for 48 hours after completing medications.
   5. Stress appropriate choice of medications if pregnant, if possibly pregnant, or if nursing
   6. Stress hygiene: cotton underwear, loose clothing, no underpants while sleeping, wipe front first and then back, no feminine deodorants or hygiene sprays
   7. Carefully review history for seizure disorders
   8. Metronidazole can cause GI upset even with no alcohol
   9. No data to suggest decreased likelihood of relapse or recurrence by treating a woman's sex partner(s). Routine treatment of sex partners is not recommended.

VIII. TREATMENT: CHRONIC, RECURRING
   A. For recurring BV, consider treatment with a different regimen
   B. If no relief, consider consultation with a specialist

C. Try metronidazole gel 0.75% twice a week for 4 to 6 months after completion of recommended regimen as mentioned previously, or oral nitroimidazole followed by intravaginal boric acid and suppressive metronidazole gel for women in remission, or monthly oral metronidazole with fluconazole as suppressive therapy per CDC 2010

IX. COMPLICATIONS

BV has been associated with PID, endometritis, cervicitis, inflammation, or atypical squamous cells (ASC) on Pap smears, possible link to low-grade squamous intraepithelial lesion (LGSIL) on Pap smears, preterm rupture of membranes, preterm labor, preterm birth, low birth weight, chorioamnitis, postpartum endometritis, and increased risk of HIV acquisition

X. CONSULTATION/REFERRAL

If no response to treatment as discussed previously

XI. FOLLOW-UP

A. None necessary unless:
   1. Symptoms persist after treatment
   2. Symptoms recur
   3. Pregnancy—asymptomatic women at high risk, consider evaluation 1 month after completion of treatment

See Appendix I and Bibliographies.
Website: http://www.cdc.gov/std/treatment/2010

CHANCROID

I. DEFINITION

Chancroid is a bacterial infection of the genitourinary tract in which a rapidly growing ulcerated lesion forms on external genitalia. Definitive diagnosis requires the identification of *Haemophilus ducreyi* using special culture media. Even with the use of these media, sensitivity is <80%. Diagnosis is usually based on clinical findings.

II. ETIOLOGY

A. Causative agent is *H. ducreyi*, a short gram-negative bacillus with rounded ends, usually found in chains and groups
B. Incubation period is 4 to 7 days after exposure (rarely <3 or >10 days); lesion appears 3 to 14 days after exposure

III. HISTORY

A. What patient may present with
   1. History of 1 to 3 painful macules on the external genitalia, which rapidly change to a pustule and then to an ulcerated

lesion; may have "kissing ulcers" from autoinoculation; can also be painless
2. Enlarged inguinal nodes
3. Abscess in inguinal region
4. A sinus formed over the healed lesion
5. New lesions forming when exposed to lesions already present
6. Pain on voiding or defecating
7. Rectal bleeding
8. Dyspareunia
B. Additional information to be obtained
1. History of STD or PID
2. Previous vaginal infections; diagnosis, treatment
3. Previous urinary tract infections
4. Sexually active
5. Last sexual contact; new partner
6. If partner complained of sores
7. LMP
8. Method of birth control; other medications (antibiotics may mask symptoms)
9. Any associated vaginal discharge; duration of ulcers
10. Any associated pain
11. Travel to Asia (Thailand especially), Africa, South America, or the Philippines in past month

IV. PHYSICAL EXAMINATION
A. Vital signs
1. Temperature
2. Blood pressure
3. Pulse
B. Inguinal nodes
1. Size
2. Tenderness
3. Nodes matted together forming a fluctuant abscess (buboes) in groin; usually unilateral inguinal lymphadenopathy
C. External examination
1. Observe labia, fourchette, clitoris, vagina, anal area for macules, papules
2. Observe for shallow, nonindurated, painful ulcers with ragged, undetermined edges, varying in size and often coalesced; base of ulcers may be gray/bluish gray; surrounding red halo
3. Observe for sinuses that may have formed when skin over abscesses has broken down
4. Look for new lesions that may be forming as a result of auto-inoculation
D. Vaginal examination (speculum); observe for lesions in vagina, on cervix
E. Bimanual examination

V. LABORATORY EXAMINATION
A. Usually based on clinical findings and history
B. Cultures to laboratory; use media containing fresh defibrinated rabbit's blood or patient's own serum
C. Dark-field exam for *Treponema pallidum* or serologic test for syphilis performed at least 7 days after onset of lesions and repeated in 3 months
D. Gonococcus (GC) culture, *Chlamydia* test
E. Herpes antibodies
F. HIV testing should be done at the time of this diagnosis and again in 3 months if initial results are negative
G. Further laboratory work as indicated
H. Polymerase chain reaction (PCR) testing for *H. ducreyi* is available in clinical laboratories that have conducted the Clinical Laboratory Improvement Amendments (CLIA) verification studies

VI. DIFFERENTIAL DIAGNOSIS
A. Herpes simplex
B. Syphilis

VII. TREATMENT
A. Medications
   1. Azithromycin 1 gram orally in a single dose OR
   2. Ceftriaxone 250 mg intramuscularly (IM) in a single dose *or*
   3. Ciprofloxacin 500 mg orally twice a day for 3 days (safety in children <18 years of age or in pregnancy or lactation has not been established) OR
   4. Erythromycin base 500 mg orally 3 times a day for 7 days
B. Medications in pregnancy
   1. Azithromycin 1 gram orally in a single dose OR
   2. Ceftriaxone 250 mg IM in a single dose OR
   3. Erythromycin base 500 mg orally 4 times a day for 7 days
C. General measures
   1. Buboes should be aspirated through adjacent intact skin, not incised
   2. No sexual contact until the course of medication is finished
   3. Stress the importance of completing the course of medication
   4. Comfort measures
      a. Tepid water sitz baths; dry carefully with cool air hair dryer, making sure to hold it away from body
      b. Avoid tight, restricting clothing
      c. Expose perineum to airflow as much as possible (wear a skirt without underpants when at home)
      d. Recommend peri-irrigation set for comfort
   5. Patient education
      a. Explain disease process and route of transmission
      b. Stress that sexual partner(s) need to be checked regularly (*see Follow-up*, **X.C**)

VIII. COMPLICATIONS
A. Phimosis in the male
B. Urethral stricture
C. Urethral fistula
D. Severe tissue destruction
E. Ulcers may take years to heal
F. Perineal fistulas

IX. CONSULTATION/REFERRAL
A. If infection is suspected
B. If no response after 7 days of treatment, treatment as outlined previously
C. Secondary infections
D. All HIV-positive persons diagnosed with chancroid

X. FOLLOW-UP
A. Patient should be reexamined 3 to 7 days after initiation of therapy. If treatment is successful, there should be symptomatic improvement within 3 days of starting therapy. Clinical improvement should be evident within 7 days. If no improvement, consultation as described previously.
B. It should be noted that it may take >2 weeks for complete healing of ulcers. The amount of time is related to the size of the ulcer.
C. All sexual partners who have had sexual contact within 10 days preceding symptoms with a person diagnosed with chancroid should be evaluated and treated even in the absence of symptoms.

See Bibliographies.
Website: http://www.cdc.gov/mmwr/pdf/rr/rr5912.pdf

CHLAMYDIA TRACHOMATIS INFECTION

I. DEFINITION
Chlamydia trachomatis infection is a parasitic STD of the reproductive tract mucous membrane of either sex

II. ETIOLOGY
A. The causative organism is a small, obligate, intracellular, bacterium-like parasite (*C. trachomatis*) that develops within inclusion bodies in the cytoplasm of the host cells
B. The incubation period is unknown

III. HISTORY
A. What the patient may present with
  1. Female
    a. Vaginal discharge
    b. Dysuria
    c. Pelvic pain
    d. Changes in menses
    e. Intermenstrual spotting in cervical os
    f. Postcoital bleeding
    g. Frequently asymptomatic
    h. Mucopurulent discharge
  2. Male
    a. Dysuria
    b. Thick, cloudy penile discharge
    c. Rarely asymptomatic
B. Additional information to be considered
  1. Previous vaginal infections; diagnosis, treatment; compliance with treatment
  2. Chronic illness
  3. Sexual activity, new partner(s)
  4. History of STD or PID
  5. Known contact
  6. Last intercourse, sexual contact, sex toys
  7. Method(s) of birth control, other medications
  8. Description of discharge
    a. Onset
    b. Color
    c. Odor
    d. Consistency
    e. Amount
    f. Constant versus intermittent
    g. Relationship to sexual contact
    h. Relationship to menses
  9. Use of vaginal deodorant sprays, deodorant tampons, panty liners, pads, perfumed toilet tissue, douches
  10. Change in laundry soaps, fabric softener, body soap
  11. Clothing: consistent wearing of tight-crotched pants
  12. Personal hygiene
  13. Any drug allergies
  14. Travel to Asia, Africa, Europe—lymphogranuloma venereum (LGV) *Chlamydia* (not detected by usual laboratory tests in the United States; *see section on LGV for symptoms and treatment*)

IV. PHYSICAL EXAMINATION
A. Vital signs
  1. Blood pressure
  2. Temperature

B. Abdominal examination: check for guarded referred pain, rebound pain
C. External examination: observe perineum for edema, ulcerations, lesions, excoriations, erythema, enlarged, tender Bartholin's glands
D. Vaginal examination (speculum)
   1. Inspection of vaginal walls
   2. Cervix (cervicitis), friability
   3. Discharge, if present, is characteristically mucopurulent
E. Bimanual examination: cervical motion tenderness, fullness in adnexa, tender uterus

V. LABORATORY EXAMINATION
A. Direct fluorescent antibody (DFA) test: secretions fixed on slide and stained with fluorescein-labeled monoclonal antibody specific for chlamydial antigens
B. Laboratory test for *Chlamydia* (sensitivities and specificities vary):
   1. Enzyme-linked immunosorbent assay (ELISA) and enzyme-linked immuno assay (EIA): detection of chlamydial antigens
   2. Nucleic acid amplification test (NAAT): vaginal, rectal, urogenital (test for both *Chlamydia* and gonorrhea) finds the genetic material of *Chlamydia* and gonorrhea bacteria—example is the PCR
   3. Nucleic acid hybridization tests (DNA probe test) for *Chlamydia* DNA; not as sensitive as NAAT
   4. DFA: quick test to find *Chlamydia* antigens
   5. *Chlamydia* culture—takes 5 to 7 days; used when child sexual abuse is suspected
   6. Rapid test with endocervical swab or brush—30 minutes for results
C. Endocervical culture (only 100% specific test) in transport media; perform in medicolegal cases—rape, child sexual abuse
D. Serology test for syphilis if history indicates
E. Consider HIV testing
F. Consider hepatitis B and C testing
G. GC culture or NAAT

VI. DIFFERENTIAL DIAGNOSIS
A. Gonorrhea
B. Appendicitis
C. Cystitis

VII. TREATMENT
A. Medication
   1. Azithromycin 1 gram orally in a single dose *or* Doxycycline 100 mg orally twice a day for 7 days
   2. Alternative regimens
      a. Erythromycin base 500 mg orally 4 times a day for 7 days OR
      b. Erythromycin ethylsuccinate 800 mg orally 4 times a day for 7 days OR

      c. Levofloxacin 500 mg orally once daily for 7 days
      d. Ofloxacin 300 mg orally twice a day for 7 days
    3. In pregnancy
      a. Azithromycin 1 gram orally in single dose OR
      b. Amoxicillin 500 mg orally 3 times a day for 7 days
    4. Alternative regimens in pregnancy
      a. Erythromycin base 500 mg orally 4 times a day for 7 days OR
      b. Erythromycin base 250 mg orally 4 times a day for 14 days OR
      c. Erythromycin ethylsuccinate 800 mg orally 4 times a day for 7 days OR
      d. Erythromycin ethylsuccinate 400 mg orally 4 times a day for 14 days
B. For sexual contacts during 60 days preceding onset of patient's symptoms or diagnosis of *Chlamydia*
    1. Offer *Chlamydia* test prior to treatment
    2. Start treatment prior to results of testing
    3. Treat same as for the woman; do follow up if symptoms persist and rescreening per CDC Guidelines 2010
C. General measures
    1. Stress that the partner(s) should be treated
    2. No intercourse for 7 days after single-dose treatment or until completion of the 7-day treatment regimen
    3. No intercourse until all sex partners are treated
    4. Condom for backup birth control method for the remainder of cycle if on oral contraceptives
    5. Stress the importance of completing medication for the woman and partner
    6. Stress that the use of feminine hygiene sprays, deodorants, or douches should be stopped
    7. Stress the possibility of increased photosensitivity with medication
    8. Inform the patient taking tetracycline that medication should be taken 1 hour before or 2 hours after meals and/or consumption of dairy products, antacids, or mineral-containing products
    9. Return for reevaluation if symptoms persist or return after treatment

VIII. COMPLICATIONS
A. Women
    1. PID
      a. Pelvic abscess (ovarian)
      b. Infertility, chronic pelvic pain, ectopic pregnancy
    2. Abnormal Pap smear with cervicitis (30%–50%)
    3. Postpartum endometritis
B. Men
    1. Epididymitis, prostatitis
    2. Reiter's syndrome

    C. Risk of acquiring HIV
    D. Newborn
       1. Conjunctivitis
       2. Pneumonia
       3. Urogenital tract, rectal infection
    E. Urethritis

IX. CONSULTATION/REFERRAL
    A. If no response to treatment as discussed previously
    B. If complications develop

X. FOLLOW-UP
    A. If no response to treatment or the possibility of reinfection is present
    B. Test of cure not routinely required per CDC Guidelines 2010. If symptoms persist or reinfection is suspected, consider retesting women after treatment (rate of reinfection). Consider rescreening all women with *Chlamydia* infection approximately 3 months after treatment. Rescreen all women treated when they next present for care within 12 months.
    C. Consider retesting 3 weeks after completion of treatment with erythromycin because the frequent GI side effects of the drug are often associated with noncompliance
    D. Repeat Pap smear if abnormal prior to treatment
    E. Gonorrhea cultures if not done
    F. Serology test for syphilis
    G. In some states, *Chlamydia* is a reportable disease

Appendix I has information on C. trachomatis *infection to photocopy or adapt for your patients. See Bibliographies.*
Website: http://www.cdc.gov/std/treatment/2010

CONDYLOMATA ACUMINATA (GENITAL WARTS)

Human Papillomavirus

I. DEFINITION
Condylomata acuminata is a sexually transmitted condition (but it may also be a fomite) caused by one or more members of the human papillomavirus (HPV) group numbering more than 150 types, and characterized by the formation of warty excrescences on the external genitalia, and on the cervix, vagina, anal area, nipples, umbilicus, and pharynx. The virus does not always cause a lesion; subclinical infection occurs on cervix and externally.

II. ETIOLOGY

A. The cause of the condition is a DNA virus of the papilloma group (HPV); more than 30 types of HPV can affect the genital tract; 17 are considered high-risk types. Ninety percent of genital warts (condylomata) are caused by HPV Types 6 and 11. Types 16, 18, 31, 33, and 35 usually are found as coinfections with Types 6 and 11.

B. Incubation period: 1 to 6 months; may be much longer (up to 30 years); up to 70% may regress spontaneously

C. Period of communicability is unknown

III. HISTORY

A. What the patient may present with
   1. "Feeling a lump" in vulvar area
   2. Increased vaginal discharge
   3. Vulvar itch, burning, pain, bleeding

B. Additional information to be considered
   1. Previous vaginitis/vaginosis; diagnosis, treatment
   2. Sexual activity, last intercourse, sexual contact
   3. LMP: any chance of pregnancy
   4. Method of birth control
   5. Previous history of genital warts, herpes simplex
   6. Known contact; consider any contact with person with warts on any body part
   7. History of STD(s) or PID
   8. Description of discharge (odor, consistency, amount, color)
   9. Any drug allergies
   10. History of abnormal Pap smear, colposcopy, treatment
   11. Reactivation of subclinical infection with sexual activity
   12. Self-infection from condyloma on any body part
   13. Lifestyle: smoking, sexual practices such as anal intercourse, sex toys, exposure to utraviolet light, nutrition

IV. PHYSICAL EXAMINATION

A. External examination
   1. Small, pink or flesh colored, soft papillomatous, or raised "warty" lesion visualized in:
      a. Periclitoral area
      b. Vestibule
      c. Posterior perineal and perianal areas
      d. Extragenital areas
   2. Confluence of many individual warts may give impression of a single, fleshy, proliferative lesion
   3. Secondary infection of lesions (from scratching)
   4. On hair-bearing skin, keratotic appearance

B. Vaginal examination (speculum); observe for same lesions as described previously
   1. Vaginal walls
   2. Cervix (more often subclinical and no visible lesions on inspection)

V. LABORATORY EXAMINATION
A. Visual examination (classic appearance, as described previously); often visible after application of 5% acetic acid (white vinegar)— not a specific test for HPV
B. GC culture
C. *Chlamydia* smear
D. Serology test for syphilis
E. Other laboratory work as indicated by history and examination
F. Colposcopy
G. Pap smear
H. DNA testing—such as the Hybrid Capture 2 DNA Test
I. Biopsy of cervix or unresponsive or unusual lesion on vulva for histologic examination
J. HIV testing

VI. DIFFERENTIAL DIAGNOSIS
Condylomata lata (associated with syphilis), molluscum contagiosum, lipomas, fibroma, adenomas, squamous cell carcinoma, nevi, seborrheic keratoses, psoriatic plaques, carcinoma in situ, micropapillometosis labialis, giant condyloma (Buschke-Löwenstein tumor), Bowenoid papulosis, malignant melanoma, skin tags, lichen nitidus, lichen planus, sebaceous Tyson's glands, herpes simplex, angiokeratoma

VII. TREATMENT
A. Medical treatment
   1. Patient applied
      a. Podofilox (Condylox) 0.5% solution or gel twice a day for 3 days; no therapy for 4 days; repeat as needed up to 4 cycles OR
      b. Imiquinod (Zyclara, Aldara; an immune response modifier inducing cytokines) 5% cream 3 times a week at bedtime for up to 16 weeks (may weaken rubber in diaphragms, condoms); needs to be washed off after 6 to 10 hours OR
      c. Sinecatechin (Veregen) 15% ointment: green tea extract with active ingredient catechins applied 3 times a day (0.5 cm strand of ointment to each wart, covering the wart with a thin layer of ointment), continuing this treatment until all warts are covered and should not be washed off. Use no longer than 16 weeks
   2. Provider applied for visible genital warts
      a. Cryotherapy with liquid nitrogen or cryoprobe with repeat application every 1 to 2 weeks OR
      b. Apply podophyllin resin (podophyllin), 10% to 25% in compound tincture of benzoin and isopropyl alcohol (10%) *or* trichloracetic acid (TCA) or bichloracetic acid (BCA; 80%–90%): allow to air dry (apply vaseline collar with podophyllin); no need to wash TCA off; wash podophyllin off in 1 to 4 hours; may burn on application; if excess amount of TCA or BCA is applied, powder treatment area with talc, sodium bicarbonate,

or liquid soap to remove unreacted acid; only use once a week for 8 to 12 weeks

   c. Inject intralesional interferon

3. Cervical warts—colposcopy/consultation; vaginal warts—cryotherapy, TCA, or BCA repeated weekly; urethral meatus—cryotherapy *or* podophyllin; oral and anal—cryotherapy, BCA, or TCA, or surgical removal
4. Pregnancy: Podofilox, imiquimod, and podophyllin should *not* be used in pregnancy

B. Surgical treatment
   1. Cryotherapy with liquid nitrogen or cryoprobe; dimethylether (Histofreezer) repeat every 1 to 2 weeks
   2. Carbon dioxide (CO_2) laser vaporization
   3. Surgical excision
   4. LEEP

C. General measures
   1. Sexual partner(s) should be checked if lesions are present; CDC Guidelines 2010 note that the role of reinfection in recurrences is probably minimal
   2. Stress the importance of personal hygiene

D. Use of condoms to help prevent further infection with partners likely to be uninfected (*Note:* precaution with imiquimod)

E. Education that even after treatment and elimination of visible warts, the potential for transmission exists

VIII. COMPLICATIONS

A. Lesions can become numerous and large, requiring more extensive treatment
B. Visible genital warts and benign low-grade cervical changes are usually caused by HPV Types 6, 11, 40, 42, 43, 44, 54, 61, 70, 72, and 81. Other HPV types in the anogenital region (Types 16, 18, 31, 33, 35, 39, 45, 51, 52, 56, 58, 59, 68, 73, and 82) have been strongly associated with low-grade and high-grade cervical changes, cervical neoplasia, and anogenital and other cancers.
C. Laryngeal papillomatosis in infant
D. Men with HPV are at incre ased risk for dysplastic changes and cancers in the penile and anorectal areas

IX. CONSULTATION/REFERRAL

A. Refer to or consult with physician
   1. After 8 to 12 treatments for evaluation
   2. If warts are present on vaginal walls or cervix or rectal mucosa (*see Treatment, VII.C*)
   3. Extensive or deep anorectal warts for proctologic examination; urethroscopy as indicated
   4. If any wart is more than 2 cm in size or for large cluster of warts

5. Abnormal Pap smear (*per ASCCP guidelines, see Cervical Aberrations, Chapter 10*)
6. For possible biopsy in older age groups; atypical appearance of lesions, poor response to treatment in younger patients
7. Pregnant women

X. FOLLOW-UP
A. Weekly for 8 to 12 weeks
B. Patient advised to check self periodically and return if warts recur
C. Consider use of HPV vaccine Gardasil (quadrivalent vaccine against HPV 6, 11, 16, and 18 and also protects against most genital warts) or Cervarix (protects against HPV 16 and 18) in preadolescent girls, adolescent girls, and young women ages 9 to 26. Gardasil and Ceravix are both licensed for boys and men ages 9 to 26 per U.S. Food and Drug Administration (FDA) approval.

See Appendix I on condylomata acuminata and for information you may want to photocopy or adapt for your patients. See Bibliographies.
Website: http://www.cdc.gov/std/treatment/2010

GENITAL HERPES SIMPLEX

I. DEFINITION
Genital herpes simplex is a chronic, life-long, recurrent viral infection of the skin and mucous membranes of the genitalia, characterized by eruptions on a lightly raised erythematous base

II. ETIOLOGY
A. Herpes simplex virus (HSV). There are two HSV strains:
1. HSV Type 1 (HSV-1): commonly causes herpes labialis (cold sores) and herpes keratitis; increasingly, the cause of anogenital herpetic infections
   a. Usually seen in childhood (as acute gingivostomatitis)
   b. May be seen in adults who engage in oral sex, kissing
   c. Incubation period: 3 to 7 days, course 1 to 3 weeks
   d. May be recurrent and has no cure
   e. Offers no protection against getting HSV Type 2 (HSV-2), but makes HSV-2 more likely to be subclinical
2. HSV-2
   a. Genital counterpart of acute gingivostomatitis; primarily sexually transmitted
   b. Incubation period: 4 to 7 days up to 4 weeks, course may last 2 to 3 weeks
   c. HSV-2 remains dormant in dorsal nerve ganglia, may be recurrent, and has no cure

d. May be present for many years with no symptoms or no recognizable symptoms

e. HSV-2 does provide immunity against HSV-1

f. 25% of population has HSV-2

3. Both HSV-1 (10%) and HSV-2 (90%) have been implicated in genital infections, but rarely is HSV-2 found orally

III. HISTORY

A. Genital herpes

1. Primary infection (may actually be caused by HSV-1 or HSV-2); mean duration of 12 days

a. Multiple lesions

i. Male: penis, buttocks, thighs

ii. Female: labia, fourchette, cervix, buttocks, thigh, nipples

b. Myalgia

c. Arthralgia

d. Malaise

e. Fever, lymphadenopathy

f. Dysuria, male and female (urinary retention may occur, especially in women with lesions close to meatus)

g. Dyspareunia

h. Headache (can be sign of herpes meningitis)

2. Recurrent genital lesions

a. Lesions less painful

b. Less or no systemic symptoms

c. Unilateral

d. Prodromal symptoms (itching, burning, and/or tingling at site where lesions then appear)

B. Additional information to be considered

1. Genital herpes: primary infection

a. Known exposure

b. Sexual preference

c. Recent participation in oral sex with partner who has herpes labialis

2. Genital herpes: recurrent infection

a. History of recent exposure to reactivating factors: physical trauma, exposure to sunlight, stress, menses

b. Prodrome

i. Pruritus

ii. Burning at site of previous lesion(s)

iii. Tingling at site of previous lesion(s)

iv. Symptoms as in A and B across nerve tract serving site of previous lesion(s); (i.e., sciatic pain with lesion on labia)

IV. PHYSICAL EXAMINATION

A. Genital herpes

1. Primary infection

a. Temperature, blood pressure

b. Examination of genitalia: vesicular lesions containing cloudy liquid on erythematous base. Vesicles break, lesions coalesce forming ulcerative lesions with irregular borders, macerated if in moist areas.

   i. Female: lesions (painful), examination will be difficult; use of speculum may be impossible. Lesions present as described in *History, III.A.* Cervicitis may be present.

   ii. Male: lesions (painful) present in areas previously described in *History, III.A.* Urethral discharge may be present.

c. Groin: inguinal adenopathy may be present

d. Abdomen: bladder distension, secondary to urinary retention, may be present; more common in women

e. Check for atypical presentation as cystitis, meningitis, encephalitis, urethritis, ocular lesions

2. Recurrent infection genital herpes

   a. As previously mentioned (*History, III.B.2*), but clinical picture is less severe

V. LABORATORY EXAMINATION (BOTH NONSENSITIVE AND NONSPECIFIC)

A. May include HSV Types 1 and 2. Scrape lesion for samples for

1. Virology culture with typing (within 7 days of first episode, 2 days of recurrence)—low sensitivity especially for recurrent lesions

2. Genital lesions: consider GC culture, serology test for syphilis, *Chlamydia* test (may need to wait until follow-up visit if infection is severe)

3. Herpes can be diagnosed through tissue culture, blood test, or antigen detection (swab or scrape a lesion)

4. HerpeSelect type-specific glycoprotein (gG) test for HSV-1 and HSV-2 can differentiate between the two types

B. Consider HIV testing

VI. DIFFERENTIAL DIAGNOSIS

A. Syphilis

B. Chancroid

C. Lymphogranuloma inguinale

D. Granuloma inguinale

VII. TREATMENT OF GENITAL HERPES

A. General therapy

1. Consider immune status of patient with frequent outbreaks and/or long duration outbreaks, plus the degree of systemic involvement

2. Consider also the potential for asymptomatic shedding

3. Comfort measures

   a. Tepid water sitz baths, plain or with Betadine solution; dry carefully with cool air hair dryer, making sure to hold it away from body

    b. If voiding over lesions is painful, instruct patient to void while sitting in water in a bathtub

    c. Stress avoidance of tight, restricting clothing. The vulva should be exposed to airflow as much as possible (patient may wear a skirt or robe without underpants when at home).

    d. Peri-irrigation for comfort

4. Patient education

    a. Explain the disease process and route of transmission to the patient (i.e., oral/genital sex during outbreaks)

        i. Ninety percent of those infected do not know they are infected

        ii. Most transmissions occur without symptoms in the infected person

        iii. Viral shedding occurs 5% to 70% of day

        iv. Condom use protects women, not men

    b. Patients should be advised to abstain from sexual activity while lesions are present

    c. Explain the dangers associated with herpes during pregnancy

    d. Discuss possible factors involved with recurrences

    e. Discuss need for yearly Pap smear

    f. Support group: alt.support.herpes (Usenet newsgroup)

B. Medication

1. Initial genital outbreak

    a. Acyclovir 400 mg orally 3 times a day for 7 to 10 days OR

    b. Acyclovir 200 mg orally 5 times a day for 7 to 10 days OR

    c. Famciclovir (Famvir) 250 mg orally 3 times a day for 7 to 10 days OR

    d. Valacyclovir (Valtrex) 1 g orally twice a day for 7 to 10 days

    e. Comfort measures: Zylocaine 2% gel or cream; apply 3 to 4 times daily (do not use around urethra) for comfort measure *or* bacitracin ointment, apply locally, for secondary infection only 2 to 5 times a day *or* add gramicidin, a topical antibiotic, to suppress replication of HSV-1 and HSV-2

2. Episodic therapy for recurrent infection—therapy should be initiated within 1 day of lesion onset or during prodrome

    a. Acyclovir 400 mg orally 3 times a day for 5 days OR

    b. Acyclovir 800 mg orally twice a day for 5 days OR

    c. Acyclovir 800 mg orally 3 times a day for 2 days OR

    d. Famciclovir 125 mg orally twice daily for 5 days OR

    e. Famciclovir 1,000 mg orally twice daily for 1 day OR

    f. Famciclovir 500 mg orally once followed by 250 mg twice daily for 2 days OR

    g. Valacyclovir 500 mg orally twice a day for 3 days OR

    h. Valacyclovir 1 g orally once a day for 5 days

3. Suppressive therapy for recurrent genital herpes: Evidence is growing showing benefits of beginning suppressive therapy

with the first episode, not waiting for chronic outbreaks to be established. Safety and efficacy have been established for as long as 6 years with acyclovir and 1 year for valacyclovir or famciclovir. Early intervention will decrease recurrences during the first year when outbreaks are the most frequent as well as decrease the likelihood of viral shedding.

    a. Acyclovir 400 mg orally twice a day OR

    b. Famciclovir 250 mg orally twice a day OR

    c. Valacyclovir 500 mg orally daily for persons with ≤9 outbreaks per year *or*

    d. Valacyclovir 1 g orally daily for persons with ≥10 outbreaks per year

4. Recommended regimens for daily suppressive therapy in persons with HIV

    a. Acyclovir 400 to 800 mg orally twice to 3 times a day OR

    b. Famciclovir 500 mg orally twice a day for 5 to 10 days OR

    c. Valacyclovir 1 g orally twice a day for 5 to 10 days

5. Recommended regimens for episodic infection in persons with HIV

    a. Acyclovir 400 mg orally 3 times a day for 5 to 10 days OR

    b. Famciclovir 500 mg orally twice a day OR

    c. Valacyclovir 500 mg orally twice a day

6. Suppressive therapy in persons infected with HIV

    a. Acyclovir 400 to 800 mg orally twice to 3 times a day OR

    b. Famciclovir 500 mg orally twice a day OR

    c. Valacyclovir 500 mg twice a day

7. In pregnancy (*see CDC Guidelines 2010*)

    a. First clinical episode or severe recurrent—treat with oral acyclovir

    b. In life-threatening, severe maternal HSV infection, treat with intravenous (IV) acyclovir

8. Unresolved herpes—herpes outbreaks lasting several weeks or more

    a. Immunologic status should be evaluated with physician consultation

VIII. COMPLICATIONS

    A. Secondary infection of lesion

    B. Keratitis (keep fingers away from eyes)

    C. Generalized herpetic skin eruptions

    D. Meningitis

    E. Encephalitis

    F. Pneumonitis

    G. Hepatitis

    H. Fetal–neonatal infection

    I. Spread to other persons at risk for developing disseminated herpes

      1. Immunosuppressed or deficient individuals including persons with HIV

2. Patients with open skin lesions (e.g., burns, atopic dermatitis)
3. Infants, small children

IX. CONSULTATION/REFERRAL
A. Secondary infections
B. Urinary retention if unable to void in bathtub
C. Suspected ocular lesion
D. Severe primary episode
E. Poor fluid intake associated with severe primary episode
F. Persistent headache, nausea, vomiting, photophobia, convulsions, pain in upper right quadrant, chest pain, shortness of breath
G. Unresolved outbreaks lasting several weeks or more
H. Life-threatening episode in pregnant women

X. FOLLOW-UP
As needed or see Appendix I for information, which you may want to photo-copy or adapt for your patients. See Bibliographies.

Websites: http://www.herpes.com; http://www.ashastd.org/herpes/ her-pes_overview.cfm; http://www.webmd.com (America Online keyword: Better Health); http://www.thrive.com; http://www.viridas.com; http://www.diagnol-ogy; American Social Health Association (ASHA) booklets, books, handouts; The Helper, 800-230-6039; ASHA patient herpes hotline, 919-361-8488; http://www.cdc.gov/mmwr/pdf/rr/rr5912.pdf, p. 58

GONORRHEA

I. DEFINITION
Gonorrhea is a sexually transmitted bacterial infection of the urethra, rec-tum, and/or cervix; the causative organism can also be cultured in the nasopharynx. As many as 80% of infected women may be asymptomatic.

II. ETIOLOGY
The causative organism is *N. gonorrhoea*, a gram-negative, intracellular, nonmotile diplococcus. Plasmid-mediated penicillinase-producing *N. gon-orrhoea* (PPNG), plasmid-mediated tetracycline-resistant *N. gonorrhoea* (TRNG), chromosomally mediated resistant *N. gonorrhoea* (CMRNG), spectinomycin-resistant, and quinolone-resistant strains exist. Incubation period: 1 to 13 days.

III. HISTORY
A. What patient may present with
    1. Females: A large percentage (perhaps 80%) of infected women are asymptomatic in the early disease stage
       a. Early symptoms
         i. Dysuria, dyspareunia
         ii. Leukorrhea; change in vaginal discharge
         iii. Unilateral labial pain and swelling

        iv. Lower abdominal discomfort

        v. Pharyngitis

   b. Later symptoms

       i. Purulent, irritating vaginal discharge

       ii. Fever (possibly high)

       iii. Rectal pain and discharge

       iv. Abnormal menstrual bleeding

       v. Increased dysmenorrhea

       vi. Nausea, vomiting

       vii. Lesions in genital area; labia pain

       viii. Joint pain and swelling

       ix. Upper abdominal pain (perihepatitis)

       x. Pain, tenderness in pelvic organs; urethral pain

  2. Males: usually symptomatic (up to 10% asymptomatic)

   a. Early symptoms

       i. Dysuria with frequency

       ii. Whitish discharge from penis

       iii. Pharyngitis

   b. Later symptoms

       i. Yellow or greenish discharge from penis

       ii. Epididymitis

       iii. Proctitis

B. Additional information to be considered

  1. Age of the woman is less than 25 years

  2. Previous vaginal infections, diagnosis, and treatment

  3. Chronic illness

  4. Sexual activity; number, new sexual partner(s)

  5. History of STD or PID

  6. Known contact

  7. Last intercourse, sexual contact

  8. Method of birth control, other medications

  9. History of cervical ectopy, friability in known patient

  10. Postcoital bleeding

  11. Description of discharge

   a. Onset

   b. Color

   c. Odor

   d. Consistency

   e. Amount

   f. Relationship to sexual contact

  12. Any change in menses (increased flow or dysmenorrhea)

  13. Any drug allergies

  14. HIV risk or exposure

  15. Travel to Asia, Africa, the Pacific, U.S. West Coast

IV. PHYSICAL EXAMINATION

A. Vital signs

  1. Blood pressure

    2. Temperature
    3. Pulse
  B. Abdominal examination
    1. Guarding
    2. Referred pain
    3. Rebound pain
    4. Upper bilateral quadrant pain
    5. Bowel sounds indicating intestinal hyperactivity
  C. External examination
    1. Inspection of Skene's glands
    2. Inspection of urethra
    3. Inspection of Bartholin's glands
  D. Vaginal examination (speculum)
    1. Vaginal walls: discharge, redness
    2. Cervix: mucopurulent discharge, ectopy, friability
    3. Vaginal discharge
  E. Bimanual examination
    1. Pain when cervix is moved by examiner
    2. Uterine tenderness
    3. Adnexal tenderness
    4. Adnexal mass
  F. Throat examination
    1. Erythema including tonsils
    2. Edema of posterior pharynx
    3. Erythema

V. LABORATORY EXAMINATION
  A. GC culture, nucleic acid hybridization tests, or NAATs from oral, endocervical, vaginal, and/or rectal swabs. Note that nonculture tests do not provide antimicrobial susceptibility data.
  B. If positive for gonorrhea and/or by history and risk factors, test for syphilis, *Chlamydia*, and HIV.

VI. DIFFERENTIAL DIAGNOSIS
  A. *Chlamydia* infection
  B. Appendicitis
  C. Ectopic pregnancy

VII. TREATMENT: CERVIX, URETHRA, RECTUM
  A. Medication
    1. Ceftriaxone 250 mg IM single dose, *if not an option*, then give Cefixime 400 mg orally in single dose (not for girls younger than 12) *or* single-dose injectable cephalosporin regimens *plus*
      a. Azithromycin 1 g orally in a single dose OR
      b. Doxycycline 100 mg a day for 7 days

2. Alternative regimens
   a. Cefpodoxime 400 mg orally for uncomplicated urogenital gonorrhea (meets minimal efficacy criteria); not recommended for pharyngeal site
   b. Cefuroxime axetil 1 g orally meets minimal efficacy as an alternative for urogenital and rectal infections, but less than those of cefpodoxime, cefixime, or ceftriaxone; Cefpodoxime is poor for pharyngeal infection
3. Pregnancy: Treat with recommended or alternative cephalosporin. Alternative: If a woman cannot tolerate a cephalosporin, then use azithromycin 2 g orally.
4. HIV-positive patients—same regimen for gonorrhea as those who are HIV negative
5. Pharynx: uncomplicated infections
   a. Ceftriaxone 250 mg IM single dose OR
   b. Azithromycin 1 g orally in a single dose OR
   c. Doxycycline 100 mg a day for 7 days
   d. Ciprofloxacin 500 mg orally single dose
   e. *Plus Chlamydia* regimen
6. Conjunctiva: 1 g IM Ceftriaxone in a single dose, plus consider lavage of infected eye with saline solution once
7. For contacts: verify if partner had diagnosed infection; after appropriate culture, treat with same regimen as the patient depending on history of sensitivities
B. General measures
1. All sexual partners should be treated if last sexual contact was within 60 days of onset of symptoms in patient or diagnosis of infection. If >60 days, treat patient's most recent sexual partner.
2. For heterosexual patients whose partners' treatment cannot be ensured, consider delivery of therapy for gonorrhea and *Chlamydia* infection by the patients to their partners, along with efforts to educate partners about symptoms and to encourage them to seek evaluation. For male patients whose partners are female, include educational materials about seeking evaluation for PID.
3. No intercourse until both partners are treated, or use condoms, but abstinence is preferred
4. Stress the importance of completing medication
5. Stress personal hygiene
6. Stress need for follow-up culture if symptoms persist, recur, or exacerbate

VIII. COMPLICATIONS
A. Females
1. PID
   a. Pelvic abscess or Bartholin's abscess
   b. Infertility

2. Disseminated gonococcal infection—gonococcal bacteremia
3. In pregnancy: spontaneous abortion, premature rupture of membranes, premature delivery, chorioamnionitis

B. Males
   1. Proctitis
   2. Infertility caused by epididymitis, prostatitis, and/or seminal vesiculitis
   3. Urethral stricture
   4. Disseminated gonococcal infection—gonococcal bacteremia

C. Newborns: ophthalmia neonatorum, sepsis, arthritis, meningitis, rhinitis, urethritis, vaginitis, inflammation at sites of fetal monitoring

D. Males and females
   1. Meningitis
   2. Endocarditis
   3. Gonococcal conjunctivitis

IX. CONSULTATION/REFERRAL
A. If no response to treatment as discussed previously
B. If complications develop

X. FOLLOW-UP
A. Test of cure not recommended by CDC (2010) unless symptoms recur, exacerbate, or do not resolve
B. Most infections are reinfections, not treatment failures
C. Serology test for syphilis in 30 days
D. *Chlamydia* test if not done at initial visit prior to treatment
E. Consider HIV and hepatitis B and C screening
F. If symptoms persist after treatment, then evaluate by culture for *N. gonorrhoeae* and test any gonococci for antimicrobial susceptibility

Appendix I has information about gonorrhea that you can photocopy or adapt for your patients. See Bibliographies.

Websites: http://www.cdc.gov/std/treatment/2010; http://www.cdc.gov/mmwr/pdf/rr/rr5912.pdf

GRANULOMA INGUINALE

I. DEFINITION
Granuloma inguinale (donovanosis) is a chronic granulomatous bacterial infection with the intracellular gram-negative bacterium *Klebsiella granulomatis* usually involving the genitalia and surrounding tissues, and probably spread by sexual contact

II. ETIOLOGY
A. Usually found in tropical and subtropical areas such as India, Papua New Guinea, the Caribbean, central Australia, and southern Africa
B. *K. granulomatis* (a difficult-to-grow, encapsulated bacillus organism)
C. Incubation period: 5 to 6 weeks (some say anywhere from 1–12 weeks)

III. HISTORY
A. What the patient presents with
   1. Female
      a. Painless papular or nodular ulcerative lesions arising on the vulva, in the vagina, urethra, anal area, inguinal region, or on the perineum with proliferation of granulation tissue and local destruction with scar tissue formation; single or multiple
      b. Beefy red proliferative lesion of fourchette with elevated rolled borders; bleeds easily
      c. Inguinal adenopathy (caused by secondary infection)—bilateral
      d. Malodorous vaginal discharge
   2. Male
      a. Lesion same as in the female and appearing on penis, scrotum, groin, or thighs
      b. In homosexual males, lesions on anus and buttocks
B. Additional information to be obtained
   1. History of STD or PID
   2. History of chronic illness
   3. Has patient recently been out of the country? Where (especially India, Papua New Guinea, the Caribbean, central Australia, southern Africa)? Is patient or patient's partner from, or has either visited, southeastern United States?
   4. Sexual preference, sexual practices (anal intercourse, sex toys)
   5. Last sexual contact
   6. Birth control method, current medications
   7. LMP

IV. PHYSICAL EXAMINATION
A. Vital signs
   1. Temperature
   2. Blood pressure
   3. Pulse
   4. Respirations
B. External examination
   1. Observe vulva for lesions (papular, nodular, or vesicular), beefy red nodules that develop into a rounded, elevated, velvety granulomatous mass; sharply defined rolled borders; signs of secondary infection

    C. Vaginal examination (speculum)
       1. Inspect vaginal walls for lesions
       2. Inspect cervix for lesions
    D. Bimanual examination

V. LABORATORY DIAGNOSIS
    A. Giemsa-stained smears of ulcer (diagnosis is confirmed by visualization of the Donovan bodies, large mononuclear cells with intracytoplasmic vacuoles containing the organism)—scrape at base of ulcer to get the tissue crush preparation or biopsy; there are no FDA-cleared PCR tests available; some laboratories have assays that have conducted a CLIA verification study
    B. Syphilis serology
    C. HSV culture

VI. DIFFERENTIAL DIAGNOSIS
    A. Syphilis
    B. Herpes simplex
    C. LGV
    D. Chancroid
    E. Carcinoma
    F. Fungal infection
    G. Genital amoebiasis

VII. TREATMENT
    A. Medication
       Doxycycline 100 mg orally twice a day for 21 days
    B. Alternative regimens
       Erythromycin base 500 mg orally 4 times a day for 21 days
    C. In pregnancy and lactation
       Erythromycin base 500 mg orally 4 times a day for 21 days
    D. General measures
       1. No sexual contact until treatment is completed
       2. Stress the importance of completing course of medication
       3. Stress the importance of examination of sexual contacts (within 60 days preceding onset of symptoms)

VIII. COMPLICATIONS
    A. Scar tissue secondary to slow healing formation
    B. Secondary infection, a common occurrence that results in gross tissue necrosis of genitalia
    C. Deformity of genitalia
    D. Dyspareunia
    E. Systemic infection
    F. Massive edema of vulva; penis (may be chronic)

IX. CONSULTATION/REFERRAL
A. Consult with physician prior to treatment if disease is suspected
B. If no response to treatment as discussed previously in 7 days—contact CDC or state health department

X. FOLLOW-UP
A. After completion of 2 to 5 days of medication
B. Follow clinically until signs and symptoms have resolved
C. Annual follow-up visits because the disease can reappear, and there is a possibility of scar carcinoma

See Bibliographies.
Website: http://www.cdc.gov/std/treatment/2010

HEPATITIS

I. DEFINITION
Hepatitis is an acute or chronic inflammation of the liver with or without permanent tissue damage and can be caused by many viruses including influenza viruses, mononucleosis, and cytomegalovirus (CMV); there are also hepatitis viruses whose only target is the liver. At least six types of hepatitis are known at present and are designated by the letters A, B, C, D, E, and G.

II. ETIOLOGY
A. Causative organisms include hepatitis viruses A to E and G, mononucleosis virus, CMV, and various influenza viruses
   1. Hepatitis A virus (HAV) is transmitted enterically—fecal–oral route (rarely parenterally) with an incubation period of 15 to 50 days, 28–day average
   2. Hepatitis B virus (HBV) is transmitted parenterally or sexually through body fluids—highest concentration in the blood, perinatally, or from saliva from human bites; incubation period of 6 weeks to 6 months
   3. Hepatitis C virus (HCV) is transmitted parenterally and permucosally, with an incubation average of 1 to 3 weeks for detection of HCV RNA in blood, and 8 to 9 weeks to seroconversion for the antibody; major cause of posttransfusion hepatitis. It is thought that sexual and perinatal transmission may be possible, the former among HIV-infected men who have sex with men; the latter is rare unless mother is coinfected with HIV.
   4. Hepatitis D virus (HDV), also known as delta virus, only affects persons who have active hepatitis B; transmitted parenterally, sexually, and perinatally. Incubation period of 3 to 13 weeks.

5. Hepatitis E virus (HEV) is transmitted enterically (rarely parenterally) with 15 to 60 days, mean of 40 days incubation. Spread by fecally contaminated water.
6. Hepatitis G, also called GB virus: Percutaneous route, posttransfusion disease; associated with chronic hepatitis C; noted especially in drug users

III. HISTORY
A. What the patient may present with
1. Right upper quadrant pain (may be intermittent)
2. Loss of appetite
3. Malaise, fatigue (increased sleep, decreased activity level, libido)
4. Fever, often low grade
5. Flulike symptoms, including headache
6. Adenopathy
7. Jaundice
8. Nausea and vomiting
9. Rash, hives
10. Joint and muscle pain
11. Darkened urine
12. Light-colored stools
13. Taste and smell peculiarities
14. Intolerance of fatty foods, cigarettes
B. Additional information to consider
1. Use of recreational drugs
2. Alcohol use, quantity, and frequency
3. Medication use (including nontraditional remedies, herbal preparations)
4. If partner is an injectable drug user
5. Recent transfusion of blood or blood products
6. Recent surgery
7. Eating raw or undercooked shellfish
8. Day care worker or has child/children in day care
9. Occupational risks including exposure to body fluids, excrement; blood, blood products
10. Sexual history and habits, especially anal intercourse; number of partners; use of sex toys; human bites
11. History of STDs
12. Sexual partner and/or household member with symptoms
13. Known exposure to someone with hepatitis
14. Military or civilian service in the Middle East; travel to Africa, Asia, Central and South America, Eastern Europe, or Alaska
15. History of hepatitis B
16. Visited or from disease-endemic areas of the world
17. Hemodialysis patient; transplant recipient; hemophiliac
18. Inmate of correctional institution
19. Contraceptive history

20. History of needlestick injury, tattoos, body piercing; acupuncture, sharing toothbrushes, razors, nail files, clippers
21. Infants of HBV and HCV mothers

IV. PHYSICAL EXAMINATION
A. Vital signs
  1. Temperature
  2. Pulse
  3. Respirations
  4. Blood pressure
B. Abdomen
  1. Liver percussion, palpation
  2. Observation of skin color, turgor
  3. Organomegaly, tenderness
  4. Masses
  5. Adenopathy
C. Complete physical examination with careful attention to
  1. Skin: rash, hives, color, turgor
  2. Joints: joint pain on range of motion; muscle pain
  3. Adenopathy

V. LABORATORY EXAMINATION
A. Feces for virus
B. Liver function tests
C. Mononucleosis screen
D. Serology to determine type of HAV: IgM (immunoglobulin M) anti-HAV in serum with acute or convalescent phase (5–10 days into incubation up to 6 months); HBV: several including HBV surface antigen (HBsAg), IgM anti-HBc; HCV: test for antibody with EIA or enhanced chemiluminescence assay, possible supplemental antibody test; HDV: HBsAg, anti-HDV; HEV: IgM anti-HEV, IgG anti-HEV; HGV: PCR testing, test for HAV, HBV, HCV, HDV, HEV
E. CMV
F. HIV testing
G. In severe hepatitis, serum albumin, prothrombin, and partial thromboplastin times, electrolytes, glucose, complete blood count (CBC), platelets
H. Pregnancy test

VI. DIFFERENTIAL DIAGNOSIS
A. Infectious mononucleosis
B. Primary or secondary hepatic malignancy
C. Ischemic hepatitis
D. Drug-induced hepatitis
E. Alcoholic hepatitis
F. Acute fatty liver (acute fatty metamorphosis) of pregnancy

VII. TREATMENT
A. As needed according to laboratory report and etiology; generally referral for medical management and follow-up
B. Supportive for symptoms
   1. No alcohol during acute phase of hepatitis and for 6 to 12 months thereafter
   2. Adequate calories; balanced diet
C. Interferon is being used for HBV and HCV
D. Gamma globulin to household and day care center contacts for hepatitis A within 2 weeks of exposure
E. Prevention for hepatitis B: for exposed persons, HBV hyperimmune globulin and then hepatitis B vaccination after antibody testing
F. Prevention for hepatitis D: hepatitis B vaccination; Twinrix
G. HAV recovery not aided by activity limitation; isolate food handlers with HAV; prevention for HAV with Havrix or Twinrix vaccine

VIII. COMPLICATIONS
A. Hepatitis A: rarely fatal, no chronic form, fulminant hepatitis, relapse
B. Hepatitis B: death; chronic disease in 5% to 10% of victims; of these, 50% get chronic liver disease leading to hepatocellular carcinoma in half of the cases; fulminant hepatitis, transmission to fetus 10% to 85%
C. Hepatitis C: >50% of cases become chronic; cirrhosis; hepatocellular carcinoma; perinatal transmission
D. Hepatitis D: chronic liver disease, fulminant hepatitis
E. Hepatitis E: high mortality in pregnancy (fetus and mother); no reported chronic cases
F. Hepatitis G: little information to date

IX. CONSULTATION/REFERRAL
For medical treatment and follow-up

X. FOLLOW-UP
A. As appropriate for type of hepatitis
B. Encourage hepatitis B vaccination of those who have not had disease; schedule three-dose administration; okay in pregnancy and lactation
C. Repeat laboratory work as indicated for monitoring liver function after illness
D. Test for chronic HBV with serum assay for HBsAg
E. Encourage HAV vaccination for persons at increased risk
F. Note availability of Twinrix—HAV and HAB combined three-dose vaccine

See Bibliographies.
Website: http://www.cdc.gov/std/treatment/2010

HIV/AIDS

Information on AIDS/HIV is ever evolving and changing. Because our role as clinicians in ambulatory settings is to identify, educate, and refer persons at high risk for the disease, the purpose of this guideline is to serve as a reference in those three areas only. Because AIDS has become the leading cause of death among young women, it has become increasingly important that women's health care clinicians keep abreast of current information by consulting professional journals and attending seminars on the subject.

I. DEFINITION
AIDS is the commonly used acronym for acquired immune deficiency syndrome, which is the name for a complex of health problems first reported in 1981. This spectrum of disease can begin with a brief acute retroviral syndrome that then morphs into the chronic, often clinically latent illness that will, without treatment in time, progress to a life-threatening immunodeficiency disease known as AIDS. If untreated, the time between infection with the virus and AIDS varies from a few months to many years, the median being 11 years.

II. ETIOLOGY
AIDS is caused by the human immunodeficiency virus (HIV); infection mainly by sexual contact (anal, vaginal, oral); contaminated blood and blood products, including needle and syringe sharing; contaminated semen used for artificial insemination; intrauterine acquisition (baby of a woman with AIDS); and, rarely, breast milk. Most cases in the United States continue to be HIV-1; HIV-2 infection is endemic in West Africa and is increasing in some European countries.

III. HISTORY
    A. What the patient may present with
        1. Rapid weight loss without known factor (>10%)
        2. Extreme fatigue; unexplained, increasing tiredness
        3. Chronic diarrhea (>1 month)
        4. Persistent dry cough, shortness of breath, dyspnea on exertion
        5. Prolonged fever, soaking night sweats, shaking chills
        6. Loss of appetite
        7. Skin rash; purple or pink, flat or raised lesions on skin or under skin, inside mouth, nose, eyelids, anus
        8. Changes in neurologic and/or cognitive function
        9. Generalized lymphadenopathy
      10. Chronic herpes simplex
      11. Recurrent herpes zoster
      12. Generalized pruritic dermatitis
      13. Oral and pharyngeal candidiasis; fungal infection of nails
      14. Persistent muscle pain

15. Fear of exposure to AIDS through sexual partner or high-risk behaviors or work-related accident (needlestick, contact with infected blood)
16. Chronic sinusitis
17. History of abnormal Pap smears
18. Persistent vulvar, vaginal, and anal condyloma
19. Seeking evaluation and treatment for STDs

B. Additional information to be considered
1. Sexual history
   a. Homosexual encounters; anal penetration
   b. Use of condoms, other methods of contraception, anal intercourse as contraception
   c. High-risk partners
   d. High-risk sexual practices
   e. History of previous STD
   f. Contact with prostitute
   g. Multiple partners or a partner with multiple partners
2. Use of injectable drugs by self or partner; other substance abuse history
3. High-risk occupation
4. History of blood transfusions or recipient of blood products particularly from 1980 to 1985
5. Duration and frequency of any presenting symptoms
6. Reason for fear of exposure to AIDS
7. Gynecologic history
   a. Recurrent STDs, vaginitis, vaginosis
   b. Widespread molluscum contagiosum, 100 or more lesions
   c. Infected with several STDs concurrently (may include gonorrhea, syphilis, *Chlamydia*)
   d. Rapidly progressing cervical dysplasia
   e. Papillomavirus on Pap smear
   f. Recurrent, recalcitrant vaginal candidiasis
   g. External condyloma unresponsive to treatment
   h. Existing pregnancy
   i. Anal discharge
   j. Pelvic, abdominal pain
8. Travel outside the United States, especially to West Africa or to European countries with known cases of HIV-2
9. Vaccination history

IV. PHYSICAL EXAMINATION

As appropriate to presenting complaint; gynecologic examination: testing for all STDs, Pap smear and wet mount or culture for *Trichomonas vaginalis*

V. LABORATORY EXAMINATION

A. Per protocol for presenting complaint, symptoms, risk status, or exposure

B. HIV testing if indicated or requested; if setting offers testing, resources must be in place for both pretest and posttest counseling for positive or negative results and follow-up; retest as needed
C. The CDC recommends HIV testing for all persons seeking evaluation for STDs; consider rapid testing if the patients are unlikely to return for results
D. All pregnant women should have HIV screening as early in pregnancy as possible and encourage screening for women planning a pregnancy (per new CDC Guidelines 2010)
E. Workplace exposures
F. Consider other blood-borne screening including HBV, HAC

VI. DIFFERENTIAL DIAGNOSIS
Widely different depending on presenting complaint.

VII. TREATMENT
A. General measures
   1. Counseling to avoid or minimize high-risk behaviors
      a. Instruction and counseling regarding safer sexual practices to protect self and partner from exchange of body fluids (e.g., by using latex condoms, female condoms, dental dams, Saran Wrap); by avoiding anal intercourse and oral–genital contact; avoiding sharing sex toys such as vibrators and dildos (or clean them with bleach or alcohol)
      b. Decreased number of sexual partners; mutual monogamy; abstinence
      c. Discourage use of injectable drugs; if patient is using injectable drugs, stress the need to avoid needle, works, or cooker sharing; offer resources on drug rehabilitation programs
      d. Avoid unsafe sexual contact with persons who are injectable drug users or fall into other high-risk groups
      e. Sexual activities with a partner with AIDS that do not involve direct passage of body fluids, such as light kissing, caressing, or mutual masturbation
      f. Empowering women to maintain equal decision-making power in their relationship(s)
      g. Avoid sharing razors, toothbrushes, nail files and clippers, and other items that could be contaminated with blood
B. Specific treatment
   1. Per guideline for specific presenting complaint
   2. Refer those patients falling into high-risk groups for further counseling and appropriate testing and follow-up if setting does not offer such services
   3. Referral for exposure so prophylactic therapy can be instituted

VIII. COMPLICATIONS
A. Opportunistic infections
B. AIDS may be fatal to some of its victims within 2 years of diagnosis

C. Transmission to unborn child or a child: definitive determination at <18 months, usually based on HIV nucleic acid testing

IX. CONSULTATIONS AND REFERRAL
A. All patients falling into high-risk groups in need of testing for presence of HIV virus unless setting offers testing and counseling
B. Referral for all patients testing positive to HIV antibody for appropriate treatment
C. Referral per guideline for all occupational exposures

X. FOLLOW-UP
A. Per referral
B. Contraceptive and gynecologic services for women with AIDS

See Appendix D for self-assessment of AIDS (HIV) risk list, which can be photocopied or adapted for your patients. See Bibliographies.
Website: http://www.cdc.gov/mmwr/pdf/rr/rr5912.pdf

LYMPHOGRANULOMA VENEREUM

I. DEFINITION
LGV is an STD characterized by a transitory primary lesion followed by suppurative lymphangitis and serious local complications

II. ETIOLOGY
A. Causative agent: *C. trachomatis*, serotypes L1, L2, and L3
B. Incubation period: 3 to 12 days up to 3 weeks
C. Found mainly in tropical or subtropical climates (Asia, Africa, South America); rare in the United States

III. HISTORY
A. What the patient may present with
1. "Sore" in genital area, mouth, anus, penis (of short duration, may go unnoticed); usually single and painless vesicle or non-indurated
2. Fever
3. Malaise
4. Headaches
5. Joint pain
6. Anorexia
7. Vomiting
8. Unilateral tender enlargement of inguinal lymph node; stiffness, aching of groin
9. Abscess in groin after 2 to 3 weeks

      10. Sinuses, scars in lower vagina or around introitus, or (in males) on penis

      11. Rectal discharge; perirectal/perianal fistulas and strictures

      12. Vaginal discharge

  B. Additional information to be considered

      1. Sexual preference; sexual practices

      2. Last sexual contact; new partner

      3. Known contact

      4. History of STD or PID

      5. LMP

      6. Method of birth control; other medications (antibiotics may mask symptoms)

      7. History of chronic infections

      8. Recent trip out of the country or new immigrant from a country where LGV is common

      9. Duration of lesion

IV. PHYSICAL EXAMINATION

  A. Vital signs

      1. Blood pressure

      2. Pulse

      3. Respiration

      4. Temperature

  B. Inguinal nodes

      1. First symptoms are unilateral tender enlargement of nodes

      2. Disease progresses for 2 to 3 weeks to form a large, tender, fluctuant mass that adheres to deep tissues and has overlying reddened skin (bubo)

      3. Multiple sinuses develop with purulent or serosanguinous discharge

      4. Healing occurs with scar formation, but sinuses persist or recur

      5. Chronic inflammation causes blockage of the lymphatic vessels leading to edema, ulceration, and fistula formation

  C. Vaginal examination (speculum)

      1. Vaginal walls: initial lesion may be on upper vaginal wall, resulting in enlargement and suppuration of perirectal and pelvic lymphatic vessels

      2. Cervix: initial lesion could be on the cervix

  D. Bimanual examination: tenderness in groin, vulva

  E. Rectovaginal examination: rectal wall may be involved, resulting in ulcerative proctitis with serosanguinous rectal discharge

V. LABORATORY EXAMINATION AND DIAGNOSIS

  A. Genital and lymph node swabs of lesion or bubo aspirate can be tested by culture, immunofluorescence, or nucleic acid detection

  B. *Chlamydia* serology complement fixation test: fourfold rise or single titer of >1:64 can support diagnosis

    C. Serology test for syphilis, gonorrhea culture
    D. Biopsy of chronic anorectal lesions and lymph nodes to rule out carcinoma
    E. Diagnosis made on clinical suspicion, epidemiologic information, and exclusion of other etiologies along with *C. trachomatis* testing

VI. DIFFERENTIAL DIAGNOSIS
    A. Syphilis
    B. Herpes simplex
    C. Carcinoma
    D. Chancroid
    E. Granuloma inguinale
    F. *Chlamydia* infection
    G. Hodgkin disease
    H. Proctocolitis
    I. Inguinal lymphadenopathy
    J. Genital or rectal ulcers

VII. TREATMENT
    A. Medications
      1. Doxycycline 100 mg orally twice a day for 21 days
      2. Alternative regimens: Erythromycin base 500 mg orally 4 times a day for 21 days
    B. Medications in pregnancy and lactation
      1. Erythromycin base 500 mg orally twice a day for 21 days
    C. General measures
      1. Sitz bath
      2. Stress the importance of completing the course of medication.
      3. All sexual partners should be treated if contact within 30 days before onset of symptoms; examine and test for *Chlamydia*/gonorrhea in urethra, cervix
      4. Comfort measures
        a. Tepid water sitz baths; dry carefully with cool air hair dryer making sure to hold it sufficiently away from body
        b. Avoid tight, restricting clothing
        c. Expose perineum to airflow as much as possible (wear a skirt or robe without underpants at home)
        d. Recommend peri-irrigation set
      5. Patient education
        a. Explain disease process and route of transmission
        b. Stress the importance of checking sexual partner(s) for urethral or cervical *Chlamydia* infection within 60 days of onset of symptoms.

VIII. COMPLICATIONS
    A. Scar formation
    B. Sinuses causing blockage of the lymphatic vessels, which leads to edema

C. Fistula formation: rectovaginal, vulvar, other
D. Suppuration of perirectal and lymphatic vessels
E. Rectal stricture
F. Systemic: phlebitis, hepatomegaly, nephropathy

IX. CONSULTATION/REFERRAL
A. Consult with physician prior to treatment if infection is suspected
B. If no response to treatment as outlined previously
C. If any of the aforementioned complications occur

X. FOLLOW-UP
A. Reevaluate 3 to 5 days after treatment
B. Then evaluate every 1 to 2 weeks until healing is complete

See Bibliographies.
Website: http://www.cdc.gov/mmwr/pdf/rr/rr5912.pdf

MOLLUSCUM CONTAGIOSUM

I. DEFINITION
Molluscum contagiosum is an infectious disease of the skin affecting the face, arms, genitals, abdomen, and thighs. It is caused by a virus and is seen in all age groups and in both sexes.

II. ETIOLOGY
A. Molluscum contagiosum virus, a member of the poxvirus family
B. Probably transmitted through direct skin contact including sexual contact with an affected partner, and through contact with contaminated objects such as toys, doorknobs, and faucet handles
C. Incubation period: 1 week to 6 months (usually 2–7 weeks)

III. HISTORY
A. What the patient may present with
  1. Fleshy growths (1–20), dome-shaped, waxy, or pearly white papules with central caseous white core, primarily in genital area, but may be found on other body surfaces; may be 1 to 5 mm in diameter (but up to 15 mm), may be pedunculated; can be single or grouped
  2. No other symptoms or complaints but occasional pruritus, tenderness, and/or pain
B. Additional information to be considered
  1. Previous episode of similar lesions
  2. History of STD
  3. Sexual activity, last intercourse
  4. Known contact

5. Method of birth control; other medications
6. Any drug allergies
7. HIV risk/exposure, especially with widespread lesions 100 or more

IV. PHYSICAL EXAMINATION
A. Observe perineum for fleshy, usually papular, skin-colored lesions with indented centers that contain white, curdlike material
B. Observe any other involved body area

V. LABORATORY EXAMINATION
A. Visual examination
B. Skin scrapings under a microscope
C. Pathology report on crushed excised lesion using Pap smear, Wright, Giemsa, or Gram stain
D. Serology test for syphilis
E. GC culture/*Chlamydia* test
F. Further laboratory work as indicated by history
G. Consider HIV screen especially with 100 or more lesions

VI. DIFFERENTIAL DIAGNOSIS
A. Genital warts (condylomata acuminata)
B. Herpes simplex
C. Pyogenic granuloma
D. Folliculitis
E. Small epidermal cysts
F. Closed comedones
G. Basal cell carcinoma
H. Furunculosis

VII. TREATMENT
A. Removal of lesion
1. Cytotoxic agents—TCA, BCA, podophyllin
2. Excision of lesions by curettage with topical anesthetic followed by application of silver nitrate
3. Destruction of lesions by cryotherapy; consider physician consult
4. Laser therapy
5. Topical 5% imiquimod daily for 5 days a week at bedtime
B. General measures
1. Return for weekly or biweekly evaluation and treatment until lesions have healed
2. Refer sexual partner(s) for evaluation

VIII. COMPLICATIONS
Secondary staphylococcus infection

IX. CONSULTATION/REFERRAL
A. For treatment as stated previously
B. Patients with extensive molluscum, lesions on face, or repeated recurrence after treatment should be reevaluated for HIV infection

X. FOLLOW-UP
Return for reevaluation if lesions persist/recur after treatment

See Bibliographies.
Website: http://www.cdc.gov/mmwr/pdf/rr/rr5912.pdf

SYPHILIS

I. DEFINITION
Syphilis is a sexually transmitted, systemic disease characterized by periods of active florid manifestations and periods of symptomless latency. It can affect any tissue or vascular organ of the body and can be passed on from mother to fetus.

II. ETIOLOGY
A. The causative organism is a motile spirochete, *T. pallidum*
B. Incubation period: 10 to 90 days; with an average of 21 days

III. HISTORY
A. What the patient may present with
1. Primary symptoms
   a. Painless lesion (chancre) at site of entry of *T. pallidum*. Chancre appears on average about 3 weeks after sexual contact and heals in 3 to 6 weeks with a small inculum—this incubation period may be as long as 90 days. Sites include the vulva, labia, fourchette, clitoris, cervix, nipple, lip, roof of mouth, tonsils, bite area, finger, urethra, rectum, and smooth, firm borders of an ulcer.
   b. Enlarged inguinal or regional nodes; trochlear
2. Secondary symptoms that may or may not occur in untreated patients within 4 to 10 weeks of resolution of primary symptoms
   a. Generalized symmetrical papillosquamous eruption of palms, soles, or mucous membrane (condylomata lata)
   b. Alopecia; may have a moth-eaten look
   c. Loss of lateral one-third of eyebrow
   d. Generalized nontender lymphadenopathy with firm, rubbery feel
   e. Symptoms of upper respiratory tract infection
   f. Low-grade fever
   g. Malaise, anorexia, and arthralgia

      h. Mild hepatitis, splenomegaly, or nephrotic syndrome in about 10% of cases

      i. Mucus patches on tongue, under foreskin, and in intertriginous areas

  3. Latent stage: No clinical symptoms, although 25% may have recurrence of cutaneous lesion; however, patients demonstrate serologic evidence

      a. Early latency: infection within the preceding year

      b. Late latency: over a year from date of initial infection. Patients may remain in latent stage for remainder of their lives; however, one-third will develop the tertiary form of disease.

      c. Tertiary stage: Osseous or cutaneous structures, cardiovascular system or nervous system becomes involved; most common developments are cardiovascular syphilis and neurosyphilis

      d. Neurosyphilis (exceedingly uncommon today) can occur at any stage from 1 to 30 or more years after original infection

B. Additional information to be considered

  1. Sexual preference

  2. Current sexual activity

  3. Last sexual contact

  4. Birth control method(s)

  5. History of known contacts

  6. History of previous STD

  7. History of recurrent infectious illness (e.g., mononucleosis)

  8. History of fever, malaise, arthralgia, or rash of unknown etiology

  9. History of cognitive dysfunction, sensory deficits, other neurologic symptoms

  10. Current medical therapy

  11. Risk for HIV exposure

IV. PHYSICAL EXAMINATION

A. Vital signs

  1. Temperature

  2. Blood pressure

  3. Pulse

B. General examination of skin

  1. Alopecia

  2. Rash including soles of feet, palms, condyloma lata

C. Pharyngeal examination

D. Examine for enlarged inguinal nodes

E. External examination of genitalia; vulvar lesions; chancre at point of inoculation

F. Internal examination (speculum)

  1. Inspection of vaginal walls for lesions

  2. Inspection of cervix for lesions

  3. Inspection of discharge

G. Bimanual examination
H. Neurologic examination per history and clinical findings

V. LABORATORY EXAMINATION

A. Nontreponemal: venereal disease research laboratory (VDRL) and rapid plasma reagin (RPR)—these are nonspecific serum tests—detect cross-reaction of antibody to syphilis with cardiolipin. Reported as reactive or nonreactive. Reactive test is reported by a quantitative titer, and reactive tests should be confirmed with treponemal testing. Use of only one type of serologic test is insufficient for diagnosis.
  1. Biological false-positives occur with cardiolipin antigens sometimes present in drug abuse and in such diseases and conditions as:
     a. Lupus erythematosus
     b. Mononucleosis
     c. Malaria
     d. Leprosy
     e. Viral pneumonia
     f. After smallpox vaccinations or other recent vaccinations
     g. Persons with HIV
     h. Narcotic addiction
     i. Arthritis
     j. Scleroderma
     k. Tuberculosis
     l. Chronic fatigue syndrome
     m. Pregnancy
B. Specific serum treponemal antibody tests (correlate poorly with disease activity; persons who have a reactive test will have it for life unless diagnosis and treatment are very early)
  1. Fluorescent treponemal antibody-absorption (FTA-ABS) test
  2. *T. pallidum* particle agglutination (TP-PA)
C. GC culture
D. *Chlamydia* test
E. Biopsy of the lesion
F. Dark-field microscopy exam (rarely available in free-standing clinics or offices)—most useful for males
G. Consider HIV testing; testing for hepatitis B and C

VI. DIFFERENTIAL DIAGNOSIS

A. Herpes simplex
B. Condylomata acuminata
C. Granuloma inguinale
D. Chancroid
E. LGV
F. Carcinoma
G. Pyoderma

VII. TREATMENT (WITH PHYSICIAN CONSULT IN SOME SETTINGS)
A. Medication (for primary and secondary syphilis)
1. Benzathine penicillin G (BiCillin) 2.4 million units IM single dose immediately. Caution regarding Jarisch-Herxheimer reaction: In 50% of cases, 6 to 12 hours after injection, the patient develops high fever, malaise, and exacerbation of symptoms lasting 24 hours. (This is a sign that the spirochete is breaking down.) Occurs most frequently among patients with early syphilis.
2. For penicillin allergy: Doxycycline 100 mg orally twice a day for 14 days *or* tetracycline 500 mg orally 4 times a day for 14 days
B. For early latent syphilis (<1 year)
Benzathine penicillin G, 2.4 million units IM in a single dose
C. For late latent syphilis or unknown duration
Benzathine penicillin G, 7.2 million units total, in three doses of 2.4 million units IM each at 1-week intervals
D. For late syphilis or unknown duration
Benzathine penicillin G, 7.2 million units total, in three doses of 2.4 million units IM each at 1-week intervals
E. In pregnancy
1. Treat with penicillin regimen appropriate for stage of syphilis
2. Hospitalize pregnant patients with history of penicillin allergies to undergo skin testing. If positive, they should be desensitized and treated with penicillin (*see CDC Guidelines 2010*).
F. General measures
1. Support, especially in regard to possible Jarisch-Herxheimer reaction
2. Stress the importance of completing all medication
3. Partner should be treated concurrently; treat all contacts exposed within 90 days of diagnosis of primary, secondary, or early latent syphilis presumptively; persons exposed >90 days before diagnosis of primary, secondary, or early latent syphilis in a sex partner should be treated presumptively if serologic test results are not immediately available and follow-up is uncertain

VIII. COMPLICATIONS
A. Progression of disease to tertiary stage
B. One hundred percent transmission to fetus with primary and secondary in pregnancy; 50% fetal mortality and 50% congenital syphilis. Early latent: 80% fetal infection (20% premature, 20% fetal death, 40% congenital syphilis). Late latent: 30% fetal transmission, 11% fetal death.

IX. CONSULTATION/REFERRAL
Positive diagnosis of disease

X. FOLLOW-UP
Quantitative serology tests for primary and secondary syphilis (non-treponemal serologic) should be obtained at 6 and 12 months (falling titer should be demonstrated if treatment is adequate—at least a fourfold drop by 6 months using the same test). If repeat titer does not decrease, patient should be followed with titers, or re-treated. For persons with persistent signs and symptoms, symptoms that recur, or a fourfold increase in non-treponemal test titer, re-treat and reevaluate for HIV. For latent syphilis, repeat testing at 6, 12, and 24 months.

See Appendix I and Bibliographies.
Websites: http://www.cdc.gov/std/treatment/2010; http://www.cdc.gov/mmwr/pdf/rr/rr5912.pdf

TRICHOMONIASIS

I. DEFINITION
Infection with *Trichomonas* is usually sexually transmitted; found in the vagina and urethra of women and the urethra of males

II. ETIOLOGY
The parasitic protozoan flagellate, *T. vaginalis*

III. HISTORY
    A. What the patient may present with:
        1. Foul-smelling, diffuse vaginal discharge, often fishy
        2. Burning and soreness of vulva, perineum, thighs
        3. Vaginal and perineal itching
        4. Dyspareunia, dysuria
        5. Postcoital bleeding
        6. Possibly no objective symptoms
    B. Additional information to be considered
        1. Previous vaginal infection, vaginosis; diagnosis, treatment; compliance with treatment
        2. Sexual activity; partner preference (do not disregard possibility of women having sex with women)
        3. History of STD or PID
        4. LMP
        5. Last intercourse, sexual contact
        6. Method of birth control; other medications
        7. History of chronic illness (especially seizure disorders)
        8. Description of discharge
            a. Color
            b. Onset
            c. Odor
            d. Consistency

e. Amount
f. Constant versus intermittent
g. Relationship to menses
h. Relationship to sexual contact
9. Whether or not partner has symptoms

IV. PHYSICAL EXAMINATION
A. External examination
Observe perineum for excoriation, erythema, edema, ulceration, or lesions
B. Vaginal examination (speculum)
1. Inspection of vaginal walls; red papules may appear
2. Inspection of cervix: strawberry appearance of cervix and upper vagina because of petechiae
3. Discharge: greenish, yellow, malodorous, frothy with a pH of >4.5 (5.0–7.0)
C. Bimanual examination

V. LABORATORY EXAMINATION
A. Wet prep microscopic examination; should see highly motile cells, slightly larger than leukocytes, smaller than epithelial cells; >10 WBCs per high-power field
B. GC culture, *Chlamydia* test, serology testing for syphilis if history indicates; culture for *T. vaginalis*; DNA probe for *T. vaginalis*
C. CBC should be done if more than two courses of metronidazole taken within a 2-month period
D. KOH whiff test: sometimes fishy but not always
E. OSOM Trichomonas Rapid Test—dipstick of vaginal swab; 83% sensitivity
F. Affirm VPIII results available in 45 minutes (noting that with this test and OSOM, false-positives can occur)
G. Modified Amplicor for *T. vaginalis* in vaginal or endocervical swabs and urine (sensitivity 88%–97%; specificity 98%–99%)

VI. DIFFERENTIAL DIAGNOSIS
A. Candidiasis
B. Bacterial vaginosis
C. Urinary tract infection
D. Gonorrhea
E. *Chlamydia* infection

VII. TREATMENT
A. Medications
1. Metronidazole (Flagyl, Metryl, Protostat, Satric) 2 g orally in single dose (review history for seizure disorder) OR
2. Tinidazole (Tindamax) 2 g orally in a single dose with food (tablets come in 250 and 500 mg; pregnancy Category C)

3. Alternative regimen: Metronidazole 500 mg orally twice a day for 7 days
4. In pregnancy at any stage: Metronidazole 2 g orally in single dose
5. *Note:* Metronidazole gel: not recommended (<50% efficacious as therapeutic levels are not achieved in the urethra or perivaginal glands)
6. Lactation: Tindamax single dose; interruption of breastfeeding for 72 hours following treatment
7. Refer sex partners for treatment
8. Treatment failure with metronidazole 2 g single dose: Exclude reinfection and treat with metronidazole 500 mg orally twice daily for 7 days; for patients failing this regimen, treat with tinidazole or metronidazole 2 g orally for 5 days
9. Consult with specialist if the previous regimens are not effective
   B. General Measures
1. Stress the importance of not drinking alcohol during treatment or for 48 hours after treatment; with Tindamax 72 hours
2. Metronidazole can cause GI upset; also causes urine to darken
3. Stress avoidance of intercourse during treatment; if intercourse does occur, condoms should be used
4. Stress the importance of completing medication
5. Stress personal hygiene; cotton underpants, no underpants while sleeping, wipe front first, and then back
6. Patient should be given informational handout to deliver to sexual partner advising need for partner's treatment
7. Comfort measures for severe symptoms: sitz baths
8. Stress that if partner is not treated before next act of unprotected intercourse, reinfection can occur

VIII. COMPLICATIONS
   A. Disease complications
1. Spread of the infection to the urethra, or prostate in the male
2. Untreated *T. vaginalis* may result in atypia on Pap smear; may also be associated with adverse pregnancy outcomes (premature rupture of membranes and premature delivery); increased susceptibility to HIV acquisition
3. Adverse pregnancy outcomes: Premature rupture of membranes, preterm delivery, low birth weight
   B. Treatment complications
1. Nausea
2. Neurologic symptoms: seizures
3. Vomiting (may be severe) if alcohol is consumed while on treatment or within 48 hours after treatment
4. Possibility of blood dyscrasia posttreatment

IX. CONSULTATION/REFERRAL
   A. Refer to physician if the woman has seizure disorder prior to initiating therapy

B. If the woman is pregnant

C. Consult if treatment (*see Treatment, VII A. 1 and 2*) fails

X. FOLLOW-UP

Consider rescreening at 3 months (because of high rate of reinfection) for sexually active women

See Appendix I and Bibliographies.
Website: http://www.cdc.gov/std/treatment/2010

NOTES

1. Adapted from material developed by R. M. C. Secor (1997). Vaginal microscopy: Refining the nurse practitioner's technique. *Clinical Excellence for Nurse Practitioners, 1*(1), 29–34; and from H. A. Carcio & R. M. C. Secor (Eds.). (2010). Vaginal microscopy. In *Advanced health assessment of women* (2nd ed., pp. 189–228). New York, NY: Springer Publishing Company.
2. Note that KOH should be used with care because it is very damaging to the microscope.

Part

IV

Appendices

APPENDIX
Patient Information and Consent Forms

(May also be used as an informational handout)

I. MECHANISM OF ACTION
    A. A systemic method of preventing conception that acts by:
        1. Suppressing ovulation
        2. Producing changes in the endometrium that make it unreceptive to implantation
        3. Producing a thickened cervical mucus; interference with sperm reaching the egg

II. BENEFITS OF THE METHOD
    A. Highly effective: 99.66% for combination hormonal contraceptives (0.1 pregnancy/year); 97% for progestin-only hormonal contraceptives
    B. Sexual spontaneity
    C. Regulated menstrual flow
    D. Lighter flow and less cramping
    E. Decreased incidence of uterine and ovarian cancers
    F. Relief of symptoms associated with perimenopause

III. RISK OF METHOD
Applies to combination oral contraceptives (OCs), patch, and ring
    A. Minor side effects (these are rare and usually subside after several months of method use; may be alleviated by changing type of hormonal contraception or by discontinuing). Listed are a few more common, although rare, side effects:
        1. Nausea (if using OC, try taking pill with a meal or with milk; with severe nausea/vomiting, use backup method of birth control such as condoms)
        2. Spotting
        3. Decreased menstrual flow and sometimes missed periods
        4. May have more problems with yeast infections or vaginal discharges
        5. Depression or mood changes
        6. Acne or increase in acne
        7. Headaches (not severe)
    B. Major side effects (rare in women younger than 40 years old who are nonsmokers)
        1. Blood clots in legs, lungs; stroke
        2. Hypertension (high blood pressure)
        3. Gallbladder disease
        4. Heart attack (smokers age 35 years and older)
        5. Smoking doubles risk factors associated with hormone use. These side effects are characterized by the following danger signals (if they occur, seek medical care *immediately*): pain, redness, or swelling of the legs or a localized tender red spot

warm to the touch may indicate a blood clot in a vein; persistent and severe headaches; chest pain and/or difficulty breathing; blurred vision, flashing vision; blindness; abdominal pain.

IV. CONTRAINDICATIONS

Women with a history of any of the following conditions may not be able to use hormonal contraceptives containing estrogen:

A. Thromboembolic disorders (blood clot) in legs, lungs
B. Impaired liver function at present time; liver problems
C. Cancer of breast or reproductive system (uterus, ovaries, cervix)
D. Hypertension (high blood pressure); uncontrolled, or smoking and high blood pressure
E. Hyperlipidemia (high cholesterol)
F. Stroke
G. Coronary artery disease
H. Major surgery on legs or with prolonged immobility
I. Age 35 years or older and currently a smoker
J. Pregnancy—known or suspected
K. Undiagnosed genital bleeding
L. Taking certain prescription drugs
M. Diabetes with vascular (blood vessel) disease
N. Headaches, migraines with neurologic symptoms

V. ALTERNATE METHODS OF BIRTH CONTROL

A. Abstinence
B. Sterilization; natural family planning
C. Condom used with contraceptive cream, jelly or foam, contraceptive suppositories or tablets, vaginal film, contraceptive gel, sponge
D. Intrauterine device (IUD)
E. Diaphragm with contraceptive cream or jelly, FemCap, Lea's Shield
F. Female condom
G. Contraceptive patch, ring (if estrogen is not a problem)
H. Progestin-only methods: progestin-only pill, Mirena IUD, etonogestrel implant (Implanon), Depo-Provera

VI. INQUIRIES ARE ENCOURAGED

Please ask us questions; a change in decision does not create a problem

VII. EXPLANATION OF METHOD

A. Ways in which hormonal contraceptives are prescribed
  1. A complete physical examination is done, including blood pressure, weight, urinalysis, and gynecologic examination with Pap smear (unless one was done within the past year)
  2. Review side effects and dangers of use; review pill packet if using OCs

3. If requested to do so by your clinician, review and sign an informed consent for hormonal contraceptives
4. You may transfer your records from another clinic or clinician's office
B. Ways in which OCs are taken
   1. Start taking your first package of pills as directed by your clinician
   2. OC pills are *usually* started initially at the same time as your period; you begin the Sunday of the week your period starts, even if you are still bleeding
   3. Swallow one pill at the *same time* daily
   4. A second form of contraception is recommended for the first 7 days after starting the pill (unless specified differently)
   5. Some medications can decrease effectiveness or cause other pill-related problems (e.g., spotting). Always mention to your clinician and pharmacist that you are on OCs and the type prior to starting any other medication. Also, tell us if you are on any medications prior to starting OCs. Use a backup method of birth control if you have any doubts about the possibility of a drug interaction.
   6. If you are taking prescribed antibiotics for an illness, you should continue your pill but use a backup method
   7. Breakthrough bleeding (spotting) is common during the first few months a woman is on an OC; do not be alarmed if the following occurs:
      a. If you experience spotting after several months of using pill, make sure that you are taking the pill correctly, as directed in the subsequent text. But make sure that you discuss this at the time of your first pill check.
      b. If the pill is taken improperly, breakthrough bleeding may occur. You must make every effort to take your pill at the same time *every day*.
         i. If you take your pill later than 6 hours, take the pill when you remember it; you are also advised to use a second method of birth control for the next 7 days
         ii. If you miss one pill, take the pill when you remember and then take the scheduled pill at the regular time. A second method of birth control is recommended for 7 days.
         iii. If you miss two pills in the first 2 weeks of a pill pack, take two pills at the regular time, and then the next day, take two pills at the regular time; use a second method of birth control for 7 days
         iv. If you miss two pills in the third week, or if you miss three or more pills at any time and you start packets on Sunday, take a pill each day until Sunday, then discard the remainder of that pack and start a new pack immediately, omitting the hormone-free week (if there is one). If you do not start a new pack on Sundays, throw away the rest of the pill pack and start a new pack that day.

A backup method of birth control should be used for the first 7 days of this new pill pack.

    v. If you miss one or more pills and used no backup method and have no period, call to discuss possible pregnancy test

    vi. If you are not sure what to do about missed pills, use a backup method any time you have sex and keep taking a birth control pill (hormone pill) each day until you can talk with your clinician

C. Occasionally, withdrawal bleeding (your period) does not occur during the week of nonhormone pills (placebos)

    1. If this happens to you and all pills have been taken properly, continue with the next pill cycle. If you miss two periods, start your third pill cycle but call your clinician for advice.

    2. If this happens to you and you have taken your pill late or forgotten to take it, and did not use a second birth control method, start your next pill packet but call your clinician for advice

D. If you experience severe vomiting and/or diarrhea, use a backup method of birth control because the pill may not have been absorbed properly

I have read the above material; it has been fully explained. I have been given the opportunity to ask questions, and I understand the information. I have chosen to use an oral contraceptive.

Signed   _____   Date _____

Witness _____   Date _____

Danger Signals Associated With Hormonal Contraceptive Use

Abdominal pain (severe)

Chest pain (severe) or shortness of breath

Eye problems such as blurred vision or loss of vision

Headaches (severe)

Severe leg pain (calf or thigh)

Contact us at ( ) _____ if you develop any of the above problems.

Note: Birth control pills can be used as emergency contraception. Ask your health care provider; check directions in pill packet; call 1-888-NOT-2-LATE; visit http://not-2-late.com. Emergency contraception (EC) Plan B is available over the counter at a pharmacy (no prescription) if you are 18 years of age or older.

Injectable Contraception (Depo-Provera)[1]

(May also be used as an informational handout)

I. DEFINITION
Depo-Provera is a hormonal substance that prevents ovulation from occurring. It is injected intramuscularly or subcutaneously every 12 weeks into the muscle of the upper arm or buttocks.

II. HOW IT WORKS
The hormones in the injection suppress ovulation (egg production) for 12 weeks.

III. HOW EFFECTIVE IS IT?
Failure rate is less than one pregnancy per 100 women per year when women return for injections every 12 weeks (Depo) and when injection is done in the first 5 days of menses (bleeding).

IV. WHY CHOOSE THIS METHOD
   A. Consider using other methods and whether their side effects make you prefer this method
   B. Desire for long-term contraceptive—12-week coverage
   C. Desire for reversible method (ability to stop injections)
   D. Desire for method disconnected from intercourse; nothing to take or put in

V. WHY YOU MIGHT NOT BE A CANDIDATE
   A. Known or suspected pregnancy
   B. Unexplained abnormal vaginal bleeding
   C. Known breast cancer
   D. Known sensitivity to Depo-Provera or any of its ingredients (have you ever had an allergic reaction to local anesthetic at the dentist)

VI. THINGS TO CONSIDER BEFORE CHOOSING DEPO-PROVERA
   A. Depression
   B. Abnormal mammogram
   C. Kidney disease
   D. Hypertension (high blood pressure)
   E. Planned pregnancy in near future
   F. Gallbladder disease
   G. Mild cirrhosis (liver disease)
   H. Do you regularly use any prescription drugs or herbals—we need to check possible interactions with Depo-Provera

VII. SIDE EFFECTS YOU MIGHT EXPERIENCE
   A. Weight gain or weight loss; change in appetite
   B. Menstrual irregularity—possibly no periods by second or third shot

C. Headaches
D. Abdominal bloating
E. Breast tenderness
F. Tiredness, weakness
G. Dizziness
H. Depression, nervousness
I. Nausea
J. No hair growth or loss or thinning of hair; increased hair growth on face or body
K. Skin rash or increased acne
L. Increased or decreased sex drive

VIII. EXPLANATION OF METHOD AND ASSESSMENT

Depo-Provera is injected intramuscularly or subcutaneously in one dose every 12 weeks for as long as contraceptive effect is desired. It is injected in the first 5 days of the menstrual cycle (after onset of menses), within 5 days postpartum.

IX. USE OF THIS METHOD AND WARNING SIGNS

A. Drug interactions are possible when using Depo-Provera with other prescription drugs. Always check with your physician or nurse practitioner and pharmacist for such possible interactions before taking any other prescription drug; Depo-Provera is a medication and you need to list it in your health history.
B. Warning signs to report to your clinician (physician or nurse practitioner):
  1. Sharp chest pain, coughing of blood, sudden shortness of breath
  2. Sudden severe headache, vomiting, dizziness, or fainting
  3. Visual disturbance (double vision, blurred vision, spots before your eyes) or speech disturbance (slurred, unable to speak)
  4. Weakness or numbness in arm or leg
  5. Severe pain or swelling in calf or leg
  6. Unusually heavy vaginal bleeding (unlike usual periods)
  7. Severe pain or tenderness in lower abdomen, pelvis
  8. Persistent pain, pus, or bleeding at injection site

X. FOLLOW-UP CARE OF YOURSELF

A. Visit your clinician every 12 weeks for injection of Depo-Provera
B. The first visit should take place during the first 5 days of your menses (period)
C. Review any side effects or danger signs with your clinician
D. Review your menstrual cycles with your clinician
E. Have a Pap smear every year along with a complete physical examination, including pelvic and breast examinations
F. Depo-Provera provides no protection against sexually transmitted diseases (STDs) (including AIDS) or vaginal infections, so consider using condoms to protect yourself

G. Depo-Provera contains no estrogen. Estrogen is needed for strong bones. While using this birth control method, you need to be sure you get enough calcium and vitamin D in your diet. Your clinician will advise you on how to do this.

I have read the above and have been given a copy of this consent form and the manufacturer's information, and I agree to have Depo-Provera.

Patient's signature   _____   Date _____
Witness's signature   _____   Date _____

(May also be used as an informational handout)

I. MECHANISM OF ACTION
A contraceptive diaphragm is a shallow rubber cup with a flexible rim that is placed in the vagina to cover the cervix. It functions as both a mechanical barrier and a receptacle for spermicidal cream or jelly or vaginal film that must be used to ensure effectiveness.

II. BENEFITS OF THE METHOD
 A. Effectiveness rate ranges from 80% to 95%: theoretically, 95%; 80% to 85% use effectiveness (because of user failure)
 B. No chemicals are taken internally

III. RISKS OF THE METHOD
 A. Allergic response to the rubber and/or spermicidal agent
 B. Foul-smelling discharge from leaving diaphragm in place too long (diaphragm should not be left in place longer than 24 hours)
 C. Toxic shock syndrome has been reported in association with diaphragm use during the menstrual period. To avoid this, do not leave your diaphragm in place for more than 24 hours and follow the use of precautions at the end of these instructions.

IV. CONTRAINDICATIONS
 A. Inability to achieve satisfactory fitting
 B. You are unable to learn correct insertion technique
 C. Allergy to rubber or spermicidal agent
 D. Inconvenience of method (e.g., lack of sexual spontaneity, timing, messiness)
 E. Repeated bladder infections (cystitis)
 F. Chronic constipation (causes discomfort for some users)

V. ALTERNATIVE BIRTH CONTROL METHODS
 A. Abstinence
 B. Sterilization
 C. OCs (birth control pills, mini pills)
 D. IUD
 E. Condom used with contraceptive cream, foam, gel, suppositories, vaginal film, or sponge
 F. FemCap, Lea's Shield
 G. Natural family planning
 H. Female condom
 I. Depo-Provera contraceptive injection
 J. Contraceptive patch, ring, etonogestrel implant (Implanon)

VI. EXPLANATION OF THE METHOD

A. How a diaphragm is prescribed
1. A complete physical examination, including Pap smear, is necessary unless one has been done within the past year. A pelvic examination (bimanual) will be done at the time the diaphragm is fitted.
2. If required by your clinician, review and sign an informed consent similar to this one prior to your initial prescription

B. How a diaphragm is used
1. How it works
   a. Inserted prior to intercourse to fit snugly in vagina
   b. Holds spermicidal cream or jelly or vaginal film against cervix and kills sperm
   c. Diaphragm is to be left in place for 8 hours after last intercourse.
   d. No douching for 8 hours after intercourse
   e. Prior to repeated intercourse, additional jelly or cream should be applied with applicator to outside of diaphragm or another vaginal film should be inserted
   f. Effective immediately upon insertion and up to 4 hours without adding more cream, jelly, or film, or for one intercourse (some sources suggest 6 hours for c., d., and f.)
2. Technique for use
   a. Empty your bladder, wash your hands carefully whenever you insert or remove your diaphragm
   b. Apply approximately 1 tablespoon of spermicidal cream or jelly into the dome of the diaphragm and spread around the dome; cream or jelly need not be spread on the rim or outside of diaphragm
   c. Fold in half and insert into vagina like a tampon
   d. With index finger, check rim at pubic arch and make sure cervix is covered
   e. To remove (at proper time), hook finger around rim and pull diaphragm out
3. Care of diaphragm
   a. Wash with warm water and mild soap after removal
   b. Dry thoroughly
   c. Store in a dry place (allowing it to dry thoroughly before putting it in a case keeps rubber in better condition longer and prevents odor; powder lightly with cornstarch)
   d. Soak in rubbing alcohol (70%) for 30 minutes after use following treatment for vaginal infection

VII. DIAPHRAGM CHECK

A. We encourage you to return to the office 1 week after fitting for diaphragm check
B. If you lose or gain 10 to 15 lbs (or if diaphragm fit seems to change)
C. If you have a miscarriage, abortion, or a baby
D. If you have any kind of pelvic surgery
E. If you experience problems urinating or trouble moving your bowels with diaphragm in place

VIII. INQUIRIES ARE ENCOURAGED

Please feel free to ask us questions at any time!

You may change your mind about a birth control method at any time.

I have read the above material; it has been explained fully. I have been given the opportunity to ask questions and I understand the information. I have chosen to use the diaphragm.

Patient's signature   _____   Date _____
Witness's signature   _____   Date _____

Toxic Shock Syndrome

Toxic shock syndrome has been reported in association with diaphragm use during menses. It is recommended that if you use your diaphragm during menses, you observe hand-washing recommendations carefully, use tampons only during heaviest days (not super-absorbent type—see tampon package labeling), and monitor yourself carefully for any signs of toxic shock syndrome.

Danger Signals Associated With Possible Toxic Shock Syndrome

Fever (temperature higher than 100°F)
Diarrhea
Vomiting
Muscle ache
Rash (sunburn-like)

Contact us at ( ) _____ if you develop any of the above problems (and do not use your diaphragm—remove at once)

If your diaphragm slips out of place or comes out, you can call 1-888-NOT-2-LATE for information about emergency contraception. Websites: http://not-2-late.com; http://www.go2planB.com

EC Plan B is available over the counter (no prescription) at pharmacies if you are 18 years old or older.

(May also be used as informational handout)

I. DEFINITION/MECHANISM OF ACTION

An IUD consists of a sterile body placed in the uterus to prevent fertilization. This is accomplished through several mechanisms of action, depending on the type of device:

    A. A local sterile inflammatory response to the foreign body (the IUD) causes a change in the cellular makeup of the uterine lining

    B. A possible increase in the local production of prostaglandins may increase endometrial activity

    C. Alteration in uterine and tubal transport of egg

    D. Change in cervical mucus causing barrier to sperm penetration

    E. Mirena may stop release of an egg but this is not the primary way it works

II. BENEFITS OF THE METHOD

    A. Encourages sexual spontaneity

    B. Effectiveness rate, theoretically, 97% to 99%

    C. Semipermanent (depending on the type of device); replacement time varies, but all devices are effective for at least 5 years; one device lasts for 10 years

III. RISKS OF METHOD

    A. Major risks

        1. Involuntary expulsion (approximately 6%)

        2. Pelvic inflammatory disease

        3. Ectopic pregnancy (outside of the uterus)

        4. Uterine perforation

        5. Pregnancy

    B. Minor risks

        1. Increased menstrual flow

        2. Increased dysmenorrhea (cramps)

        3. String may cause some discomfort to partner

IV. REASONS FOR NOT USING AN IUD

    A. Active pelvic infection (acute or subacute), including known or suspected gonorrhea or *Chlamydia*

    B. Known or suspected pregnancy

    C. Recent or recurrent pelvic infection

    D. Purulent cervicitis, untreated acute cervicitis, or vaginosis

    E. Undiagnosed genital bleeding

    F. Uterine cavity not suitable for IUD insertion

    G. History of ectopic pregnancy (pregnancy outside uterus)

    H. Diabetes mellitus can use ParaGard IUD

I. Allergy to copper (known or suspected) or diagnosed Wilson's Disease; can use Mirena IUD
J. Abnormal Pap test result; cervical or uterine cancer, precancer
K. Impaired response to infection (diabetes, steroid treatment, immunocompromised patients such as those with HIV/AIDS)
L. Previously inserted IUD
M. Genital actinomycosis; chronic infection of genital area

V. REASONS IUD MAY NOT BE THE BEST CHOICE OR REQUIRE CAREFUL MONITORING WITH CLINICIAN

A. Multiple sexual partners or partner has multiple partners
B. In very rural areas, emergency treatment difficult to obtain
C. Cervical opening resistant to inserting IUD
D. Impaired blood clotting response
E. Uterine cavity too small, too large
F. Endometriosis
G. Fibroids in uterus
H. Polyps in uterine lining (endometrium)
I. Severe dysmenorrhea (Mirena IUD may help)
J. Heavy or prolonged menstrual bleeding without anemia; consider oral iron or nutritional changes to prevent anemia
K. Unable to check for IUD string
L. Concerns for future fertility
M. Postpartum or infected abortion within the past 3 months
N. History of pelvic uterine infection
O. Valvular heart disease infection

VI. ALTERNATIVES

A. Abstinence
B. Sterilization
C. Birth control pills
D. FemCap, Lea's Shield, contraceptive sponge
E. Natural family planning
F. Depo-Provera
G. Female condom
H. Contraceptive ring, patch, implant
I. Diaphragm and spermicidal cream or jelly, film, sponge
J. Condom used with contraceptive cream, foam, suppositories, gel, or vaginal film

VII. EXPLANATION OF THE METHOD

A. How the IUD may work (no one is quite sure), but there are several theories:
   1. Motility of the egg in fallopian tube is altered
   2. A sterile inflammatory response to the IUD causes a change in the cells of the uterine lining
   3. A change in the cervical mucus causing a barrier to sperm

B. What you should know about caring for your IUD
  1. Know the type of device you have in place
  2. Know when your device should be replaced
  3. Learn how to check the string that extends from the center of the cervix into the vaginal canal
  4. Check the string frequently the first few months and then after each period
  5. Do not let your partner pull on the string
  6. Never try to remove IUD yourself
  7. Return for your 6-week checkup after insertion of the device
  8. Get a checkup every year, including a Pap smear
  9. Depending on your normal menstrual cycle, if you miss a period, consult your clinician for possible pregnancy
C. What to expect
  1. Possible increase in menstrual flow, menstrual cramping

Remember: If this condition becomes intolerable, you have the option of having your IUD removed by a clinician.

D. Side effects to be reported *immediately*
  1. Late period or absence of period
  2. Abdominal or pelvic pain (severe)
  3. Elevated temperature, chills (not caused by illness)
  4. Unpleasant vaginal discharge (smelly, foul, bloody, or greenish color)
  5. Unusual vaginal bleeding (heavy period, clotting)
E. Insertion
  1. IUDs are usually inserted within 7 days of menses
  2. Should have negative gonococcus and *Chlamydia* cultures prior to insertion (within 30 days); consider culture for Group B *Streptococcus*
  3. Must have recent (within the year) normal Pap smear
  4. May have some discomfort and dizziness with insertion
  5. May have spotting for several months after insertion
  6. Although the IUD is effective immediately, it is recommended that intercourse not take place for 24 hours

VIII. INQUIRIES ARE ENCOURAGED—ASK US QUESTIONS AT ANY TIME

I have read the above material; it has been explained fully. I have been given the opportunity to ask questions and I understand the information. I have chosen to use the IUD _____ type.

Signed _____   Witness _____
Date   _____

Danger Signals Associated With the Use of the IUD

Late period or absence of period
Abdominal pain (severe)
Elevated temperature, chills (not caused by illness; e.g., flu)
Unpleasant vaginal discharge (smelly, foul, bloody, or greenish color)
Unusual vaginal bleeding (heavy period, clotting)
    Contact us or a clinician immediately if the danger signs develop.

I. DEFINITION

EC, often known as the morning after pill, is the use of birth control pills to prevent pregnancy after a contraceptive method has failed or because there was no contraception. Currently, in the United States, there is one product available just for EC—Plan B.

II. HOW IT WORKS

If used within the first 120 hours after unprotected sexual intercourse, EC probably works because of one or more of the following reasons:

    A. Progestational hormones in Plan B pills interfere with the sperm's ability to travel up through the uterus and into the fallopian tube to fertilize the egg; also, they affect the growth of the ovary's follicles

    B. Combination hormones are thought to interfere with or disrupt ovulation (release of an egg by the ovary).

III. HOW EFFECTIVE IS IT?

If used within the first 72 hours after sex without birth control protection, EC is greater than 90% effective. EC literature says that EC may be used up to 120 hours after unprotected sex; however, the earlier the pills are taken, the more effective they will be.

IV. BENEFITS

    A. Pregnancy prevention
    B. Inexpensive
    C. Relatively noninvasive

V. DISADVANTAGES

    A. May not be appropriate for women with certain medical conditions
    B. Pregnancy may occur because of the following:
        1. Fertilized egg already implanted in the uterus
        2. Too much time between unprotected sex and taking EC
        3. Failure of the emergency contraception
        4. Must be used within 72 or at most 120 hours of unprotected sex

VI. RISKS AND SIDE EFFECTS

    A. Nausea and/or vomiting
    B. Breast tenderness
    C. Irregular bleeding
    D. Headache

VII. YOU MAY NOT BE ABLE TO TAKE COMBINATION BIRTH CONTROL PILLS SUCH AS EC IF YOU HAVE:

    A. An active liver disease
    B. Unexplained bleeding from the vagina

C. An already established pregnancy
D. History of blood clots, inflammation in the veins, or cancer of the breast, uterus, or ovaries

VIII. ALTERNATIVE EC
A. Progestin-only OCs used as EC
B. Insertion of an IUD

IX. HOW EC IS PRESCRIBED
A. Pelvic examination as appropriate (to be determined by you and your clinician)
B. If rape or sexual assault occurred, specimens can be collected if desired by you and your clinician
C. Pregnancy test
D. Testing for STDs if desired or if recommended by clinician
E. Blood pressure

X. WAYS IN WHICH EC IS TAKEN
A. Take one Plan B pill within 72 to 120 hours of unprotected intercourse and follow directions from D to F. Take second pill 12 hours later or you can take both pills at the same time. (EC is indicated in the packet for up to 120 hours; however, the earlier you take it, the greater the efficacy.)
B. Take _____ birth control pills within 72 to 120 hours of unprotected intercourse. Do not take the pills on an empty stomach: eat a snack such as juice or milk and crackers and take the pills 20 minutes later. Take _____ birth control pills 12 hours after the first dose.
C. If you vomit within an hour after taking the birth control pills, follow the instructions your clinician gives you
D. Talk with your clinician about methods of contraception you might be interested in for ongoing protection. EC is just for emergencies and is not recommended for routine use. Some birth control methods can be started immediately or the day after using EC. Methods vary in how soon they become effective.
E. Report any of the warning signs listed subsequently to your clinician at once
F. After using EC, return to your clinician as directed for a checkup, particularly if you have not had a normal menstrual period

Note: Plan B is now available over the counter if you are 18 years old or older. Check with your pharmacy.

I have read the above material. I have been given the opportunity to ask questions and I fully understand the information. I have chosen to use emergency contraception.

Signed   _____   Date _____
Witness _____   Date _____

Danger Signals Associated With EC

Abdominal pain (severe)
Chest pain (severe), arm pain, or shortness of breath
Eye problems such as blurred or double vision, loss of vision
Headaches (severe)
Severe leg pain (calf or thigh)

Contact us at ( ) _____ if you develop any of the above danger signals.
Emergency contraception hotline: 1-800-584-9911, 1-888-NOT-2-LATE; websites: http://not-2-late.com; http://www.go2planB.com
Copyright Hawkins, J. W., Roberto-Nichols, D. M., & Stanley-Haney, J. L. (2012). *Guidelines for nurse practitioners in gynecologic settings* (10th ed.). New York, NY: Springer Publishing Company.

NOTE

1. Boxed warning from the U.S. Food and Drug Administration (FDA): Prolonged use of medroxyprogesterone contraceptive injection may result in a loss of bone mineral density (BMD). Loss is related to the duration of use and may not be completely reversible on discontinuation of the drug. The impact on peak bone mass in adolescents should be considered in treatment decisions. U.S. boxed warning: Long-term use (i.e., more than 2 years) should be limited to situations where other birth control methods are inadequate. Consider other methods of birth control in women with (or at risk for) osteoporosis.
Websites: http://www.drugs.com/pro/depo-provera.html; http://www.fda.gov/bbs/topics/ANSWERS/2004/ANS01325.html

Consent Form for Antidepressants

Your physician or nurse practitioner has prescribed an antidepressant medication. It is most important that you carefully follow the directions provided by your physician. Antidepressants are safe and helpful medications when taken correctly. When you start your prescription, you may exhibit some mild side effects. These may differ with medications and will be discussed on an individual basis with you by your provider.

To ensure that you are progressing well on the prescribed medication, you will be required to return to the office for medication monitoring. Your provider will decide on the timing of the visits.

INITIAL MEDICATION CHECK WILL BE IN _____ WEEKS. FOLLOW-UP MEDICATION CHECK WILL BE DECIDED DEPENDING ON YOUR RESPONSE TO THE MEDICATION(S). THIS WILL NEVER BE LESS THAN EVERY 6 MONTHS.

All patients on ongoing antidepressant medications will be required to return at 6-month intervals.

You must keep this appointment or reschedule in a timely fashion. If you do not keep your follow-up appointment, your prescription will not be refilled.

PLEASE BE ADVISED: ABRUPT DISCONTINUATION OF AN ANTIDE-PRESSANT MEDICATION MAY LEAD TO UNPLEASANT (ALTHOUGH NOT DANGEROUS) SIDE EFFECTS. THESE SYMPTOMS INCLUDE THE FOLLOWING: DIZZINESS, ANXIETY, IRRITABILITY, DECREASED CONCENTRATION, MOOD CHANGES, INSOMNIA, PANIC ATTACKS, NAUSEA, INTESTINAL CRAMPING, AND VOMITING.

I have read and understood that I will be expected to comply with the above policy.

Signature of Patient _____

Date: _____   Provider: _____

Signature: _____

B

APPENDIX
Abuse Assessment Screen

ABUSE ASSESSMENT SCREEN

1. Have you **EVER** been emotionally or physically abused by your partner or someone important to you? YES/NO
2. **WITHIN THE LAST YEAR,** have you been hit, slapped, kicked, or otherwise physically hurt by someone? YES/NO
   If YES, by whom? _____
   Total number of times: _____
3. **SINCE YOU HAVE BEEN PREGNANT,** have you been hit, slapped, kicked, or otherwise physically hurt by someone? YES/NO
   If YES, by whom? _____
   Total number of times: _____
   Mark the areas of injury on a body map (Figure B.1)
   Score each incident according to the following scale
   > 1 = Threats of abuse, including use of a weapon
   > 2 = Slapping, pushing; no injuries, and/or lasting pain
   > 3 = Punching, kicking, bruises, cuts, and/or continuing pain
   > 4 = Beating up, severe contusions, burns, broken bones
   > 5 = Head injury, internal injury, permanent injury
   > 6 = Use of weapon; wound from weapon

   If any of the descriptions for the higher number apply, use the higher number.
4. **WITHIN THE LAST YEAR,** has anyone forced you to have sexual activities? YES/NO
   If YES, by whom? _____
   Total number of times: _____
5. **ARE YOU AFRAID** of your partner or anyone in your life? YES/NO

Developed by the Nursing Research Consortium on Violence and Abuse. Readers are encouraged to reproduce and use this assessment tool. Adapted by Pregnancy Support Project, Boston College, William F. Connell School of Nursing. Spanish translation available in *Violence Against Women*, July 2003, pp. 859–878.

Website for this and other screening tools: http://www.nnvawi.org/page .cfm/assessment-tools

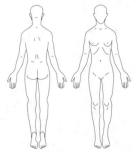

FIGURE B.1. Body map.

C

APPENDIX
Danger Assessment

DANGER ASSESSMENT

Several risk factors have been associated with increased risk of homicides (murders) of women and men in violent relationships. We cannot predict what will happen in your case, but we would like you to be aware of the danger of homicide in situations of abuse and for you to see how many of the risk factors apply to your situation.

Using the calendar, please mark the approximate dates during the past year when you were abused by your partner or ex-partner. Write on that date how bad the incident was according to the following scale:

1 = Slapping, pushing; no injuries and/or lasting pain
2 = Punching, kicking; bruises, cuts, and/or continuing pain
3 = "Beating up"; severe contusions, burns, broken bones
4 = Threat to use weapon; head injury, internal injury, permanent injury, miscarriage, choking
5 = Use of weapon; wounds from weapon

(If **any** of the descriptions for the higher number apply, use the higher number.)

Mark **Yes** or **No** for each of the following:

("He" refers to your husband, partner, ex-husband, ex-partner, or whoever is currently physically hurting you.)

Yes   No

1. Has the physical violence increased in severity or frequency over the past year?
2. Does he own a gun?
3. Have you left him after living together during the past year?
    3.a.   (If have *never* lived with him, check here: _____)
4. Is he unemployed?
5. Has he ever used a weapon against you or threatened you with a lethal weapon?
    5.a.   (If yes, was the weapon a gun? _____)
6. Does he threaten to kill you?
7. Has he avoided being arrested for domestic violence?
8. Do you have a child that is not his?
9. Has he ever forced you to have sex when you did not wish to do so?
10. Does he ever try to choke you?
11. Does he use illegal drugs? By drugs, I mean "uppers" or amphetamines, speed, angel dust, cocaine, "crack," street drugs, or mixtures.
12. Is he an alcoholic or problem drinker?
13. Does he control most or all of your daily activities? (For instance, does he tell you who you can be friends with, when you can see your family, how much money you can use, or when you can take the car?) (If he tries, but you do not let him, check here: _____)

14. Is he violently and constantly jealous of you?
    (For instance, does he say "If I can't have you, no one can"?)
15. Have you ever been beaten by him while you were pregnant?
    (If you have never been pregnant by him, check here: _____)
16. Has he ever threatened or tried to commit suicide?
17. Does he threaten to harm your children?
18. Do you believe he is capable of killing you?
19. Does he follow or spy on you, leave threatening notes or messages on answering machine, destroy your property, or call you when you don't want him to?
20. Have you ever threatened or tried to commit suicide?

Total "Yes" Answers

Thank you. Please talk to your nurse, advocate, or counselor about what the Danger Assessment means in terms of your situation.

D

APPENDIX
Self-Assessment of HIV Risk

SELF-ASSESSMENT OF HIV RISK

1. Do you use injectable drugs? Does your sexual partner(s)? Do you or your partner(s) have a partner(s) who uses injectable drugs? How about in the past?
2. If you or your partner(s) use injectable drugs, do you ever share needles/syringes or works such as cooker, swabs, cotton, or barrel? How about in the past? Have you ever used intranasal drugs (snorted)?
3. Did you or your partner(s) have a blood transfusion between 1975 and 1985 or have sexual exposure to partners who did? Have you shared needles or syringes with these same partners?
4. Do you have or have you had a hemophiliac partner(s) who received blood or blood products between 1975 and 1985?
5. Do you or your partner(s) use latex condoms/female condoms whenever you have vaginal or anal sex?
6. Do you use whips or knives or anything that would break the skin during sex?
7. Do you have oral/anal sex?
8. Do you actively use fisting or fingering in sex?
9. Do you ever let your partner(s) ejaculate (cum) in your mouth? Do you ever have oral sex with a female partner during menses?
10. Have you ever had unprotected sex with a man who has had sex with another man?
11. Do you ever share sex toys (such as a vibrator)?
12. If you are a clinician, have you ever experienced a needle stick, exposure to a patient's blood, or exposure to amniotic fluid on your unprotected hands or face?
13. Are you and your partner mutually monogamous? How long have you been?
14. Have you ever traded sex for money, shelter, food, or drugs?
15. Have you ever had unwanted or forced (nonconsensual) sex?
16. How many sexual partners have you had in the past 12 months?
17. How many sexual partners in your whole life?
18. Have you ever exchanged money for sex in the past 12 months?
19. Have you ever had sex with somebody you did not know about at the time (casual sex)?
20. How often do you use drugs?
21. How often do you use alcohol?
22. Have you ever been tested for HIV?
23. Have you ever had a tattoo?
24. Have you ever had a piercing on your body?
25. Have you ever had a sexually transmitted infection (STI) such as gonorrhea, syphilis, *Chlamydia*, trichomonas, HPV or genital warts, herpes, and so forth?
26. Have you ever had hepatitis?
27. Have you ever had sex with someone who is HIV positive?

If your answer to any of the Yes/No questions except 5 and 10 is yes, you may be at risk and might consider being tested.

Assessment tool courtesy of Richard S. Ferri, PhD, ANP, ACRN; and updated by Rosanna DeMarco, PhD, PHCNS-BC, ACRN, FAAN, associate professor of Public Community Health, William F. Connell School of Nursing, and affiliate faculty of African and African Diaspora Studies, College of Arts and Sciences, Boston College.

E

APPENDIX
Women and Heart Disease:
Risk Factor Assessment

WOMEN AND HEART DISEASE: RISK FACTOR ASSESSMENT

I. NONMODIFIABLE

A. Age: leading cause of death in women older than 40 years old; risks increase after menopause

B. Race or ethnicity: Black women have a higher rate of death than White women; 5-year survival rate is lower, and Black women younger than 55 years old have greater than 2 times the death rate of White women. Rates of diabetes and hypertension in Black women are higher than those in White women.

C. Family history of the disease, especially heart attack at age younger than 50 years old

D. Gender: attenuating advantage of being a woman, especially pre-menopausally (premenopausally, women's risk is lower than men's)

E. Socioeconomic status: inverse association with morbidity and mortality

II. MODIFIABLE

A. Lifestyle

1. Exercise: Aerobic exercise can increase high-density lipopro-teins (HDLs; e.g., brisk walking, jogging) >30 minutes daily or most days; sedentary life increases risk for heart disease almost twofold

2. Chronic diseases: diabetes increases risk to 57.3% by age 75 years old compared to 16.3% risk without diabetes; obesity—risk with BMI >25 kg/m² and risk escalates >30; blood pressure ideal <120/80; interventions with ≥140/90 or 130/80 in women with diabetes or chronic kidney disease

3. Nutrition: dyslipidemia elevated low-density lipoprotein (LDL)-cholesterol, elevated triglycerides, low HDL cholesterol (HDL-C); high- versus low-fat diet; <20% of all calories from fat; <2.4 g/day of sodium and maintain BMI between 18.5 and 24.9 kg/m², modifying effects of antioxidants (vegetables/fruits, five to nine servings/day; whole grain foods, six servings/day; dietary fiber, 25 g/day; oily fish twice a week; alcohol, one serving/day; sodium, <2.3 g/day; saturated fats, <7% of calories)

4. Cigarette smoking

   a. Smoking and oral contraceptive (OC) use (combination hormonal contraception) increases rate of atherosclerosis

   b. Women (younger than 40 years old) who have myocardial infarction (MI) are mainly smokers

   c. Older women who smoke have a 50% greater chance to experience sudden death than older nonsmokers

   d. Acts synergistically with hyperlipidemia

   e. Women with hypertension using hormonal contraception with estrogen or estrogen therapy postmenopausally increase risk 10 to 15 fold

B. Internal and external environmental factors
   1. Comorbidities: hypertension, diabetes, obesity; poor management of these chronic diseases increases risk while good management decreases risk. Blood pressure maintain at <120/80.
   2. Psychosocial concerns: stress and social support; high stress and low social support increase morbidity and mortality. Lower level employees (such as clerks, cashiers) have two times the likelihood of heart disease than do women in white collar jobs.
   3. Access to health care: Unequal access appears to be a factor in morbidity and mortality

Websites: http://www.americanheart.org/presenter.jhtml?identifier=4786; http://www.whi.org/; http://www.nih.gov/news/health/feb2010/nhlbi-15.htm

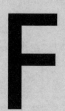

APPENDIX
Complementary and
Alternative Medicine

Complementary and alternative medicine (CAM)[1] therapies are diverse group of medicines, devices, providers of care, and health care systems not generally considered part of the mainstream conventional medicine, defined in the United States as allopathic or Western medicine, as practiced by those whose designation is medical doctor (MD) or doctor of osteopathy (DO) and other licensed and/or credentialed health care professionals, including nurse practitioners, nurse midwives, nurses, physical therapists, occupational therapists, speech and language therapists, psychologists, mental health therapists, and psychiatric social workers. The two categories are not mutually exclusive as a patient might, for example, be seeing a massage therapist or chiropractor as well as an orthopedic medical doctor. This is an example of complementary medicine. Another term is *mind–body medicine*, comprised of practices and therapies that focus on interactions among the brain, mind, body, and behavior. Some examples of CAM and of mind–body medicine include the following:

1. Acupuncture: stimulation of specific points on the body using various techniques such as penetrating the skin with needles or using electrical stimulation
2. Acupressure: stimulation of specific points on the body using external pressure only without penetrating the skin
3. Naturopathic medicine: a branch of the healing sciences focusing on enhancing the body's ability to heal itself. Naturopathic physicians are licensed in some of the United States. Their education for the first 6 years is identical to that of allopathic physicians, and the last 2 years focus on healing strategies for the body and use of a pharmacopia of supplements, herbs, and other natural botanicals and biologicals.
4. Chinese medicine: Traditional Chinese medicine includes the use of Chinese herbs, acupuncture, meditation, Chinese massage therapy, nutritional therapy, and mental and physical disciplines such as Tai Chi and Qigong.
5. Chiropractic medicine: manipulation of the spine and other joints to achieve relief of pain, spasms, pressure on nerves and to align the body parts
6. Homeopathic medicine: Homeopathic remedies are generally based on natural ingredients. Homeopathy works in harmony with the body's immune system. Homeopathy is holistic, treating all the symptoms as one, which in practical terms means that it addresses the cause, not the symptoms.
7. Osteopathic medicine: osteopathic physicians practice the entire scope of modern medicine, bringing a patient-centered, holistic, hands-on approach to diagnosing and treating illness and injury. These physicians can choose any specialty, prescribe drugs, perform surgeries, administer anesthesia, and practice medicine anywhere in the United States. They often use manipulative techniques to diagnose and treat patients and focus on health education, injury prevention, and disease prevention.

8. Herbal medicine: dietary supplements that come from plants and other botanical sources and are supplied in liquid or powdered forms as tablets, teas, capsules, extracts and dried or fresh plants

9. Dietary supplements: vitamins, minerals, herbs and other botanicals, amino acids, enzymes, organ tissues, glandulars, and metabolites. These come as tablets, liquids, softgels, capsules, powders, and other forms such as a bar.[2]

10. Meditation: specific postures, focused attention, music, and/or an open attitude toward distractions; increases calmness, relaxation, and enhances overall health and feelings of well-being. There are many practices of meditation each with its own rituals and benefits.

11. Yoga: various styles combining physical postures, breathing techniques, meditation, and/or relaxation.

12. Ayurvedic medicine: A whole medical system that originated in India. It aims to integrate the body, mind, and spirit to prevent and treat disease. Therapies used include herbs, massage, and yoga.

13. Massage therapy: The massage therapist presses, rubs, and otherwise manipulates muscles and other soft tissues of the body and may use heat or cold to complement the therapy.

14. Movement therapy: Feldenkrais method, Alexander technique, Pilates, and Trager psychophysical integration

15. Magnet therapy: use of static magnetic fields

16. Electromagnetic therapy: use of electromagnetic energy, including electricity, microwaves, radio waves, infrared rays, and electrically generated magnetic fields to diagnose or treat disease

17. Light therapy: a way to treat seasonal affective disorder (SAD) by exposure to artificial light. Using a light therapy box may also help with other types of depression, sleep disorders, and some other conditions. Light therapy is also known as bright light therapy or phototherapy.

18. Qigong: various Chinese systems of physical and mental training for health, martial arts, and self-enlightenment.

19. Reiki: a Japanese technique for stress reduction and relaxation that also promotes healing. The Reiki practitioner lays hands on the patient. Reiki is based on the idea that a life force energy flows through each person and causes that person to be alive.

20. Healing touch: a form of energy healing in which the practitioner lays hands on the patient. Proponents believe that gentle healing touch helps the recipient to achieve physical, mental, emotional, and spiritual well-being.

NOTES

1. See National Center for Complementary and Alternative Medicine (NCCAM) at hccam.nih.gov

2. http.//www.fda.gov/food/dietarysupplements/consumerinformation/ucm110417.htm

G

APPENDIX
Constipation

CONSTIPATION

Constipation is a common problem for women, especially as they age. It can be related to a number of factors. First, though, it is important to clarify what is meant by the term. Irregularity is another related term—it implies that there is some standard of regularity. Although many of us have been taught that daily bowel elimination (having at least one bowel movement [BM] daily) is normal, for many persons, normal is every 2 or 3 days. Beyond that time frame, the feces become harder and thus more difficult to pass.

Constipation occurs when one's regular pattern (whatever is normal for that person) changes; so when the time between BMs lengthens, pain and/or straining are associated with them and/or the BMs are very hard. Sometimes, bleeding occurs because the fecal material (the stool) is hard, and the person has to strain so much that there is damage to the rectum (lowest part of the bowel) or to the opening of the intestinal track (called the *anal opening*). There are other causes of bleeding, too; so if you ever have bleeding with a BM, you should not ignore it.

Some causes of constipation are:

> *Stress* can cause spastic constipation, meaning tightening or spasm of the muscles in the large intestine; stress can also mean not taking time to eat properly, drink enough fluids, and/or go to the bathroom when your body signals you.
>
> *Diet.* More about this later, but lack of roughage or fiber in the diet can cause constipation, as can lack of sufficient fluids, notably water.
>
> *Lack of exercise.* Having no active exercise on a regular basis can cause constipation.
>
> *Medications* such as diuretics (water pills), iron pills, calcium pills, and laxatives can cause constipation in some people, so pay attention to your body and to changes in your BMs when taking any medication. So can narcotic pain medications, antidepressants, anticonvulsants, iron supplements, calcium channel blocking drugs, and antacids containing aluminum.
>
> *Hormones.* Too little thyroid hormone, too much parathyroid hormone, and the hormones that women's bodies produce at the time of menstrual periods and during pregnancy (estrogen and progesterone) also contribute.
>
> *Diseases.* Many diseases contribute to constipation. These include diabetes, multiple sclerosis, and Parkinson's disease.
>
> *Symptoms.* Some diseases have constipation as a symptom, so be sure to tell your clinician if you continue to be constipated after trying the suggestions here.

What You Can Do About Constipation

1. Eat right. Select foods from those in the table below, including lots of roughage or fiber in each day's diet. You can also add coarse bran to a bowl of cereal or to other foods.

2. Time. Take time when your body signals you; do not put off bowel evacuations.
3. Fluids. Fluid intake is very important to your general good health and especially for good bowel and bladder and kidney health. Six to eight glasses of water a day are recommended to prepare fecal material at the proper consistency for bowel elimination. In addition to water, add fruit juices, coffee, tea, and soda; the latter three can be irritating to your bladder or stomach or both (if caffeinated), so try to keep amounts limited and do not substitute these for water. An easy rule of thumb is that we should drink our weight in water; for example, if you weigh 125 lbs, you should drink 125 oz of water daily, as well as other fluids such as juices, teas, coffees, and so on.
4. Exercise. Regular exercise (4–7 times a week) is important to general good health and also helps us to keep our regular (usual for us) bowel evacuation schedule. Walking, running, bicycling, swimming, working out, doing an active work routine (walking a lot, lifting and moving things), dancing, skating, playing sports such as tennis, soccer, touch football, basketball, volleyball, handball, and racquetball all help keep our bodies and their functions in shape.
5. Flavored or unflavored Metamucil or store brand psyllium hydrophilic mucilloid fiber is useful if diet, exercise, and fluids do not work for you. Mix a tablespoon in 8 or more ounces of water. Metamucil also comes in wafers (cookies) in several flavors. You can also try over-the-counter stool softeners such as Dialose, Kasof, and Colace.

TABLE G.1.   Preventing Constipation; Promoting Intestinal Health

Food Group	Foods to Emphasize	Servings per Day
Breads, cereals, grains	Whole grain and multigrain breads, whole grains, bran cereals, rice, wheat germ, whole wheat pasta, popcorn, oats, rice cakes, corn cakes, granola, wheat bran	3–4 servings 1 cup or more
Fruits, fruit juices	Dates, raisins, figs, apples, berries, melons, whole oranges, pears	3 or more fresh fruits
Vegetables	Broccoli, cauliflower, peas, green and wax beans, Brussels sprout, lettuce, spinach, cabbage, celery, asparagus, artichokes, carrots, squash, turnips	3 or more, some raw vegetables
Miscellaneous	Legumes (dried peas, kidney beans, navy beans)	Varies with diet
Seeds, nuts	Various seeds and nuts (not tropical)	Some each day

Follow directions carefully on how to use; it is best to discuss with your clinician before using any of these products. Stool softeners and sources of fiber are not harmful or habit forming, but you should try diet, fluids, and exercise first.

6. Laxatives. Laxatives, enemas, and drugs that cause you to evacuate your bowels can be harmful in the long run. It should be used only after consulting a health care provider to rule out bowel disease as the cause of the constipation and after trying the measures discussed here.

Websites:http://www.medicinenet.com/constipation/page2.htm;http://www.webmd. com/digestive-disorders/digestive-diseases-constipation; http://www.mayoclinic.com/ health/constipation/DS00063/DSECTION=causes

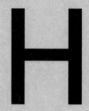

APPENDIX
Body Mass Index Table

BODY MASS INDEX TABLE

BMI	Normal						Overweight					Obese					
	19	20	21	22	23	24	25	26	27	28	29	30	31	32	33	34	35
Height (inches)	Body Weight (pounds)																
58	91	96	100	105	110	115	119	124	129	134	138	143	148	153	158	162	167
59	94	99	104	109	114	119	124	128	133	138	143	148	153	158	163	168	173
60	97	102	107	112	118	123	128	133	138	143	148	153	158	163	168	174	179
61	100	106	111	116	122	127	132	137	143	148	153	158	164	169	174	180	185
62	104	109	115	120	126	131	136	142	147	153	158	164	169	175	180	186	191
63	107	113	118	124	130	135	141	146	152	158	163	169	175	180	186	191	197
64	110	116	122	128	134	140	145	151	157	163	169	174	180	186	192	197	204
65	114	120	126	132	138	144	150	156	162	168	174	180	186	192	198	204	210
66	118	124	130	136	142	148	155	161	167	173	179	186	192	198	204	210	216
67	121	127	134	140	146	153	159	166	172	178	185	191	198	204	211	217	223
68	125	131	138	144	151	158	164	171	177	184	190	197	203	210	216	223	230
69	128	135	142	149	155	162	169	176	182	189	196	203	209	216	223	230	236
70	132	139	146	153	160	167	174	181	188	195	202	209	216	222	229	236	243
71	136	143	150	157	165	172	179	186	193	200	208	215	222	229	236	243	250
72	140	147	154	162	169	177	184	191	199	206	213	221	228	235	242	250	258
73	144	151	159	166	174	182	189	197	204	212	219	227	235	242	250	257	265
74	148	155	163	171	179	186	194	202	210	218	225	233	241	249	256	264	272
75	152	160	168	176	184	192	200	208	216	224	232	240	248	256	264	272	279
76	156	164	172	180	189	197	205	213	221	230	238	246	254	263	271	279	287

BODY MASS INDEX TABLE

	Obese				Extreme Obesity														
BMI	36	37	38	39	40	41	42	43	44	45	46	47	48	49	50	51	52	53	54
Height (inches)					Body Weight (pounds)														
58	172	177	181	186	191	196	201	205	210	215	220	224	229	234	239	244	248	253	258
59	178	183	188	193	198	203	208	212	217	222	227	232	237	242	247	252	257	262	267
60	184	189	194	199	204	209	215	220	225	230	235	240	245	250	255	261	266	271	276
61	190	195	201	206	211	217	222	227	232	238	243	248	254	259	264	269	275	280	285
62	196	202	207	213	218	224	229	235	240	246	251	256	262	267	273	278	284	289	295
63	203	208	214	220	225	231	237	242	248	254	259	265	270	278	282	287	293	299	304
64	209	215	221	227	232	238	244	250	256	262	267	273	279	285	291	296	302	308	314
65	216	222	228	234	240	246	252	258	264	270	276	282	288	294	300	306	312	318	324
66	223	230	235	241	247	253	260	266	272	278	284	291	297	303	309	315	322	328	334
67	230	236	242	249	255	261	268	274	280	287	293	299	306	312	319	325	331	338	344
68	236	243	249	256	262	269	276	282	289	295	302	308	315	322	328	335	341	348	354
69	243	250	257	263	270	277	284	291	297	304	311	318	324	331	338	345	351	358	365
70	250	257	264	271	278	285	292	299	306	313	320	327	334	341	348	355	362	369	376
71	257	265	272	279	286	293	301	308	315	322	329	338	343	351	358	365	372	379	386
72	265	272	279	287	294	302	309	316	324	331	338	346	353	361	368	375	383	390	397
73	272	280	288	295	302	310	318	325	333	340	348	355	363	371	378	386	393	401	408
74	280	287	295	303	311	319	326	334	342	350	358	365	373	381	389	396	404	412	420
75	287	295	303	311	319	327	335	343	351	359	367	375	383	391	399	407	415	423	431
76	295	304	312	320	328	336	344	353	361	369	377	385	394	402	410	418	426	435	443

Source: Adapted from Clinical Guidelines on the Identification, Evaluation, and Treatment of Overweight and Obesity in Adults. The Evidence Report.

APPENDIX
"For Your Information":
Patient Education Handouts

I. DEFINITION

Overgrowth of various anaerobic bacteria, genital mycoplasmas, and/or *Gardnerella vaginalis*

II. TRANSMISSION

The condition is considered sexually associated rather than sexually transmitted, and it may also be identified in the nonsexually active female

III. SIGNS AND SYMPTOMS

  A. In the female
    1. Fishy, musty odor with a thin, milky white to dark or dull gray watery vaginal discharge
    2. Discharge may cause vaginal and vulvar itching and burning
    3. Burning and swelling of genitals after intercourse
    4. No symptoms in some women
  B. In the male: No male version of bacterial vaginosis (BV) has been identified

IV. DIAGNOSIS

  A. Female evaluation may include
    1. Vaginal examination to check for BV
    2. Further laboratory work to rule out *Candida, Trichomonas,* gonococcus, or *Chlamydia*
    3. Blood test for syphilis
  B. Male evaluation: Rule out other infections such as *Trichomonas,* gonococcus, or *Chlamydia*

V. TREATMENT

  A. Treatment may be by mouth or with a vaginal cream or gel
  B. Treatment of partners is not recommended because studies have not shown that their treatment decreases the number of recurrences unless partner is a woman also
  C. It is very important to report any medical conditions you may have or medications you take regularly (especially for a seizure disorder) before taking any treatment
  D. If treated with vaginal cream (clindamycin, brand name Cleocin), the mineral oil in the medication may weaken latex or rubber products such as condoms and vaginal diaphragms for 5 days after use

VI. PATIENT EDUCATION

  A. Sexual partners should be alerted to the diagnosis and referred for evaluation and possible treatment if the patient has other concurrent infections
  B. Sexual partners should be protected by condoms until patient's treatment is over. Check with your clinician if you use condoms or a vaginal diaphragm as per section *Treatment,* *V.D.*

C. Alcoholic beverages should not be consumed during or for 48 hours after oral treatment
D. Minor side effects of oral treatment may include nausea, dizziness, and a metallic taste
E. No douching with or after treatment; douching is never recommended

VII. FOLLOW-UP
Return to clinician for a reevaluation if symptoms persist or new symptoms occur

Special notes: _____

Clinician: _____

For more information call Centers for Disease Control and Prevention (CDC) Sexually Transmitted Disease (STD) hotline: 1-800-CDC-INFO: Phone numbers of free (or almost free) STD clinics are listed in the Community Service Numbers in the government pages of your local phone book.
Website: http://www.cdc.gov/std/phq.htm

Candidiasis (Monilia)
Yeast Infection

I. DEFINITION
Candidiasis, or monilia, is a yeastlike overgrowth of a fungus called *Candida albicans* (may also be caused by *Candida tropicalis* or *Candida torulopsis glabrata* and rarely by other *Candida* species). *Candida* can be found in small amounts in the normal vagina, but under some conditions, it gets out of balance with the other vaginal flora and produces symptoms.

II. TRANSMISSION
    A. Usually nonsexual
    B. Some common causes of *Candida* overgrowth are the use of hormonal contraceptives such as birth control pills, patches, rings, implants; antibiotics; diabetes; pregnancy; stress; deodorant tampons and other scented and deodorant menstrual products; use of vaginal deodorant sprays, and perfumed toilet tissue

III. SIGNS AND SYMPTOMS
    A. In the female
        1. Vaginal discharge: thick, white, and curdlike
        2. Vaginal area itch and irritation with occasional swelling and redness
        3. Possibly itching, burning, and swelling around and outside the vaginal opening
        4. Burning on urination
        5. Possibly, pain with intercourse
    B. In the male
        1. Itch and/or irritation of penis
        2. Cheesy material under foreskin, underside of penis
        3. Jock itch; athlete's foot

IV. DIAGNOSIS
    A. Female evaluation may include vaginal examination to check for *Candida* and rule out trichomoniasis, bacterial vaginosis, *Chlamydia* infection, and gonorrhea
    B. Male evaluation may include:
        1. Examination of penis to check for irritation and/or cheesy material
        2. Culture for ruling out gonorrhea and *Chlamydia*
        3. Urinalysis

V. TREATMENT
Prescription medicine: _____; over-the-counter medication recommendation _____ _____

VI. PATIENT EDUCATION

A. No intercourse until symptoms subside

B. Continue prescribed treatment even if menses occurs, but use pads rather than tampons

C. Ways to prevent recurrent *Candida* (yeast) infections
1. Bathe daily (with lots of water and minimal soap)
2. To minimize the moist environment that *Candida* favors, use:
   a. Cotton-crotched or cotton underwear/pantyhose (or cut out the crotch of pantyhose)
   b. Loose-fitting slacks
   c. No underwear while sleeping
3. Wipe the front first and then the back after toileting
4. Avoid feminine hygiene sprays, deodorants, deodorant tampons/minipads, colored or perfumed toilet paper, tear-off fabric softeners in the dryer, and so forth—any of which may cause allergies and irritation
5. Some women have found that vitamin C 500 mg 2 to 4 times each day helps, or taking oral acidophilus tablets 40 million to 1 billion units a day (1 tablet)

D. Over-the-counter medication. Many women choose to try an over-the-counter preparation before seeking an examination. If symptoms do not subside after one course of treatment (one tube or one set of suppositories), having an examination for diagnosis is recommended.

VII. FOLLOW-UP

Return to the clinician for reevaluation if symptoms persist or new symptoms occur after treatment is completed

Special Notes: _____

Clinician: _____

For more information call CDC STD hotline: 1-800-CDC-INFO. Phone numbers of free (or almost free) STD clinics are listed in the Community Service Numbers in the government pages of your local phonebook.
Website: http://www.cdc.gov/ncidod/dbmd/diseaseinfo/candidiasis_gen_g.htm

I. DEFINITION
Chlamydia infection is a sexually transmitted disease of the reproductive tract. It is currently believed to be the most common cause of sexually transmitted diseases in males and females, more common than gonorrhea. It is caused by a parasite *Chlamydia trachomatis.*

II. TRANSMISSION
Sexual contact with an unknown incubation period before symptoms present

III. SIGNS AND SYMPTOMS
  A. In the female
1. Often no symptoms
2. Possibly, increased vaginal discharge, change in menses
3. Cervicitis or an abnormal Papanicolaou smear
4. Possibly, frequent uncomfortable urination
5. Pelvic pain
6. Bleeding after intercourse

  B. In the male
1. Possibly, thick and cloudy discharge from the penis
2. Possibly, painful urination and/or frequent urination
3. Rarely no symptoms

IV. DIAGNOSIS
  A. Evaluation may include tests to rule out candidiasis, trichomoniasis, bacterial vaginosis, gonorrhea, syphilis, and urinary tract infection

  B. Vaginal and urethral smears are examined for the *Chlamydia trachomatis* organism

V. TREATMENT
Prescription medicine: *Take all the prescribed medicine as directed,* even though the symptoms may decrease early in treatment. Incomplete treatment gives the causative organism a chance to lie dormant and reinfect later.

VI. PATIENT EDUCATION
  A. Patients who had any sexual contacts from the previous 60 days prior to the onset of symptoms should be advised to seek evaluation and treatment

  B. Do not have intercourse for 7 days after single-dose treatment or until you and any sex partner(s) have completed treatment; no intercourse until all sex partners are treated; condom as backup for birth control for the rest of the cycle if on oral contraceptives

  C. In an untreated male or female, the disease may progress to further reproductive infection with possible tissue scarring and infertility risks

D. Wash all sex toys, diaphragm, and cervical cap with soap and water or soak in rubbing alcohol or Betadine scrub. Be sure to rinse thoroughly.

VII. FOLLOW-UP

Return to clinician if symptoms persist or new symptoms occur

Special notes: _____

Clinician: _____

For more information call CDC STD hotline: 1-800-CDC-INFO. Phone numbers of free (or almost free) STD clinics are listed in the Community Service Numbers in the government pages of your local phone book. *Website: http://www.cdc.gov/std/Chlamydia/STDFact-Chlamydia.htm*

I. DEFINITION/MECHANISM OF ACTION

The contraceptive *implant* Implanon is a single-rod, implantable polymer contraceptive device impregnated with 68 mg of etonogestrel (a synthetic estrogen). It is effective for up to 3 years. The device is inserted subdermally (under the top layer of skin—the dermis) on the inner side of the woman's upper arm and releases a low, steady dose of the synthetic progestin etonogestrel.

II. EFFECTIVENESS

  A. +99% effective

  B. Women weighing 198 lbs (>90 kg), with a body mass index (BMI) of >30 are at an increased risk for pregnancy. An alternative method is recommended.

III. SIDE EFFECTS AND DISADVANTAGES

  A. Minor side effects (numbers 1–5 related to insertion)

    1. Pain, irritation, swelling, or bruising

    2. Scarring including a thick scar called keloid

    3. Infection

    4. Implanon breaks, making it difficult to remove

    5. Expulsion of the implant (occurs rarely)

    6. Decreased menstrual flow (withdrawal bleeding), no bleeding

    7. Depression, mood changes

    8. Headaches

    9. Abdominal pain

  B. Risk factors

    1. Blood clots in legs, lungs, stroke

    2. Hypertension (high blood pressure)

    3. Gallbladder disease

    4. Heart attack (smokers 35 and older)

    5. Smoking increases the risk of complications. Women with Implanon in place should not smoke.

IV. CONTRAINDICATIONS

  A. Women with a history of any of the following conditions may not be able to use the implant:

    1. Known or suspected pregnancy

    2. History of serious blood clots in legs (deep vein thrombosis), lungs (pulmonary embolism), eyes (retinal thrombosis), heart (heart attack), or head (stroke)

    3. Unexplained vaginal bleeding

    4. Liver disease

    5. Breast cancer

    6. Allergy to anything in the implant

    7. Diabetes

8. High cholesterol or triglycerides
9. Headaches
10. Seizures or epilepsy
11. Gallbladder disease
12. Kidney disease
13. Depression
14. High blood pressure
15. Allergic reaction to anesthetics or antiseptics
16. Taking certain prescription drugs
17. Smoking
18. Weight equal to or greater than 198 lbs (90 kg); weight decreases effectiveness of patch
19. Skin disorders that may predispose to application site reactions
20. Breastfeeding—not yet approved

V. ALTERNATIVE METHODS OF BIRTH CONTROL
A. Abstinence
B. Sterilization
C. Natural family planning
D. Condoms with contraceptive gel, foam, cream, jelly, suppositories, vaginal film
E. Intrauterine contraceptive device
F. Diaphragm with contraceptive jelly, cream
G. FemCap
H. Female condom
I. Depo-Provera injection
J. Progestin-only oral contraceptives
K. Contraceptive sponge

VI. EXPLANATION OF METHOD
A. Ways in which the implant works
1. Withdrawal bleed (period) will occur during the fourth week
2. If you forget to apply a new patch and less than 48 hours have passed, you can apply a new patch as soon as you remember, and then apply that next patch on the usual renewal day
3. If more than 48 hours have elapsed, you should stop the current cycle and immediately begin a new 4-week cycle by applying a new patch. The day for patch renewal will now change. Use backup contraception for 1 week
4. If missed change day occurs at the end of the 4-week cycle, remove the patch and apply a new patch on the usual change day to begin a new cycle

VII. DANGER SIGNALS ASSOCIATED WITH IMPLANON
A. Visual problems: Loss or blurring of vision, double vision, spots before eyes, flashing lights
B. Numbness or paralysis in any parts of body or face, even temporary
C. Unexplained chest pain, coughing blood, or shortness of breath

D. Painful inflamed areas along veins or severe calf pain
E. Severe recurrent headaches or new headaches or worsening of migraines
F. Heavy vaginal bleeding
G. Breast lumps
H. Severe pain, swelling or tenderness in abdomen

Contact us at _____ if you develop any of the above problems.

I. DEFINITION/MECHANISM OF ACTION

The contraceptive *patch* is a three-layer transdermal polyethylene/polyester device about the size of a matchbook with an adhesive on one side. It is impregnated by a synthetic progestin and a synthetic estrogen, and releases 150 µg of the progestin and 20 µg of the estrogen every 24 hours. The patch is changed weekly for 3 weeks, then is left off for 1 week. The patch causes suppression of ovulation, changes the lining of the uterus so it is not receptive to an egg, changes the cervical mucus so sperm cannot get through, changes the transportation of the egg down the fallopian tube, and possibly makes sperm less able to penetrate the egg.

II. EFFECTIVENESS

A. 99% effectiveness

B. Women weighing 90 kg or 198 lbs with a body mass index (BMI) of >30 kg/m^2 are at an increased risk for pregnancy. An alternative method is recommended.

III. SIDE EFFECTS AND DISADVANTAGES

A. Minor side effects
  1. Local irritation from patch
  2. Dislocation of patch
  3. Breast discomfort, tenderness
  4. Nausea
  5. Spotting
  6. Decreased menstrual flow (withdrawal bleeding), no bleeding
  7. Depression, mood changes
  8. Headaches
  9. Abdominal pain

B. Risk factors
  1. Blood clots in legs, lungs, stroke
  2. Hypertension (high blood pressure)
  3. Gallbladder disease
  4. Heart attack (smokers 35 and older)
  5. Smoking increases risk associated with patch use. Women should not smoke and use the patch.

IV. CONTRAINDICATIONS

A. Women with a history of any of the following conditions may not be able to use the patch:
  1. Thromboembolic disorders—blood clots in legs, lungs
  2. Coronary artery disease
  3. Heart disease involving the heart valves with complications
  4. Severe hypertension (high blood pressure)
  5. Diabetes with vascular (blood vessel) involvement

6. Headaches, migraines with neurologic symptoms
7. Major surgery on legs or with prolonged immobility
8. Cancer of the breast or reproductive system
9. Undiagnosed genital bleeding
10. Impaired liver function, liver problems
11. Known or suspected pregnancy
12. Taking certain prescription drugs
13. Smoking
14. Weight equal to or greater than 198 lbs (90 kg); weight decreases effectiveness of patch
15. Skin disorders that may predispose to application site reactions
16. Breastfeeding—not yet approved

V. ALTERNATIVE METHODS OF BIRTH CONTROL
A. Abstinence
B. Sterilization
C. Natural family planning
D. Condoms with contraceptive gel, foam, cream, jelly, suppositories, vaginal film
E. Intrauterine contraceptive device
F. Diaphragm with contraceptive jelly, cream
G. FemCap, Lea's Shield
H. Contraceptive implant
I. Female condom
J. Depo-Provera injection
K. Progestin-only oral contraceptives
L. Contraceptive sponge

VI. EXPLANATION OF METHOD
A. Ways in which the patch is used
1. Apply patch on first day of menses or on the first Sunday after bleeding begins; postpartum nonnursing 4 weeks or with resumption of menses. Apply to clean, dry, healthy skin on buttocks, abdomen, upper outer arm, or upper torso. Patch should not be applied to breasts. If applied to the pubic area, it may cause swelling of the genital area.
2. Do not use lotions, cosmetics, creams, powders, or other topical products in area where patch will be applied
3. Press down firmly on the patch for at least 10 seconds and then check if the edges adhere
4. Check patch daily
5. If patch detaches, immediately apply a new patch. Supplemental tapes or adhesives should not be used.
6. Apply a new patch the same day of the week, 7 days after first patch. Repeat this in Week 3.
7. No patch is applied in Week 4
8. Begin a new cycle on the same day of the week for Week 1 and repeat cycle of 3 weeks on and 1 week off

9. Withdrawal bleed (period) will occur during fourth week
10. If you forget to apply a new patch and less than 48 hours have passed, you can apply a new patch as soon as you remember and then apply that next patch on the usual renewal day
11. If more than 48 hours have elapsed, you should stop the current cycle and immediately begin a new 4-week cycle by applying a new patch. The day for patch renewal will now change. Use backup contraception for 1 week.
12. If missed change day occurs at the end of the 4-week cycle, remove the patch and apply a new patch on the usual change day to begin a new cycle

VII. DANGER SIGNALS ASSOCIATED WITH PATCH USE
A. Visual problems: loss or blurring of vision, double vision, spots before eyes, flashing lights
B. Numbness or paralysis in any part of the body or face, even temporary
C. Unexplained chest pain
D. Painful inflamed areas along veins or severe calf pain
E. Severe recurrent headaches or new headaches or worsening of migraines

Note: Concerns have been raised because of the higher exposure to estrogen as compared to most birth control pills. The U.S. Food and Drug Administration (FDA) warning has been changed to indicate this. At this time, the patch has not been recalled nor has there been an FDA warning to discontinue patch use. If you have concerns regarding this, consult your clinician.

Contact us at _____ if you develop any of the aforementioned problems.

Contraceptive Shield: Lea's Shield[1]

I. DEFINITION/MECHANISM OF ACTION

Lea's Shield is a silicone device similar to a diaphragm that is used to hold spermicide and to provide a partial barrier to sperm when placed over the cervix. It is an elliptical bowl in shape and the posterior end has a reservoir for spermicide. There is a valve in the middle to allow cervical secretions to drain and also to relieve pressure against the cervix. There is a molded loop to aid in removal. Insertion is similar to using a diaphragm.

II. EFFECTIVENESS AND BENEFITS

A. 86% effectiveness—has not been in use long, so information is scarce
B. May be inserted before intercourse and left in place for up to 48 hours
C. Latex free
D. Reusable for more than a year

III. SIDE EFFECTS AND DISADVANTAGES

A. Minor side effects
   1. Vaginal irritation from the device
   2. Vaginal irritation from the spermicide used with the device
   3. Sensation of something in the vagina
   4. Difficulty in removing
   5. Requires prescription

IV. CONTRAINDICATIONS

A. Allergy to spermicide
B. Allergy to silicone
C. Partner allergy to silicone or spermicide
D. Device is expelled repeatedly during use
E. Cannot be used during menses
F. Known or suspected uterine or cervical cancer
G. History of toxic shock syndrome
H. Current infection of vagina or cervix, pelvic inflammatory disease
I. Cannot be used during postpartum or after an abortion for 6 weeks

V. ALTERNATIVE METHODS OF BIRTH CONTROL

A. Abstinence
B. Sterilization
C. Natural family planning
D. Condoms with contraceptive gel, foam, cream, jelly, suppositories, vaginal film
E. Intrauterine contraceptive device
F. Diaphragm with contraceptive jelly, cream, FemCap, sponge
G. Female condom
H. Depo-Provera injection
I. Contraceptive patch, ring, implant
J. Oral contraceptives

VI. TYPES

Available in one size

VII. FITTING

A. Pelvic examination to rule out any problems that might occur with use and to evaluate size and position of cervix

B. Follow-up for any concerns, problems; annual examination

NOTE

1. Discontinued in the United States, available at http://www.barriermethods .com

Contraceptive Vaginal Ring
(Nuvaring)

I. DEFINITION/MECHANISM OF ACTION

The contraceptive vaginal ring is flexible, transparent, colorless, and about 2 in. in diameter. It is impregnated with a synthetic progestin and a synthetic estrogen, and releases 120 µg of progestin and 15 µg of estrogen every 24 hours over a period of 3 weeks. The ring is removed at the end of the third week and a new ring is inserted at the beginning of a new cycle, 1 week later. The ring causes suppression of ovulation, changes the lining of the uterus so it is not receptive to an egg, changes the cervical mucus so sperm cannot get through, changes the transportation of the egg down the fallopian tube, and possibly makes sperm less able to penetrate the egg.

II. EFFECTIVENESS

98% to 99% effectiveness

III. SIDE EFFECTS AND DISADVANTAGES

A. Minor side effects
1. Vaginal irritation from the ring
2. Dislocation of the ring
3. Sensation of something in the vagina
4. If ring is out for more than 3 hours, then the woman will need to use backup contraception for 7 days

IV. CONTRAINDICATIONS

A. Women with a history of any of the following conditions may not be able to use the ring:
1. Blood clots in legs (thrombosis), lungs (pulmonary embolism), or eyes (now or in the past)
2. Chest pain (angina pectoris)
3. Heart attack or stroke
4. Severe high blood pressure
5. Pregnancy or suspected pregnancy
6. Diabetes with complications of the kidney, eyes, nerves, or blood vessels
7. Headaches with neurologic symptoms
8. Need for a long period of bed rest following major surgery
9. Known or suspected cancer of the breast or cancer of the lining of the uterus, cervix, or vagina (now or in the past)
10. Unexplained vaginal bleeding
11. Yellowing of the whites of the eyes or of the skin (jaundice) during pregnancy or during past use of oral contraceptives (birth control pills)
12. Liver tumors or active liver disease
13. Disease of the heart valves with complications
14. Allergic reaction to any of the components of the rings
15. Smoking and age older than 35 (15 cigarettes a day or more)

16. Weight greater than or equal to 198 lbs (90 kg); excess weight decreases effectiveness of the ring
17. A prolapsed (dropped) uterus, dropped bladder (cystocele), or rectal prolapse (rectocele)
18. Younger than age 35 and a heavy smoker (15 cigarettes a day or more)
19. Breastfeeding—not yet approved for use

V. ALTERNATIVE METHODS OF BIRTH CONTROL
A. Abstinence
B. Sterilization
C. Natural family planning
D. Condoms with contraceptive gel, foam, cream, jelly, suppositories, vaginal film
E. Intrauterine device
F. Diaphragm with contraceptive jelly, cream
G. FemCap
H. Lea's Shield (discontinued in the United States, available at http://www.barriermethods.com)
I. Female condom
J. Depo-Provera contraceptive injection
K. Contraceptive patch
L. Oral contraceptives
M. Contraceptive implant
N. Contraceptive sponge

VI. EXPLANATION OF METHOD
A. Ways in which the ring is used
   1. Insert ring into vagina between Day 1 and Day 5 of menstrual cycle and note the start day
   2. Keep ring in place for 3 weeks in a row
   3. Remove ring for 1 week for withdrawal bleeding
   4. If ring is removed from the vagina and is out for more than 3 hours, use backup contraception for the next 7 days, except for the week with no ring

VII. DANGER SIGNALS ASSOCIATED WITH RING USE
A. Visual problems
   1. Loss or blurring of vision, double vision
   2. Spots before eyes, flashing lights
B. Numbness or paralysis in any parts of body or face, even temporary
C. Unexplained chest pain
D. Painful inflamed areas along veins or severe calf pain
E. Severe recurrent headaches or new headaches or worsening of migraines

Contact us at _____ if you develop any of the above problems.
Website for ring information: http://www.organoninc.com; http://www.nu-varing.com

Cystitis (Bladder Infection)

I. DEFINITION

Cystitis, a bladder infection, is usually caused by bacteria. Women are more prone to cystitis because the urethra (connection between the bladder and the outside through which we urinate) is short and the vagina and rectum are close to the opening of the urethra, called the urethral meatus. However, men can also develop cystitis.

II. SIGNS AND SYMPTOMS

A. Frequent urination of small amounts of urine; often you will experience an urgent feeling of needing to urinate and then just urinating a little
B. Burning, pain, or difficulty in urinating
C. Blood in the urine
D. Pain in the lower part of the abdomen (pelvic pain) around the pubic bone
E. Chills, fever

III. TREATMENT

Treatment of cystitis is with an antibiotic. It is important that you tell your clinician if you are allergic to any antibiotics so that you are given a suitable medication.

You may be asked to give what is called a clean catch urine specimen prior to the diagnosis (as opposed to just urinating in a paper cup for the specimen). For the clean catch specimen, you will be given special wipes to use on your perineal area and instructions on collecting the urine specimen in a sterile container. This specimen will be sent to the laboratory to evaluate the bacteria in the urine and to see what antibiotics will be effective against the bacteria.

It is important to take the entire prescription given to you even if symptoms disappear quickly. Follow the directions for times to take the medication and try not to skip a dose because this may allow the bacteria to increase in number. You may also be given a prescription for a bladder pain medication or information about over-the-counter medication (AZO Standard, Uristat) to take away the bladder pain. These bladder pain medications are to be used with, and not instead of, the prescribed antibiotic because they only relieve bladder pain and have no effect on the bacteria causing your cystitis.

IV. PATIENT EDUCATION

There are several things you can do to avoid cystitis and to help your body heal when you have cystitis, more commonly known as a bladder infection.

A. After going to the bathroom, wipe from front to back, or wipe the front first and then the back, so as not to carry bacteria from your rectal area to the vaginal area where your urethral opening (opening into the bladder) is located. A woman's urethra is quite short, so bacteria can travel into the bladder quite easily.

B. If sexual intercourse includes vaginal or oral contact after anal contact, you might consider washing off your genitals and those of your partner before proceeding with vaginal and/or oral sex

C. During a tub bath, it is better not to use bath oils and bubble bath, because these help bacteria travel up your urethra

D. Try to empty your bladder before sex, and after sex, empty your bladder as soon as you can to wash bacteria from your urethra, particularly if you seem to get cystitis easily (several times a year)

E. Tight clothing, especially clothes made of synthetic fabrics such as polyester, helps bacteria grow more easily by creating a warm, dark, moist environment. Cotton underpants and loose clothing help your body breathe and discourage bacterial growth.

F. Always urinate when you have the urge; do not put it off until you are desperate. Bacteria grow better in urine that is sitting in your bladder for a long period.

G. Drink 6 to 8 glasses of water and juice a day; cranberry juice helps to decrease cystitis. Cranberry is also available as AZO Cranberry juice capsules with 450 mg of cranberry juice concentrate; the dose is 1 to 4 capsules per day with meals.

H. Caffeine is a bladder irritant, meaning it can cause bladder pain or spasms (cramps), so the less caffeine you take in, the less bladder irritation you will experience. Caffeine is in coffee, tea, chocolate, and many carbonated beverages even if they are not colas. Check the labels.

I. Smoking (nicotine) is also very irritating to the bladder

J. A well-balanced diet, including six or more servings of fresh fruits and vegetables a day and three to four servings of whole grain breads, cereals, and pasta, will increase your resistance to infection

Cystitis is the least serious of the urinary tract infections. If left untreated, it can lead to infection of the rest of the urinary tract including the ureters (connecting the bladder and kidneys) and the kidneys. Prompt and correct treatment of cystitis will help you avoid having a more serious urinary tract infection. If your symptoms worsen or do not get better with the treatment prescribed by your clinician, call or return to the health care setting for further help.

Websites: http://www.mayoclinic.com/health/cystitis/DS00285; http://www. niddk.nih.gov/health/urolog/pubs/cystitis/cystitis.htm

I. DEFINITION/MECHANISM OF ACTION
The contraceptive FemCap is a prescription-only contraceptive device that is used to hold spermicide and to provide a partial barrier to sperm when placed over the cervix. Available in three sizes: 22 mm, 26 mm, and 30 mm. Your clinician will examine you and advise on size.

II. EFFECTIVENESS
96% to 98% effectiveness

III. SIDE EFFECTS AND DISADVANTAGES
  A. Minor side effects
    1. Vaginal irritation from the device
    2. Vaginal irritation from the spermicide used with the device
    3. Sensation of something in the vagina
    4. Requires a pelvic examination and prescription for the device

IV. CONTRAINDICATIONS
  A. Allergy to spermicide
  B. Allergy to material the device is made of
  C. Partner allergy to device or spermicide
  D. Device is expelled repeatedly during use
  E. Cannot be used during menses
  F. Known or suspected uterine or cervical cancer
  G. History of toxic shock syndrome
  H. Current infection of vagina or cervix
  I. Abnormality of cervix, uterus, or vagina
  J. Cannot be used during postpartum or after an abortion for 6 weeks

V. ALTERNATIVE METHODS OF BIRTH CONTROL
  A. Abstinence
  B. Sterilization
  C. Natural family planning
  D. Condoms with contraceptive gel, foam, cream, jelly, suppositories, vaginal film
  E. Intrauterine contraceptive device
  F. Diaphragm with contraceptive jelly, cream, sponge
  G. Female condom
  H. Depo-Provera injection
  I. Contraceptive patch, ring, implant
  J. Oral contraceptives

VI. EXPLANATION OF METHOD
  A. Ways in which the device is used (FemCap comes with instructional video)
    1. Insert spermicide into the device according to directions by the manufacturer and place in the vagina over the cervix before any sexual arousal

2. Keep device in place for at least 6 hours after last act of intercourse
3. Add additional spermicide to outside of device for each repeated act of intercourse within the next 48 hours. Do not remove device to add spermicide.
4. Remove FemCap by squatting and bearing down. Slip finger between the dome and the removal strap and pull gently.
5. Wash device thoroughly with antibacterial hand soap, rinse thoroughly in clear water, and allow to air dry

Contact us at _____ if you have any questions or develop any problems. You will need to return for a Pap smear after the first 3 months of use.

Website for FemCap information: http://www.femcap.com

I. DEFINITION

The herpes *simplex* virus (HSV) is one of the most common infectious agents of humans. It is transmitted only by direct contact with the virus from an active infected oral or genital lesion. The HSV is of two types:

    A. HSV Type 1: Usually affects body sites above the waist (mouth, lips, eyes, fingers); increasingly the cause of herpetic infections in the anal/genital regions

    B. HSV Type 2: Usually involves body sites below the waist, primarily the genitals

Genital herpes may be caused by either HSV-1 or HSV-2. If oral sex is practiced, remember that cold sores are herpes lesions and can be spread to the genital area. The cause, symptoms, complications, diagnosis, treatment, and patient education are the same for both males and females.

II. SYMPTOMS

    A. Painful, itchy sores similar to cold sores or fever blisters surrounded by reddened skin that appear around the mouth, nipples, buttocks, thighs or genital areas 4 to 7 days up to 4 weeks after contact

    B. Fever or flu-like symptoms

    C. Tenderness or pain in muscles

    D. Burning sensation during urination

    E. Swollen lymph nodes in the area of the lesions—neck, underarms, groin

    F. Joint pain

    G. Painful urination in both males and females; retention of urine especially in females

    H. Pain on intercourse

    I. Headache

    J. Symptoms may last 2 to 3 weeks

III. DIAGNOSIS

    A. Examination based on your clinical symptoms and history

    B. Laboratory analysis of discharge from the lesions to identify virus

    C. Blood test for HSV-1 and HSV-2 antibodies

    D. Consider HIV testing; being tested for other sexually transmitted diseases (STDs)

IV. TREATMENT

    A. Tepid bath with or without the addition of iodine solution

    B. Unrestrictive clothing

    C. Prevent secondary infection

    D. Medication for pain

    E. There are topical and oral medications that do not cure the infection but can shorten the duration and severity of symptoms and decrease recurrence; these medications may, in some cases, be taken on a long-term basis to suppress the virus

V. COMPLICATIONS
   A. Secondary infection of herpes lesions
   B. Severe systemic and life-threatening infections in infants born vaginally during an episode of herpes in the mother

VI. RECURRENCES
Herpes sores may never recur after the first episode, or there may be occasional flare-ups, which are not as painful as the initial infection, lasting up to 7 days. Recurring infections may be related to stress (physical or emotional), illness, fever, overexposure to the sun, or menstruation. Recurrences are caused by a reactivation of the virus already present in the nerve endings of your body.

VII. PATIENT EDUCATION
   A. After urinating, wash the genital area with cool water
   B. If urinating is difficult, sit in a tub of warm water to urinate
   C. Cool, wet tea bags applied to the lesions may offer some relief
   D. Avoid intercourse when active lesions are present. If intercourse does occur, condoms should be used
   E. Women with chronic herpes should have a Pap smear yearly

Medication: _____

Special notes: _____

Clinician: _____

For more information call Centers for Disease Control and Prevention (CDC) STD hotline: 1-800-CDC-INFO. Phone numbers of free (or almost free) STD clinics are listed in the Community Service Numbers in the government pages of your local phone book, or seek out local support groups. The American Social Health Association (ASHA) has booklets, books, handouts that can be used as resources, or you may call The Helper at 800-230-6039; or the ASHA patient herpes hotline at 919-361-8488. *Websites: http://www.herpes.com; http://www.ashastd.org/herpes/hrc.html; http://www.webmd.com (America Online keyword: better health); http://www .viridas.com; http://www.diagnology*

Genital Warts
(Condylomata Acuminata)

I. DEFINITION

Genital warts, or condylomata acuminata, may occur on either the male or female genital areas. The virus family causing the warts is believed to be sexually transmitted, although warts have been found on individuals whose partner has no history or sign of warts. The human papilloma virus (HPV) family has more than 150 types, some of which cause warts on the genitals (more than 30 types), nipples, umbilicus, hands, soles of the feet, cervix, vagina, penis, scrotum, and rectal area. Some HPV types are associated with cancers of the cervix, penis, mouth, anus, lungs, and other parts of the body.

II. SIGNS AND SYMPTOMS

Warts may not appear until 2 weeks (average is 1–6 months) to many months (or even years after exposure)

A. In moist areas, the warts are small, often itchy bumps or lumps, sometimes with a cauliflower-like top, appearing singly or in clusters

B. On dry skin (such as the shaft of the penis), the warts commonly are small, hard, and yellowish gray, resembling warts that appear on other parts of the body

C. On the female, the warts are commonly found on or around the vaginal opening, vaginal lips, in the vagina, around the rectum, and on the cervix. Symptoms include increased vaginal discharge, itching or burning of the vulva, pain and bleeding, and feeling a lump in the vulvar area or groin.

D. On the male, the warts can be found on any part of the penis, scrotum, or rectal area

III. DIAGNOSIS

A. The diagnosis is usually obvious based on the appearance of the warts, but sometimes a microscopic examination is necessary to identify minute lesions

B. Laboratory tests may include checking for gonorrhea, *Chlamydia*, syphilis, HIV/AIDS, and a Pap smear if none within a year

IV. TREATMENT

A. If small, the warts may be treated by several weekly applications of medication by you or your clinician

B. Patients with large, persistent warts or warts in the vagina or on the cervix may be referred to a physician for treatment. Some treatments include cryotherapy (freezing) and laser removal of the warts.

V. PATIENT EDUCATION

A. Always advise sexual partners to see a clinician for examination

B. Having warts may increase vaginal discharge; have it checked and treated

C. Treatment medication is applied weekly by the clinician in his or her office or clinic. Some of the drugs used must be rinsed off in 4 hours. Your clinician will advise you. Certain treatment medication should never be used in pregnant patients. If pregnancy is suspected, tell your clinician.

D. You may be given medication for self-treatment and separate instructions on how to do this

E. Recurrence is possible without reinfection, because treatment does not always eradicate very small warts. Microscopic examination and treatment by a specialist may be necessary.

F. A woman with a history of warts, especially if on the cervix, is encouraged to have an annual gynecologic examination with a Pap smear as recommended by her clinician (often twice a year)

G. A vaccine (Gardasil) is now available for girls and boys who are preadolescent, adolescents, and young women. It protects against several types of HPV—those associated with genital warts and also associated with cervical cancer

Special notes: _____

Clinician: _____

For more information call Centers for Disease Control and Prevention (CDC) Sexually Transmitted Disease (STD) hotline: 1-800-CDC-INFO. Phone numbers of free (or almost free) STD clinics are listed in the Community Service Numbers in the government pages of your local phone book.

Websites: *http://www.cdc.gov/std/hpv/*; *http://www.cdc.gov/vaccines/pubs/vis/default.htm#hpv*

Self-Treatment for Genital Warts

Podofilox (Condylox) is a prescription treatment for genital warts that you can use at home. Fill your Condylox prescription at any drugstore or the pharmacy in a department store. The Condylox package contains directions for use of the medication. Please read these carefully and use the medication as directed. It is important to follow these directions and those of your clinician to ensure the maximum possible effect from the medication.

Podofilox works by destroying the wart tissue. This does not happen all at once, but gradually. The wart will change in color, from skin color to a dry, crusted, dead appearance, and then disappear. You may feel some pain or burning when applying podofilox as these changes occur. You may also see some redness, may have some soreness or tenderness at the wart sites, and may even see small sores in that area. These symptoms usually disappear within a week after you have completed the treatment. If any of these changes are severe or concern you, stop the treatment and contact your clinician.

Use sinecatechin (15% ointment green tea extract with active ingredient catchechins) for no longer than 16 weeks.

Treating Your Warts

Treat your warts twice a day with podofilox. It is all right to do so even if you get your menstrual period during the time you are treating your warts. Plan a time in the morning and again in the evening to apply the medication. Repeat the twice-a-day treatments for 3 days, and then do not treat the warts again for 4 days. You can repeat this pattern of treatment—3 days of medication and then 4 days off—for up to 4 weeks. Stop the treatment, however, as soon as the warts disappear. It is important that you do not treat the warts in any week for more than 3 days, because such treatment will not help them to disappear faster and may cause you to have side effects from the medication.

If you have completed 4 weeks of treatment and still have warts, return to your clinician for further evaluation, and do not use Podofilox until you have this check-up.

Remove any clothing over the affected area and wash your hands before treating your warts. Open the bottle of podofilox and place it on a flat surface so it will not spill while you are treating your warts. It may be helpful to use a hand mirror to locate the warts so that you can treat them. Good light is also important so that you do not get medication on skin that is free of warts.

Holding onto the bottle to steady it, dip the tip of one cotton tip applicator (Q-tip) into the medication. The tip should be wet with the medication, but not dripping. Remove any excess medication by pressing the applicator tip against the inside of the bottle. Apply the podofilox only to those areas you and your clinician have identified as warts.

Try not to get any podofilox on any area of your skin that is not a wart. If the wart is on a skinfold, gently spread the skin with one hand to flatten out the wart and touch the medication applicator to the area with the other hand. Allow the podofilox to dry before letting the skinfolds to relax into the normal position and before putting clothing over the affected area.

After application, throw away the Q-tip. Close the bottle tightly to prevent evaporation of the medication and wash your hands carefully when you are finished with the treatment.

If you are using podofilox gel, follow the same treatment schedule as for the liquid. Wash your hands before treating your warts. Squeeze out a small amount of gel (about half the size of a pea) onto your fingertip. Dab a small amount of the gel onto the warts or the areas your clinician has instructed you to treat. Try not to get any of the gel on normal skin areas. For warts in skinfolds, spread the folds apart and apply the gel to the wart, letting the area dry before you return the skinfolds to their normal position. Wash your hands carefully after completing the treatment.

The area you have treated may sting when you apply the gel. It may also become red, sore, itchy, or tender after treatment.

Precautions in Self-treatment

Podofilox is intended only for treatment of venereal warts and only on the outside of the body. It is not safe to use podofilox on any other skin condition. If you have severe pain, bleeding, swelling, or itching, stop the treatment and contact your clinician. Avoid contact of this medication with your eyes. If you do so accidentally, flush your eyes immediately with running water and call your clinician. The effects of podofilox on pregnancy are unknown, so it is not safe to use this medication during pregnancy.

Apply sinecatechins (Veregen) 15% ointment 3 times a day (0.5-cm strand of ointment to each wart, covering the wart with a thin layer of ointment), continuing this treatment until all warts are covered. The ointment should not be washed off. Do not use the treatment for longer than 16 weeks.

Follow-up Care

It is important to return for a checkup as suggested by your clinician, or if you have completed 4 weeks of treatment and still have warts. If the warts reappear after you have completed the treatment, contact your clinician prior to restarting treatment. Your partner should also be checked and treated for any warts; otherwise, you can be reinfected.

Self-Treatment With Imiquimod Cream 5% (Aldara, Zyclara)

Imiquimod creams (Aldara and Zyclara) are prescription treatments for genital warts that you can use at home. Fill your prescription at any drugstore or pharmacy in a department store. The package contains directions for use of the medication. Please read these carefully and use the medication only as directed.

Imiquimod probably works by boosting your body's immune response to the wart virus (there are more than 150 types of wart virus, called human papilloma virus or HPV). Imiquimod should be used only on warts outside the vagina, on the labia, and on the area around your anus

Treating Your Warts
Careful hand washing before and after application of the cream is recommended so that you do not experience a secondary bacterial infection in the wart area and get the cream on other parts of your body. Apply imiquimod 3 times a week just prior to your normal sleeping hours. Apply a thin layer of the cream to all external genital warts and rub it in until it is no longer visible. Leave imiquimod on the skin for 6 to 10 hours. Do not cover the treated area. Following this treatment period, remove the cream by washing the treated area with mild soap and water. Continue treatment until the warts disappear. Do not continue treatment past 16 weeks without consulting your clinician.

Precautions in Treatment
Imiquimod cream may weaken condoms and vaginal diaphragms, so do not use these while you are treating your warts. Sexual (genital) contact should be avoided while the imiquimod cream is on the skin. Common reactions to imiquimod include redness, burning, swelling, itching, rash, soreness, stinging, and tenderness. If any of these occur, wash the cream

off with mild soap and water. Do not re-treat until these symptoms are gone. A very small percentage of persons have flu-like symptoms—fever, fatigue, headache, diarrhea, and/or achy joints. If you experience any of these and for any questions, call your clinician.

Websites: http://www.drugs.com/condylox.html;   http://www.rxlist.com/ veregen-drug.htm; http://www.cdc.gov/std/hpv/; http://www.cancer.gov

I. DEFINITION

Gonorrhea is an acute infection that is spread by sexual contact and involves the genitourinary tract, throat, and rectum of both sexes. It is caused by the organism *Neisseria gonorrhoeae*.

II. IMPORTANT INFORMATION

  A. The highest incidence of gonorrhea occurs in males between the ages of 20 and 24 and in females from 18 and 24. Gonorrhea is usually contracted from an infected person who has ignored symptoms or has no symptoms. This source can reinfect the patient, or possibly infect others unknowingly.

  B. Incubation: 1 to 13 days; symptoms can occur 3 to 30 days after sexual contact; average is 2 to 5 days after exposure

III. USUAL SIGNS AND SYMPTOMS

  A. Females
1. Up to 80% have no symptoms
2. Abnormal, thick green vaginal discharge; change in vaginal discharge
3. Frequency, pain on urination, urethral pain
4. Pain with intercourse
5. Urethral discharge
6. Rectal pain and discharge
7. Unilateral labial pain and swelling
8. Abnormal menstrual bleeding; increased dysmenorrhea (menstrual cramps)
9. Lower abdominal discomfort and pelvic pain and tenderness
10. Sore throat
11. Fever, possibly high
12. Nausea, vomiting
13. Sores in genital area
14. Joint pain and swelling
15. Upper abdominal pain

  B. Males
1. 4% to 10% have no symptoms
2. Frequency, pain on urination
3. Burning sensation in the urethra
4. Whitish discharge from the penis (early); may appear only as a drop during erection
5. Yellow or greenish discharge from the penis (late)
6. Sore throat

IV. DIAGNOSIS (FOR BOTH SEXES)

  A. History of sexual contact with a person known to be infected with gonorrhea

  B. Smears and cultures taken from infected areas (cervix, penis, rectum, and throat)

V. TREATMENT FOR MALES AND FEMALES

Antibiotics will be prescribed and are effective if taken according to directions. Be sure to tell your clinician if you are allergic to any antibiotic.

VI. COMPLICATIONS

A. Females: If gonorrhea goes untreated, it may lead to pelvic inflammatory disease (PID). PID involves severe abdominal cramps, pelvic pain, and high fever that will lead to scarring and possible blockage of the fallopian tubes, tubal pregnancy risk, and infertility.
B. Males: If gonorrhea goes untreated, scar tissue may form on the sperm passageway causing pain and sterility
C. Females and males: The infection may spread throughout the body causing arthritis, sometimes with skin lesions

VII. PATIENT EDUCATION (FOR BOTH SEXES)

A. All medications must be taken as directed
B. No intercourse until treatment of self and partner(s) is completed
C. Return to the clinician for reevaluation if symptoms persist or new symptoms occur after treatment is complete
D. Important: All sexual partners of the patient should be informed immediately upon finding out about exposure to sexually transmitted disease so that all persons involved can be evaluated adequately and treated immediately

Special notes: _____

Clinician: _____

For more information, call the Centers for Disease Control and Prevention (CDC) Sexually Transmitted Disease (STD) hotline: 1-800-CDC-INFO. Phone numbers of free (or almost free) STD clinics are listed in the Community Service Numbers in the government pages of your local phone book.

Websites: http://www.cdc.gov; http://www.cdc.gov/std/Gonorrhea/STDFact-gonorrhea.htm

I. DEFINITION

Hormone therapy is the use of traditional hormones or bioidentical hormones (estrogen, progesterone, and/or testosterone) by postmenopausal women. Now known as HT, the use of hormones after menopause was once known as estrogen therapy (ET) because women were given synthetic estrogen only.

II. REASONS FOR TAKING HORMONE THERAPY

A woman's body produces declining amounts of estrogens, progesterones, and androgens during the perimenopausal period, culminating in the cessation of menstrual cycles (ovulation and bleeding). After 12 months without any bleeding (periods), you can consider that you are postmenopausal. A woman is said to have gone through surgical menopause if she has had her fallopian tubes, ovaries, and uterus removed.

Some natural estrogen production does continue after natural menopause; heavier women produce more estrogen because fat cells convert body chemicals called *precursors* to *estrone*, the most common form of natural estrogen in menopause.

Decline in natural estrogen production contributes to such menopausal symptoms as loss of elasticity of the vagina, a less lush vaginal lining causing a feeling of itching or burning or dryness, and pain around the urethra (the opening to the urinary bladder). Hot flashes (or hot flushes), including night sweats, characterize menopause for some women. There may also be a relationship between menopause and loss of bone density leading to osteoporosis.

III. WHAT YOU SHOULD KNOW WHEN CONSIDERING HORMONE THERAPY

HT should never be taken by women who have vaginal bleeding after menopause until the cause of the bleeding is discovered. Pregnant women or perimenopausal women who suspect pregnancy cannot take HT. If you have ever had a stroke, heart attack, or a blood clot in your legs or lungs, liver disease, or any problems with the function of your liver, you may not be an HT candidate. Women with known or suspected cancer of the breast, ovaries, uterus, or cervix may not be good candidates for HT.

Several conditions require special evaluation to determine whether taking HT will be safe. These include undiagnosed vaginal bleeding, known or suspected pregnancy, a history of blood clots in lungs or legs, known or suspected cancer of the breast or reproductive tract or malignant melanoma, history of a bleeding disorder treated with blood transfusion, active gallbladder disease, family history of breast cancer, migraine headaches, untreated elevated lipids that are of concern, and endometriosis.

Considering HT is a decision that is yours to make if you and your clinician decide that you have no contraindications to its use. To make the best decision, you and your clinician will need to discuss whether you are at greater risk of bone density loss leading to osteoporosis because of your family or personal history, whether you have risk factors for developing osteoporosis, and your personal and family medical history including heart disease. Your desire for taking HT as well as your access to health care for monitoring HT will be considered.

IV. EVALUATING YOUR PHYSICAL RISKS AND BENEFITS IN TAKING HORMONE THERAPY

In addition to a careful personal and family history, your clinician will recommend that you need to have a complete physical exam including a pelvic (internal) exam and possible Pap smear, and testing for infections such as vaginitis and sexually transmitted diseases as indicated. Testing might also include a mammogram if you have not had one in the past year, examination of hormone levels, a lipid profile to determine your cholesterol level and the ratio of low-density lipoproteins (LDL—the bad ones) to high-density lipoproteins (HDL—the good ones), a hematocrit and/or hemoglobin to see if you are anemic, vitamin D levels, and a bone density scan. Other testing will depend on the findings from the physical exam and your personal and family health history. For some women, the benefits of taking HT outweigh the risks. For others, the risks and benefits balance, and for still others, the risks outweigh the benefits.

V. TAKING HORMONE THERAPY

If your uterus has been removed (hysterectomy), you will take estrogen only without progestin. You and your clinician will decide which estrogen is best for you, both the amount and the way you take it (in pill form, patches, or as a vaginal cream, suppository, or vaginal ring). If you still have your uterus, you may take both estrogen and a progestin patch, pill, or intrauterine device. Some women bleed when taking progestin, so you and your clinician will need to decide what is best for you.

As androgen levels drop with menopause, some women also take a small amount of male hormone (androgen), which may help women whose menopausal symptoms are not resolved with estrogen or estrogen and progestin alone, have a decreased sense of well-being, lower libido (sex drive), and/or generalized loss of energy (lethargy).

VI. CONSIDER ALTERNATIVES AND ADJUNCTS TO HORMONE THERAPY

All women need a diet with at least six to eight servings of fruit and vegetables a day; several servings of complex carbohydrates such as breads and pasta; sources of protein including dairy products, eggs, meat, fish, and poultry, and legumes such as beans and peas; and calcium. Women also need to decrease fat to 30% or less of total calories daily by using nonfat dairy products (rich in protein and calcium), limiting red meat, and eating lean meat, poultry, and fish. Whole grain pastas, cereals and breads, bran, vegetables, and fruits add roughage to the diet. Most women need calcium supplements. Postmenopausal women need a total of 1,200 mg of calcium each day as well as 600 to 800 IU of vitamin D. Six to eight 8-oz glasses of water daily will help keep all tissues healthy and promote both bowel and bladder health. Consider adding phytoestrogens to diet and essential fatty acids in recommended amounts.

Regular weight-bearing exercise and strength training are critical to the maintenance of bone density; 30 to 45 minutes, 4 to 6 times a week is recommended. Some women build this exercise into their daily routines by walking on errands and at work, and using stairs instead of elevators. Botanicals; Chinese remedies; vitamins; nonhormonal vaginal lubricants such as KY jelly, KY liquid, Lubrin, Vagisil, Replens, and Astroglide; naturalistic interventions; and homeopathic preparations can be helpful supplements or alternatives to HT. Because herbs and homeopathic remedies can interact with each other and with prescription and over-the-counter medications, it is best to consult a practitioner who specializes in their use. Your local library, health food store, bookstore, and health care providers are all sources of information about caring for yourself after menopause.

Websites about menopause: http://www.nia.nih.gov/HealthInformation/ Publications/Menopause/; http://www.nlm.nih.gov/medlineplus/hormonereplacementtherapy.html; http://www.nia.nih.gov/HealthInformation/Publications/healthyeating.htm

Lice (Pediculosis)

I. DEFINITION
Pediculosis means having the skin infested with lice, particularly on hairy areas such as the scalp, underarms, and the pubic area. Three types of lice prey on humans: head lice (*Pediculus capitis*), body lice (*Pediculus humanus corporis*), and pubic lice or crab lice (*Phthirus pubis*).

II. TRANSMISSION
Lice are transmitted by lice-infected shared clothing, bedding, brushes, combs, batting helmets, headphones, hats, stuffed animals, car seats, towels, pillows, and upholstered furniture, or by close personal contact with an infected person. Head lice move from head to head. Adult pubic lice probably survive no more than 24 hours off their host.

III. SIGNS AND SYMPTOMS
A. Intense itching
B. Observing the lice or, more easily, their nits (eggs), which are greenish white ovals attached to hair shafts in eyebrows, eyelashes, scalp hair, pubic hair, and other body hair
C. Known exposure to a household member or intimate partner with lice
D. Crusts or scabs on body from scratching
E. Enlargement of lymph nodes (swollen glands) in the neck or groin (for pubic lice), an allergic response to the lice
F. Body lice found on clothing, especially in the seams, as lice are rarely found on the body
G. Black dots (representing excreta) on skin and underclothing

IV. DIAGNOSIS
Lice can best be detected by using a magnifying glass or microscope

V. TREATMENT
A. General measures
    1. Wash clothing, towels, and so forth with hot water, or dry-clean contaminated items or run them through a dryer on heat cycle to destroy nits and lice; wash combs and hairbrushes in hot, soapy water. Items can also be sealed in a plastic bag for 2 weeks; lice will suffocate. Or items can be put outside in cold weather for 10 days.
    2. Spray couches, chairs, car seats, and items that cannot be washed or dry-cleaned with over-the-counter products (A-200 Pyrinate, Triplex, RID, or store brand products); alternative is to vacuum carefully to pick up lice and nits
B. Specific measures
    1. Head lice
        a. Thoroughly wet hair with permethrin 1% cream rinse applied to affected areas and washed off after 10 minutes or Triplex Kit (piperonyl butoxide [Pronto]), RID shampoo or

R&C shampoo, or End Lice; work up lather, adding water as necessary; shampoo thoroughly leaving shampoo on head for 5 minutes and rinse, or use Pronto shampoo/conditioner or Clear lice-killing shampoo and lice egg remover per directions on product or Klout per directions on product.
   b. Rinse thoroughly, towel dry
   c. Remove remaining nits with fine-tooth metal comb or tweezers (use of vinegar solution and hair conditioner or olive oil make combing easier)
   d. Consider buying and using a LiceMeister comb to remove nits and to check hair periodically for prevention
2. Body lice
   a. Bathe with soap and water if no lice are found
   b. Wash with warm water and dry in dryer all clothing, bedclothes, towels, and so forth
   c. Dry-clean items that cannot be washed; for items that cannot be washed or dry-cleaned, seal in a plastic bag for 1 week: lice will suffocate (in cold climates, put bags outside for 10 days; temperature change kills lice)
   d. If evidence of lice is found or the first two previously mentioned measures are not effective, use malathion 0.5% lotion applied for 8 to 12 hours, and thoroughly rinse off
3. Pubic lice
   a. Permethrin 1% cream (Nix) rinse applied to affected area and washed off after 10 minutes; *or*
   b. Pyrethrins with piperonyl butoxide (RID, Clear, A-200, Pronto, generics) applied to affected area and washed off after 10 minutes; *or*
   c. Malathion 0.5% lotion applied for 8 to 12 hours, and thoroughly rinsed off
   d. If pregnant or breastfeeding, use same products as previously mentioned
   e. Inform any sexual partners within past month that they need to be treated, too
   f. Wash in warm water and thoroughly dry on heat cycle or dry-clean all clothing, bed linen, towels, and so on, or remove from body contact for at least 72 hours
C. Carefully check family and household members and close contacts for evidence of lice contamination and if found, treat as previously mentioned or see clinician for advice
D. Call your clinician if signs of infection from scratching occur (redness, swelling of skin, discharge that looks like pus, bleeding, fever)
E. Stop using the treatment and call your clinician if you or your family members experience sensitivity to the treatment (pain, swelling, rash)
F. Consult with your clinician if you have lice on the eyelashes as the treatments cannot be used near the eyes. Ophthalmic (eye) ointment must be applied to the eyelashes twice a day for 10 days.

VI. FOLLOW-UP

Contact your clinician if itching, redness, or other problems listed previously persist or recur

Special notes: _____

Clinician: _____

Websites: http://www.health.state.ny.us/diseases/communicable/pediculosis/ fact_sheet.htm; http://www.headlice.org

Modern natural family planning (NFP) methods use normally occurring signs and symptoms of ovulation for both the prevention and achievement of pregnancy. No drugs or devices are used. The couple that uses one of the natural methods to prevent pregnancy makes the choice not to have intercourse during the method-defined fertile phase. Natural methods of family planning are 75% to 99% effective in preventing pregnancy, depending on the method used and on how well the information is taught and applied. The national NFP office uses 85% to 99% as the efficacy range based on "research typically cited." The monitoring of fertility signs also provides invaluable information for couples who are seeking pregnancy or struggling with infertility. Successful use of natural methods depends on competent instruction and follow-up, correct and consistent charting, and patient compliance with rules. NFP can be a pleasant, healthy way to avoid or achieve pregnancy and become aware of your individual fertility pattern.

I. COMMONLY USED METHODS OF NATURAL FAMILY PLANNING

    A. Cervical mucus method based on detectable changes in cervical mucus throughout the cycle

    B. Basal body temperature (BBT) method based on changes in the temperature of the woman's body at rest

    C. Sympto-thermal method is based on the changes in the body temperature, cervical mucus, and other bodily signs

    D. Sympto-hormonal method is based on the changes in cervical mucus and also makes use of the ClearBlue Easy Fertility Monitor. The fertility monitor detects rising estrogen and luteinizing hormone (LH) levels in the woman's urine and provides information on three levels of fertility (i.e., low, high, and peak).

    E. Standard Days Method makes use of CycleBeads (a plastic ring of colored beads) to track the fertility in a woman's cycle. The Standard Days Method provides a formula for woman who has cycles between 26 and 32 days in length. The days of the cycle that are considered fertile are days 8 to 19.

    F. The TwoDay Method is based on the presence or absence of cervical mucus. It makes use of two simple questions: (a) Do I have secretions today? (b) Did I have secretions yesterday? If the woman answers "no" to both questions, she can consider herself infertile that day.

    G. Terminology used in an NFP class

        1. *Abstinence:* not having vaginal sexual intercourse

        2. *Fertile days:* the days in the menstrual cycle when pregnancy (conception) is possible

        3. *Genitals or genitalia:* organs of the reproductive system in both male and female

4. *Genital-to-genital contact:* penis *touching* or coming into close contact with the vaginal area
5. *Hormone:* a substance that causes special changes in the body; may be naturally occurring or synthetically produced
6. *Infertile days:* the days in the menstrual cycle when pregnancy (conception) cannot occur
7. *Menstruation:* bleeding that occurs when the lining of the uterus breaks down and is released; this happens about 12 to 16 days after ovulation
8. *Menstrual cycle:* the time from the first day of menstrual bleeding to the day *before* the next menstrual bleeding begins; may vary normally from 21 to 40 days in length
9. *Ovulation:* release of the egg (ovum) from the ovary about 12 to 16 days before the onset of the next menstrual period (the day bleeding begins)
10. *Ovum:* female sex cell, egg
11. *Sperm:* male sex cell (spermatozoa) found in the semen

II. REVIEW OF THE MENSTRUAL CYCLE

The menstrual cycle is controlled by hormones. The cycle begins on the *first* day of menstrual bleeding and ends the day *before* menstrual bleeding begins again. Following menstruation, eggs (ova) are usually maturing in the follicles of the ovaries. As they grow, estrogen (a hormone known as the female sex hormone) is produced in increasing amounts, and the following certain changes take place:

A. The lining of the uterus builds up the blood supply needed for pregnancy to occur
B. Cervical mucus is produced and changes in character to become more hospitable to sperm so sperm can live and travel through the cervix, uterus, and fallopian tubes
C. The cervix becomes higher in the pelvis and softens as the cervical os opens to allow sperm to enter the uterus
D. BBT is low
E. As the time of ovulation nears, some women may experience one or more of the following changes:
   1. Clearer complexion and less oily hair
   2. Increase in energy level
   3. Spotting of blood
   4. Pain or aching in the pelvic area
   5. Breast tenderness and/or fullness
F. Once ovulation has occurred, there is an increase in the production of progesterone (another hormone important to the menstrual cycle and to pregnancy), and the following changes occur during the 12 to 16 days before menstruation begins:
   1. BBT rises
   2. Mucus becomes inhospitable to sperm so they cannot live and travel through the cervix, uterus, and fallopian tubes
   3. Cervix becomes lower, firmer, and the opening closes to prevent sperm from going into the uterus

4. Increased progesterone maintains the lining of the uterus in place for 12 to 16 days. As menstruation approaches, women may also experience one or more of the following changes:
   a. Cramps
   b. Headaches
   c. Oily hair and complexion, acne, or increase in acne
   d. Mood changes
   e. Decrease in energy level
   f. Desire to eat foods with sugar and/or salt
   g. Breast tenderness
   h. Pelvic aching or pain
   i. Low back pain; joint pain or aches

III. CERVICAL MUCUS METHOD

Cervical mucus is produced by tiny cells in the cervix. As the ovum is maturing, the mucus will change in a special way that helps keep sperm alive and makes it easier for sperm to travel into the uterus. The mucus loses this quality within a day after the ovum leaves the ovary. The quality or condition of the cervical mucus is an excellent indicator of the days in the menstrual cycle when the woman can become pregnant.

A. How to check the cervical mucus
   1. Begin checking for cervical mucus when the menstrual bleeding ends or becomes light enough to let you be able to determine its presence and traits
   2. As you go through the day, note mentally whether the area around the vaginal opening feels dry, moist, or wet
   3. Check sensation and for the presence of mucus each time you use the bathroom because the character of the mucus can change during the day. Cervical mucus should be checked before and after urination.
   4. Fold a piece of toilet tissue and wipe over the vaginal opening. If the tissue slides across the vaginal opening, the sensation is wet. If the tissue drags, pulls, or chafes across the vaginal opening, the sensation is dry. If the tissue sticks a little to the vaginal opening or if the sensation is neither wet nor dry, it is a moist sensation.
   5. After wiping, observe the tissue for the presence of cervical mucus. Note the color, texture, and stretchiness of the mucus. The best way to observe its characteristics is to place it between two fingers and slowly open the two fingers. The woman who does not want to touch the mucus can assess its traits by holding the tissue in both hands, then pulling it apart (see Figure I.1).

B. How to chart information about the mucus
   1. A new cycle starts the first day of the menstrual bleeding, regardless of the time of the day the flow begins. Write the date when bleeding begins in the space on the NFP chart.
   2. Record each day of bleeding with a star
   3. When the period ends, if the vaginal sensation is dry, chart a dry day using the letter D

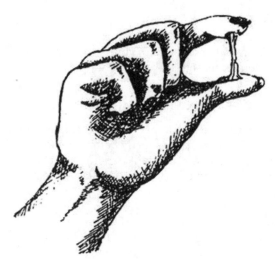

FIGURE I.1 Mucus check.

4. Continue to use the letter D each day until a moist or wet sensation is experienced. Chart a moist sensation using the letter M and a wet sensation by using the letter W.
5. Note the color and texture of any mucus found or observed on toilet tissue
6. Write an X through the W on the last day of wet vaginal sensation and/or slippery or stretchy mucus. The last day of slippery or stretchy mucus and/or wet sensation is called the *peak day*. This day will not be noted until the following day when the mucus will no longer be slippery or stretchy and the vaginal sensation will have changed to moist or dry.

C. Summary of mucus descriptions

	D	M	W	W
1. menses	dry sensation	moist sensation	wet sensation	peak day

2. Colors
   a. Yellow
   b. White
   c. Cloudy
   d. Clear
3. Texture
   a. Pasty like toothpaste or craft paste
   b. Creamy like hand lotion
   c. Slightly stretchy: stretches less than a half inch
   d. Stretchy: stretches more than a half inch
   e. Slippery like raw egg white
4. Always chart the most fertile sensation and the most fertile characteristics of the mucus.

D. How to chart other symptoms
   1. Record intercourse by a check mark
   2. Record any other changes in your body (e.g., pain with ovulation, breast tenderness) in the column under

IV. BASAL BODY TEMPERATURE METHOD

BBT is the temperature of the body at rest. As the ova are maturing, the temperature is low. At some time shortly before, during, or after the ovum leaves the ovary, the temperature will usually rise about three tenths to one full degree higher than it had been. A sustained temperature rise tells you that ovulation has taken place.
   A. How to take BBT
      1. Begin taking temperature on the first day of menstrual bleeding
      2. Take temperature about the same time every day, in the morning when you first awake. The thermometer can be placed in the mouth.
      3. Take temperature before eating, drinking, smoking, and doing any physical activity
      4. Record temperature on the NFP chart (see Figure I.2)
   B. Change in daily events
      Occasionally, a woman may become ill, drink alcoholic beverages, or change the usual time she takes her temperature. Because such events or any change in lifestyle may affect the temperature, when and if they happen, take and record the temperature anyway. In the "Notes" column on the NFP chart, record the possible reason for any change in the usual temperature. Circle your temperature each day on the NFP chart and connect the circles with a line (see Figure I.3).
   C. To adjust temperatures not taken at usual or base time
      1. Pick a base time
      2. For every *half hour* earlier than the base time, *add* one tenth of a degree to thermometer reading before it is recorded on the temperature graph
      3. For every *half hour* later than the base time, *subtract* one tenth of a degree from the thermometer reading before it is recorded on the temperature graph

V. THE CERVIX

After menses, the cervix is low in the vaginal canal, the opening is closed, and it feels firm or pointed, like the tip of a nose. As the ovum is developing and being released, the cervix will rise, soften, and the opening will become wide. These changes help sperm travel into the uterus. Within a few days after the ovum leaves the ovary (ovulation), the cervix will lower in the vaginal canal; it will feel firm or pointed and the opening will close up. These changes help prevent sperm from traveling into the uterus. It is not necessary to check the cervix in order to use a natural method. However, observing and charting the cervical changes can give interested women additional information about their fertile and infertile

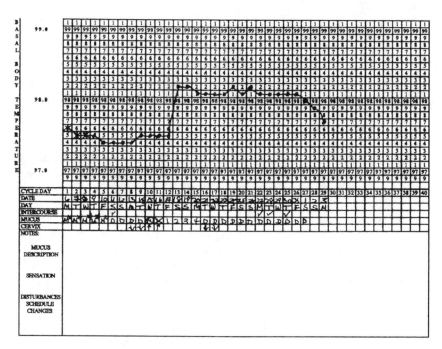

FIGURE I.2 Natural family planning chart.

To record your temperature . . .
Circle your temperature each day on the
Natural Family Planning Chart
and connect the circles with a line.

TEMPERATURE		1	2	3	4	5	6	7	8	9	10	11	12	13	14	15	16	1
	98.0	98	98	98	98	98	98	98	98	98	98	98	98	98	98	98	98	9
		9	9	9	9	9	9	9	9	9	9	9	9	9	9	9	9	
		8	8	8	8	8	8	8	8	8	8	8	8	8	8	8	8	
		7	7	7	7	7	7	7	7	7	7	7	7	7	7	7	7	
		6	6	6	6	6	6	6	6	6	6	6	6	6	6	6	6	
		5	5	5	5	5	5	5	5	5	5	5	5	5	5	5	5	
		4	4	4	4	4	4	4	4	4	4	4	4	4	4	4	4	
		3	3	3	3	3	3	3	3	3	3	3	3	3	3	3	3	
		2	2	2	2	2	2	2	2	2	2	2	2	2	2	2	2	2
		1	1	1	1	1	1	1	1	1	1	1	1	1	1	1	1	1
	97.0	97	97	97	97	97	97	97	97	97	97	97	97	97	97	97	97	9
		9	9	9	9	9	9	9	9	9	9	9	9	9	9	9	9	
CYCLE DAY		1	2	3	4	5	6	7	8	9	10	11	12	13	14	15	16	1

FIGURE I.3 Natural family planning chart (fragment).

days. The information can be particularly useful for the breastfeeding or premenopausal woman.

    A. How to check the status of the cervix

       1. Begin checking the cervix after the menstrual bleeding ends

       2. Check the cervix while in a comfortable position such as squatting or standing with one foot on a stool or chair. Use the same position each time you check the cervix.

       3. Check in the evening

       4. Wash your hands before placing a finger in the vagina

       5. When feeling the cervix, check for its position in vagina: high (may be difficult to feel) or low (usually easy to feel) softness or firmness opening: open or closed

       6. Chart the most fertile cervical sign of the day

    B. How to chart information about the cervix

       1. Use circles to represent the sizes of the cervical opening. Place the circles in different positions in the boxes on the NFP chart to represent the rising and lowering of the cervix. Another way the position of the cervix can be noted is through using arrows:

         a. Rising cervix

         b. Lowering cervix

       2. You can also use the letter F to represent a firm cervix and the letter S to represent a soft cervix (see Figure I.4)

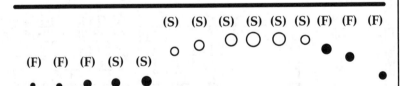
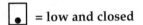
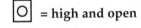

FIGURE I.4 Cervix chart.

C. Sympto-thermal method
   Combining use of all the information described to this point
D. Sympto-hormonal method
   Combining use of the cervical mucus information and the ClearBlue Easy Fertility Monitor
E. Two-day Method
   A woman observes for the presence or absence of cervical mucus secretions starting at noon. She observes for cervical mucus secretions by looking, touching, or feeling.
F. Looking observation
   When visiting the bathroom, the woman wipes and observes before urinating. She looks for cervical mucus secretions on the toilet paper. She can also look for the secretions on her underwear.
G. Touching observation
   When visiting the bathroom, the woman can touch the genital area with clean fingers or touch the surface of the toilet tissue for the presence or absence of secretions
H. Feeling observation
   As the woman goes about her daily activities, she pays attention to whether she feels moisture in her genital area

A woman marks daily on her client card whether she has or does not have secretions.

If she has her period or has had 2 days in a row without secretions, pregnancy is unlikely that day.

I. Standard Days Method
   This method is suitable for women with cycles between 26 and 32 days. The woman uses CycleBeads to keep track of her cycle. On the first day of her period, she puts the movable rubber ring on the red bead. She moves the ring from one bead to another each day in the direction of the arrow. Brown beads are infertile days and white beads are fertile days.

VI. NATURAL FAMILY PLANNING RULES

By following the NFP rules, women will know on which days they are fertile and infertile during each menstrual cycle. It is important for women to check with their instructor or health care provider before following any of the rules.

A. Ovulation method (observing and charting cervical mucus)
   1. To avoid pregnancy
      a. Avoid intercourse during menses
      b. Every other dry day rule (to determine which days before ovulation are infertile)
         i. Intercourse can take place on the evening of every other dry day. Fertility begins when mucus is observed or the sensation changes to moist or wet.
         ii. Intercourse is restricted to the evening so that the woman can observe her cervical mucus during the day undisturbed by intercourse

iii. It is common for some of the man's semen to be in the woman's vagina on the day after intercourse. If cervical mucus starts to be produced on that day, the presence of semen may prevent the woman from seeing or feeling the presence of mucus. This is the reason intercourse should not take place on consecutive evenings.

Dry Day	Abstinence	Dry Day	Abstinence
Intercourse in the evening	No Intercourse the next day	Intercourse in the evening	No Intercourse the next day

iv. When the fertile phase begins, the couple should not have vaginal intercourse until the fertile phase ends

c. Peak day rule (to determine which days after ovulation are infertile)

The fertile phase ends on the evening of the fourth day after peak day. This infertility lasts until the beginning of the next menses.

Remember: The peak day is the last day of wet sensation and/or slippery or stretchy mucus.

i. Mark the peak day on the chart with an "X"

ii. Number the days after peak day 1, 2, 3, 4. The sensation on these days must be moist or dry. There may be no mucus present or it may be pasty, sticky, or creamy. It may be cloudy, white, or yellow in color.

2. To achieve pregnancy

a. Follow the every other dry day rule until the mucus sign indicates fertility. This allows the woman to accurately chart her mucus sign and to identify the start of the fertile phase.

b. Intercourse should occur on days identified as fertile by the cervical mucus. Particular attention should be paid to the days of wet sensation *and* clear or slippery/stretchy mucus. It is important for the couple to begin intercourse at the first signs of fertility because the fertile phase is limited in length.

VII. BASAL BODY TEMPERATURE METHOD (OBSERVING AND CHARTING BASAL BODY TEMPERATURE)

A. To avoid pregnancy

1. Shortest cycle rule (to determine which days before ovulation are infertile days). This rule cannot be used until there is a record of at least six normal menstrual cycles.

Shortest Past Cycle	Assume Infertile	Fertility Begins	Abstinence Begins
26 days or longer	first 6 days of cycle	Day 7	Day 7
23–25 days	first 5 days of cycle	Day 6	Day 6
22 days or fewer	0 day	Day 1	Day 1

2. Earliest temperature rise rule (to determine which days before ovulation are infertile days)
   a. This rule cannot be used until there is a record of at least 12 normal menstrual cycles
   b. Subtract 7 days from the earliest recorded day of temperature rise. The result is the first day of fertility/abstinence.
   Example: Earliest recorded day of temperature rise Day 15: $15 - 7 = 8$.
   The first 7 days of the menstrual cycle are infertile, beginning with the first day of menstrual bleeding. Intercourse can take place at any time during these days. Fertility/abstinence begins on Day 8. If a shorter cycle is recorded, the formula needs to be recalculated.
3. Thermal shift rule (to determine which days after ovulation are infertile). Fertility ends after ovulation on the evening of the fourth consecutive temperature above the temperature cover line.
   a. Identify the temperature rise. Watch for the temperature rise—four temperatures in a row that are higher than the six preceding temperatures. Find the highest of the six temperatures immediately preceding the rise.
   b. Draw the temperature cover line. Draw a line across the chart one tenth of the degree above the highest of the six temperatures immediately preceding the rise. Number the first four temperatures above the temperature cover line.
B. To achieve pregnancy
   Previous charts can be reviewed to predict when a temperature rise might occur. Intercourse should occur on the days before an anticipated temperature rise.

VIII. SYMPTO-THERMAL METHOD (OBSERVING AND CHARTING BASAL BODY TEMPERATURE, CERVICAL MUCUS, AND OTHER BODILY SIGNS)

A. To postpone pregnancy (to determine which days before ovulation are infertile days).
   Use any of the following rules:
   Shortest cycle rule
   Earliest temperature rise rule
   Abstinence should begin if mucus appears at any time during the days that are determined infertile by the aforementioned rules
   Sympto-thermal method (to determine which days after ovulation are infertile)
   Fertility ends after ovulation on the evening of the fourth day after peak day or on the evening of the fourth day of temperature above the cover line, whatever occurs last
   1. Identify peak day. Peak day is the last day of wet sensation and/or slippery stretchy mucus. Mark peak day with an "X" and number the 4 days after peak day 1, 2, 3, and 4.

2. Identify the temperature rise. Watch for the temperature rise—four temperatures in a row that are higher than the six preceding temperatures. Find the highest of the six temperatures immediately preceding the rise.
3. Draw the temperature cover line. Draw a line across the chart one tenth of the degree above the highest of the six temperatures immediately preceding the rise. Number the first four temperatures above the temperature cover line.

B. To achieve pregnancy

Intercourse should occur on days that are identified as fertile by the cervical mucus. Particular attention should be paid to the days of wet sensation *and* clear or slippery/stretchy mucus. It is important for the couple to begin intercourse at the first signs of fertility because the fertile phase is limited in length. Previous charts can also be reviewed to predict when a temperature rise might occur. Intercourse should occur on the days before an anticipated temperature rise.

Websites: *http://nfp.marquette.edu; http://www.irh.org; http://www.cyclebeads.com*

I. DEFINITION

Osteoporosis is characterized by decreased bone mass (loss of bone density), deterioration of bone microarchitecture, and an increase in bone fragility and risk for bone fractures (broken bones).

II. ETIOLOGY

Humans have two types of bone—cortical and trabecular. Cortical bone is very compact; it forms the outer shell of bones and makes up 80% of the skeletons of adults. Trabecular bone, also called spongy or cancellous bone, makes up the remaining 20% and forms the interior of bones. For bones to develop properly and maintain bone mass, we need adequate calcium and phosphorus and other minerals in our diets. We also need other vitamins and adequate vitamin D for our bodies to absorb calcium from our diets and enable the body to maintain our bones.

We reach our peak bone mass at about 35 years of age. Estrogen seems to play a role in enabling women's bones to retain calcium and the other minerals necessary to build bone and preserve bone mass. From 35 years of age or so, some sources say that we lose about 2% of bone density each year. After menopause, the loss of bone mass may accelerate during the first 5 or 6 years. Thereafter, rate of loss returns to previous level. If bone mass loss becomes too great, the woman becomes very susceptible to fractures.

III. RISK FACTORS

The risk of developing osteoporosis is greater for women than for men (women begin with less bone mass), and increases with age. Women who have never had children, had early menopause (before the age of 50), are of northern European or Asian descent, have a thin body frame, blond or red hair, fair skin and freckles, curvature of the spine (scoliosis), are unable to digest milk or dairy products, smoke, have a high alcohol intake, low calcium diet, high salt diet, not enough vitamin D, drink more than two or three cups of caffeinated beverages a day, do not exercise or exercise excessively, live in a northern climate, have little fluoride in their drinking water, and have a family history of osteoporosis are at greater risk than women with none of these risks.

IV. PREVENTION

We cannot change our heritage, family history, gender, body build, hair or skin color, the time at which we go through natural menopause, or our inability to drink milk or eat milk products. However, we can exercise an appropriate amount, stop or never start smoking, limit alcohol intake, decrease or eliminate caffeine, decrease daily salt intake, and choose a diet with the amount of calcium we need. Current recommendations for calcium are 1,000 mg for women 19 to 50 years of age and 1,200 mg starting at the age of 51.

Calcium-rich foods include broccoli; bok choy; collard, mustard, and turnip greens; kale; and oranges. Dairy products, sardines, salmon with bones, shrimp paste, dried anchovies, soy products (tofu, soy milk, etc.), and almonds are all high in calcium. Vitamin D recommendation is no more than 4,000 IU daily. This can be obtained from 5 to 10 minutes in the sun each day, drinking the equivalent of a quart of vitamin D fortified milk, or taking a vitamin D supplement. Foods rich in vitamin D include fatty fish, butter, vitamin D–fortified margarine, egg yolks, and liver. Your clinician may choose to do a vitamin D blood level.

We can help prevent osteoporosis by changing what we can change in our lifestyles and by considering hormone therapy after menopause. Hormone therapy, known as HT, is not for every woman and is a decision each should make very carefully with her health care provider.

If you do not choose to use HT, in addition to all the lifestyle changes that are discussed previously, you may also consider the use of vitamins—especially 400 U of vitamin E each day, and exploring botanicals or other homeopathic products with knowledgeable persons.

V. TREATMENT FOR OSTEOPOROSIS

If you have osteoporosis, you can prevent further loss of bone mass and, in some cases, actually restore bone mass with a regimen of exercise prescribed by a clinician specializing in osteoporosis therapy.

Calcium supplements, adequate vitamin D, hormonal and nonhormonal drug therapy, changes in lifestyle including smoking cessation, decreasing or eliminating caffeine, and lowering alcohol intake can also improve the health of your bones.

Making your home as safe as possible will help you avoid fractures. Nurses and physical therapists specializing in working with persons with osteoporosis can help you reduce or eliminate those hazards.

Website: http://www.mayoclinic.com/health/osteoporosis/DS00128

I. DEFINITION

Polycystic ovary syndrome (PCOS) is a complex condition of the endocrine system (including the ovaries). It is one of the most common reproductive tract problems in women younger than 30 years of age. Some women, when examined with laparoscopy (a lighted scope for viewing the inside of the abdominal and pelvic areas), have ovaries with a thickened capsule and multiple cysts of the follicles (that develop and release eggs).

II. SIGNS AND SYMPTOMS (ONLY 20% TO 30% OF WOMEN HAVE THESE)

    A. Menstrual cycles without ovulation
    B. Infertility—inability to conceive
    C. No menses (periods) or very scanty menses
    D. Prolonged menses, sometimes unpredictable or irregular menses
    E. Increase in body and facial hair
    F. Increase in or appearance of acne
    G. Loss of hair especially at the crown
    H. Whitish breast discharge
    I. Change in body shape—increased waist to hip ratio
    J. Increase in skin pigment at the nape, in axillae (under arms), and in the groin area

III. DIAGNOSIS

    A. The diagnosis is made based on the signs and symptoms, laboratory tests, ultrasound of the ovaries, and imaging of the adrenal glands
    B. Refer for testing or test for metabolic syndrome based on criteria of the World Health Organization, the International Diabetes Federation, or the National Cholesterol Education Program. These include central obesity, hypertension, glucose uptake, and triglyceride level (see websites for criteria for each).
    C. Laboratory testing can include measures of androgens (male hormones), function and hormone level tests for thyroid, adrenal, and pituitary glands

IV. TREATMENT

    A. Weight loss and exercise program
    B. Low-dose combination oral contraceptives with a low-androgenic progestin to restore menstrual cycles and have a beneficial effect on hyperandrogenism
    C. Possibly prescription drugs to reduce excessive hair growth and acne
    D. Medications for Type 2 (noninsulin dependent) diabetes seem to help symptoms
    E. Electrolysis and/or depilatories for excessive hair
    F. Medications to induce ovulation when pregnancy is desired

V. PATIENT EDUCATION
  A. Education about PCOS and lifestyle alterations
  B. Education about pharmacologic (prescription drug) interventions
  C. Education about fertility

Special Notes: _____

Clinician: _____

Websites: For more information, visit http://www.pcosupport.org; criteria for the diagnosis of metabolic syndrome include the World Health Organization criteria that can be found at http://www.medicinenet.com/metabolic_syndrome/article.htm

The International Diabetes Foundation criteria can also be found at http://www.idf.org/idf-worldwide-definition-metabolic-syndrome

For National Cholesterol Foundation criteria, visit http://www.medscape.com/viewarticle/552000

1. It is helpful to have someone accompany you when you are evaluated for a medical abortion
2. Follow directions from the caregiver in taking pain medication as recommended
3. Seek emergency treatment if you are bleeding (soaking through two thick full-sized sanitary pads per hour for two consecutive hours); you have pelvic pain uncontrolled with medication regimens recommended; you have a fever higher than 100.4°F that lasts for more than 4 hours; severe abdominal pain; weakness; nausea; vomiting; and/or diarrhea for more than 24 hours after taking misoprostol
4. Normal physical activities may be resumed as soon as you feel ready
5. You may experience some uterine cramping (similar to menstrual cramps). It is okay to take acetaminophen (Tylenol, Datril, Tempra, Valadol, Valorin, Acephen) for cramps, or ibuprofen 800 mg (Motrin, Advil; every 8 hours).
6. Consult your clinician if you experience any of the following signs of incomplete abortion or infection:
   a. Uncontrolled bleeding
   b. Continued pregnancy symptoms (nausea/vomiting or breast tenderness 1 week after the medical abortion)
   c. Unexplained fever
   d. Failure to return to how you felt before you became pregnant
   e. Because of the risk of infection, it is important not to have intercourse or to insert anything into the vagina for 2 to 3 weeks. Other forms of sexual activity or orgasm will not be harmful to your body. Do not douche at all and do not use tampons for 2 to 3 weeks after the procedure, or until you stop bleeding.
7. Bleeding will probably cease after 3 to 4 days, but may last up to 3 weeks. There may be no bleeding at all. If bleeding exceeds two sanitary pads an hour or if you have a fever, call your clinician or the facility where the procedure was performed.
8. Menstruation (period) should resume in 4 to 6 weeks but may take as long as 8 weeks and as short as 2 weeks
9. You will be given an appointment with a clinician 2 to 3 weeks after your abortion. The clinician will check to see whether your body is back to normal and will provide you with your desired form of contraception or schedule an appointment for a diaphragm or cap fitting 6 weeks after the abortion. An intrauterine device (IUD) can be inserted immediately after or within 3 weeks of a first-trimester miscarriage or abortion. Depo-Provera may be given the day of the abortion or within 5 days of the procedure. This appointment will also give you an opportunity to discuss your feelings. A friend or partner is welcome to see the clinician with you if you wish.

10. If you have chosen to use a hormonal contraceptive method, begin on the Sunday following the abortion procedure. If not, be sure to use another form of contraception such as spermicide and condoms when you resume sexual relations. Remember, you will probably ovulate before you resume menses; you can become pregnant any time after your abortion. If you received Depo-Provera after your abortion, it is still important to return for your postabortion checkup 2 to 3 weeks after the procedure. You can then schedule your next Depo-Provera shot.

If you have a problem or concern, call the clinician or office at _____.

Website: http://www.fwhc.org/abortion/medical-ab.htm

The purpose of preconception self-care is to help you be at your healthiest as you plan a pregnancy. Advanced planning can help reduce your risk of having a low birth weight or premature baby. Working with your clinician, you can identify any medical condition or medications you are taking that need to be considered when contemplating a pregnancy. You may also wish to have a genetic consultation if you or your partner has a family history of inherited disorders such as cystic fibrosis, Tay-Sachs disease, hemophilia, or birth defects in the family. Infections such as sexually transmitted diseases (STDs) and tuberculosis may affect the health of a pregnancy, or even your ability to conceive.

Good health is important for a successful pregnancy and healthy baby. A complete health history and physical examination including a Pap smear, pelvic exam, and screening for STDs, as well as other communicable diseases such as hepatitis B and C and HIV prior to conception, will ensure that your body is in an optimal state for a pregnancy. Having your immunizations up-to-date will protect you and your baby. Evaluation of your nutritional state, diet and exercise patterns, and your toxin exposure at work and at home will help you prepare your body for conception.

Smoking and using alcohol and/or street drugs can have serious consequences for the health of a pregnancy and baby. At least one month before attempting to conceive, women who smoke, drink alcohol, or use street drugs should stop. If you use prescription or over-the-counter drugs, limit them to those your clinician approves of. In addition, check with your clinician about the use of herbals, homeopathics, and vitamins.

Protect yourself from exposure to toxins as much as possible. These include pesticides, household cleaning products, gases, lead, solvents, and radiation. Modify, undertake, or continue your program of exercise. Bring your immunizations up-to-date (although some are contraindicated in pregnancy, it is best to do this at least one month before trying to conceive).

Eat a balanced diet, paying particular attention to fresh fruits and vegetables (five–nine or more servings a day); whole grain breads, cereals, and pasta; protein (especially fish, poultry, legumes, eggs, and nonfat dairy products); and drink six to eight glasses of water a day. Avoid eating raw fish or raw meat. Decrease or eliminate caffeine from your diet (including coffee, tea, and carbonated soft drinks). Begin taking 400 μg of folic acid a day; a prenatal vitamin that includes at least 400 μg of folic acid is fine. Increase your calcium intake to the equivalent of 1 qt of milk a day (1,200–1,500 mg of calcium). In general, avoid food with plenty of preservatives and artificial sweeteners.

Avoid hot tubs and saunas because these bring your body temperature higher than 102°F, which can limit or eliminate sperm production. Avoiding such excessive heat will also protect the baby once conception has occurred.

If you are on hormonal contraceptives, stop using them at least one month before you plan to conceive to allow your body to resume cycling.

Several months are advised, because it often takes that long to resume ovulatory (fertile) cycles. You can use spermicides and condoms until you wish to try to conceive.

To maximize the health of their sperm, men who are planning to have children should stop smoking and using street drugs, drink only in moderation (one glass a day), and avoid toxin exposure at least three months before attempting conception. They should also have their infectious disease status checked through an STD screen and hepatitis B and C and HIV testing. One half of the baby's genetic material comes from the father, so he needs to be in good health.

Discuss with your partner your feelings about parenting, your expectations of him or her, and what parenting means to you. How do you expect your life to change? How will having a child change your relationship, the way your household functions, your work schedule, your expectations, and those of your partner? Who will be the primary parent? Will one or both of you have parenting leave? How will your finances be affected by having a child? How do you plan to integrate a new baby into the household with other children, extended family, and other members of the household?

Planning for a pregnancy will help you be at your best when you conceive. It will also help you consider the changes that pregnancy and a baby will have on your life and the lives of those close to you.

For resources on genetic counseling, nutrition, prenatal care, and prenatal classes, as well as information on conception and pregnancy, ask your clinician and check your community library, your local bookstore, and online such as the March of Dimes Birth Defects Foundation, http://www.modimes.org; information on preconception care can be found at http://www.womenshealth.gov/pregnancy/before-you-get-pregnant/preconception-health.cfm

I. DEFINITION

The premenstrual syndrome (PMS) consists of a group of behavioral and cognitive dysfunctions and physical symptoms that are associated with the menstrual cycle

II. SIGNS AND SYMPTOMS

A. Usually appear 1 week prior to menses but may also appear up to 2 weeks or just several days before menses, and include:
 1. Mood fluctuations—anxiety, crying, persistent anger
 2. Depression, feeling hopeless
 3. Fatigue, lethargy; joint or muscle pain
 4. Weight gain
 5. Headache
 6. Irritability
 7. Breast tenderness
 8. Increased appetite, craving for sweets and/or salt
 9. Insomnia/sleep disturbance
 10. Inability to concentrate, reduced interest in usual activities
 11. Constipation
 12. Palpitations
 13. Hot flashes
 14. Abdominal bloating
 15. Acne
 16. Changes in sex drive
B. If you are bothered by these changes, make an appointment with your clinician for a consultation. A complete history will be taken, and a diet and exercise regimen will be suggested. You will also be scheduled for a complete physical examination.

III. TREATMENT

Treatment consists of alleviating the signs and symptoms that are described previously with a diet and exercise plan and/or medication

A. Diet recommendations
 1. Limit your salt intake to 3 g or less per day (i.e., avoid using the saltshaker)
 2. Limit your intake of alcohol
 3. Avoid caffeine (e.g., coffee, tea, chocolate, soft drinks)
 4. Increase your intake of complex carbohydrates (e.g., fresh fruit, vegetables, whole grains, pasta, rice, potatoes)
 5. Consume moderate protein and fat. Limit your red meat consumption to 2 times weekly.
B. Exercise recommendations
 1. Exercise 3 times per week for 30 to 40 minutes. Examples are brisk walking, jogging, aerobic dancing, martial arts, swimming, and bicycling.

C. Medications
  1. Take vitamins, calcium supplements, and other medications such as antidepressants, as prescribed or recommended by your clinician
D. Consider complementary therapies such as meditation, botanicals, aroma or muscle therapy, energy healing, massage therapy, naturopathy, and acupuncture. Talk with your clinician about these.

You may be evaluated monthly for 3 months to determine the effects of diet, exercise, vitamins, and your symptoms. If there is no improvement at that time, a more extensive workup may be done with possible referral.

I. DEFINITION

Scabies is a highly contagious skin rash whose chief symptom is itching. Scabies is caused by the scabies mite (*Sarcoptes scabiei*), which burrows into the skin and deposits its eggs along the tunnel it has made. The eggs hatch in 3 to 5 days and gather around hair follicles. Newly hatched female mites burrow into the skin, mature in 10 to 19 days, then mate and start a new cycle. Norwegian scabies (crusted scabies) is an aggressive infestation of the scabies mite.

II. TRANSMISSION

A. Scabies among adults may be sexually transmitted
B. Persons living in proximity with others, in dormitories, and in crowded living spaces are more likely to incur scabies if one person among them becomes infested with the mite. Persons sharing clothing or towels are at increased risk. So are persons with blood malignancies such as leukemia, persons who are HIV positive, and those persons with other conditions in which their immune systems are compromised or have a history of atopic dermatitis.

III. SIGNS AND SYMPTOMS

A. May appear 4 to 6 weeks after contact with scabies from another person, because it takes several weeks for sensitization to develop. In persons who are previously infected, symptoms may appear within 24 hours after repeat exposure to the scabies mite.
B. Itching becoming worse at night or at times when the body temperature is raised such as after exercise. Itching begins first, before other signs and symptoms.
C. Lesions are usually on the webs between fingers, the inner aspects of the wrists and elbows, areas surrounding the nipples, umbilicus (belly button), belt line, lower abdomen, genitalia, and cleft between the buttocks. It can be all over the body, especially in persons whose immune systems are compromised. These lesions look like little burrows about 0.5 to 0.75 in. in length, ending in a raised red area (papule) or a raised area filled with fluid (vesicle). These lesions can become scaly and become crusted over. When scratched, the areas become raw looking and become infected.

IV. DIAGNOSIS

A. Diagnosis is made through examination of lesions and of those areas of the body that are most frequently involved
B. Linear burrows can be seen in the affected area
C. Scaling, crustation lesions, furuncles (boils), and/or scratches may be visible with secondary infection
D. When scrapings from the lesions are examined under low power with a microscope, the mites can sometimes be seen

V. TREATMENT
A. Treatments to kill mites
1. 5% permethrin cream (Elimite), applied to all areas of the body from neck down and washed off after 8 to 14 hours, *or*
2. Ivermectin 200 μg/kg *orally*, repeated in 2 weeks (not for children younger than 2 years old or less than 33 lbs or for pregnant or breastfeeding women)
3. Do not use lindane (Kwell) without consulting a clinician because it can be toxic
B. Treatments to relieve symptoms. Antihistamines may be taken to relieve itching (these do not kill the mites but may make you feel better).
C. General measures to decrease the risk of reinfestation
1. Clothing, towels, and bed linens should be laundered (hot cycle) and dried on heat cycle or dry-cleaned on day of treatment with medication
2. If clothing items cannot be washed or dry-cleaned, separate them from the cleaned clothes and do not wear for at least 72 hours. Mites cannot exist for more than 2 to 3 days away from the body. You can decontaminate mattresses, sofas, and rugs with over-the-counter sprays or powders.
3. Sexual partner and close personal or household contacts within the past month should be informed and referred to a clinician for examination and treatment

VI. PATIENT EDUCATION
A. Follow the treatment regimen carefully
B. Itching may persist for several weeks. If you do not respond to therapy and if itching persists after 1 week, contact your clinician to decide whether further therapy is necessary.
C. Call your clinician if the infested areas bleed, do not seem to be healing, are swollen or warm to the touch, or have drainage that looks like pus. You may have a secondary infection and need additional treatment.
D. Discontinue treatment and call your clinician if you develop a rash after using medication

VII. FOLLOW-UP
A. Call your clinician if:
1. Lesions do not begin to resolve with treatment or you are getting new lesions
2. The treatment has brought out another skin condition, the one that you had previously, such as eczema or psoriasis
3. Lesions appear to be spreading and increasing in size
4. Lesions appear crusted
B. Return to your clinician if symptoms persist or new symptoms occur
C. Return to your clinician for evaluation of the success of the treatment, or the need for retreatment

Website: http://www.cdc.gov/NCIDOD/DPD/parasites/scabies/factsht_scabies.htm

Spermicides

I. DEFINITION/MECHANISM OF ACTION

Spermicides are a barrier method of birth control. All spermicides contain an inert base or vehicle and an active ingredient, most commonly a surfactant such as nonoxynol-9 that disrupts the integrity of the sperm membrane (acts as a spermicide).

II. EFFECTIVENESS AND BENEFITS
    A. Method: 96% effectiveness rate
    B. User: 60% effectiveness rate
    C. Inexpensive and readily available

III. SIDE EFFECTS AND DISADVANTAGES
    A. Local irritation from spermicide
    B. Can necessitate the interruption of intercourse
    C. Emotional difficulty with touching one's own body

IV. TYPES
    A. Creams, jellies, gels
    B. Foams
    C. Foaming tablets
    D. Suppositories
    E. Vaginal film

V. HOW TO USE
    A. Instructions should be read prior to using any spermicide. Method of insertion, time of effectiveness, time needed prior to intercourse, and so forth will vary with each type.
    B. Use new insertion of spermicide with each intercourse
    C. After each use, wash the applicator with soap and water
    D. When using a spermicide, your partner should always use a condom unless you use a female condom

VI. FOLLOW-UP
    A. Yearly physical examination with Pap smear is recommended

Condoms

I. DEFINITION/MECHANISM OF ACTION

Condoms are thin sheaths, most commonly made of latex (female condoms are made of polyurethane; male polyurethane condoms are now on the market), that prevent the transmission of sperm from the penis to the vagina

II. EFFECTIVENESS AND BENEFITS

    A. Method: 97% to 98% effectiveness rate, providing the method is used correctly

    B. User: 70% to 94% effectiveness rate

    C. Inexpensive and readily available

    D. Offer protection against sexually transmitted disease. Only latex condoms provide protection against the AIDS (HIV) virus. The female condom is made of thick polyurethane so it does offer protection.

    E. Encourage male participation in birth control

III. SIDE EFFECTS AND DISADVANTAGES

    A. Allergic reaction to latex (rare). (Female condom is made from polyurethane as are some male condoms.)

    B. Use necessitates the interruption of intercourse for application

    C. May decrease tactile sensation

    D. Psychological impotency with male condom

    E. If latex allergy is a problem, double condom use is an option. If the woman is allergic, the male can wear a latex condom with a skin or polyurethane condom covering it. If the man is allergic, he can wear a polyurethane or skin condom with a latex condom over it. Skin condoms should not be worn alone because they do not offer protection from HIV.

IV. TYPES

Condoms vary in color, texture (smooth, studded, or ribbed), shape, and price; they come lubricated and plain; some have spermicide; some are extra strength; some are sheerer and thinner; some have a unique shape; and some are scented or flavored

V. HOW TO USE MALE CONDOM

    A. Always pull the male condom on an erect penis and before there is any sexual contact. Use for every act of intercourse

    B. Do not pull the male condom tightly over the end of the penis; leave about an inch extra for ejaculation fluid and to avoid breakage; some condoms have a reservoir tip

    C. Withdraw before the penis becomes limp and hold the open end of the condom tightly while withdrawing

    D. Partner should always use a contraceptive spermicide along with condom

    E. Condoms should be used only once

VI. HOW TO USE FEMALE CONDOM

The female condom comes prelubricated

    A. Pinch ring at closed end of the pouch and insert like a diaphragm covering the cervix; adding one to two drops of additional lubricant makes insertion easier and decreases or eliminates squeaking noise and dislocation during intercourse

    B. Adjust other ring over the labia

C. Can be inserted several minutes to 8 hours prior to intercourse
D. Remove before standing up by squeezing and twisting the outer ring and pulling out gently

If the condom breaks or slips off, check the website http://not-2-late.com for emergency contraception information. Plan B is now available over the counter for women 18 years of age and older.

Smoking is the leading cause of preventable illness and early death in the United States. If you stop, you can expect an increase in your life expectancy and an improvement in your health.

Smokers are at greater risk for:
- Strokes
- Cancer of the larynx
- Oral cancers—tongue, lip, gum
- Lung disease
- Chronic obstructive pulmonary disease
- Heart disease and heart attack
- Possibly breast cancer

Smokers may also develop other smoking-related problems:
- Pregnancy complications and losses
- Sinus infections
- Cataracts
- Impotence and infertility
- Osteoporosis and bone density problems
- Premature skin wrinkling
- Gum disease and dental cavities
- Stained teeth and bad breath
- Poor circulation
- Poor tolerance for exercise
- High blood pressure

Family members are at greater risk for:
- Lung cancer and heart disease
- Children of smokers have higher incidences of sudden death syndrome, asthma and other lung problems, ear infections, colds, and learning delays
- The rewards of quitting are experienced quickly and long term

Within several weeks of quitting smoking:
- Blood pressure drops, circulation improves
- Lung function improves
- Coughing, sinus infections, fatigue, and shortness of breath improve
- Number of colds decreases
- Energy level improves

The risk of lung cancer is increased for both current and former smokers compared with those who never smoke and declines for former smokers with increasing duration of abstinence.

Other long-term benefits include decrease in heart disease; cancer of the mouth, throat, and esophagus; stroke risk; and coronary heart disease.

Do you think you have a dependence on nicotine? Ask yourself the following questions:

- Do you smoke a cigarette first thing in the morning?
- Do you wake up to smoke a cigarette during the night?
- Do you smoke five or more cigarettes a day?
- Do you find it hard not to smoke in places where it is forbidden? Do you leave such places to smoke?
- Do you smoke more cigarettes in hours after you wake up than during the rest of the day?
- Do you smoke when you are ill?

If you answer "yes" to any of these questions, you can consider yourself as having a nicotine problem.

If you want to quit, the following suggestions may help:

1. Make the decision to stop smoking
2. Think about why you want to stop smoking. Make a list of those reasons and the rewards associated with quitting. Keep this list with you and review it when you feel the urge to smoke.
3. Talk to your friends and family; ask for their support and encouragement.
4. Keep a journal. You can start it when you are making the decision to quit. Record each cigarette smoked, the time, the place, the intensity of the craving, and the reward of the cigarette. Think about the social cues associated with smoking and about how you will deal with these after you stop smoking. Record your thoughts and feelings. Doing this can help you identify your smoking "triggers" and assist you in adapting strategies and skills to get past those triggers. Continue recording your feelings in the journal after you have quit smoking.
5. Avoid drinking alcohol. Alcohol will weaken your resolve.
6. Clean your clothes, car, drapes, and furniture to rid them of the smell of smoke.
7. Throw out all cigarettes, ashtrays, and smoking paraphernalia.
8. Avoid being around other smokers.
9. If possible, establish living space as "no smoking."
10. Increase exercise level (walking, weight lifting, yoga, tai chi). This assists in weight management, stress reduction, and general sense of well-being.
11. Change your daily routine to avoid smoking triggers.
12. Keep oral substitutes handy. Use low calorie vegetables and fruits; sugarless gum; toothpicks.
13. Engage in activities that make smoking difficult, such as exercising, gardening, or washing the car.
14. Spend time in places where smoking is prohibited.
15. Join a support group. Such groups are offered by Nicotine Anonymous, American Cancer Society, the American Lung Association, and your local hospital or health care center.

16. Make an appointment with your clinician to talk about your desire to stop smoking. Your clinician can help you choose the most appropriate method to assist in breaking your habit. Choices available include:
    - Nicotine replacements: gum, transdermal patches, nasal sprays, inhaler
    - Zyban or Wellbutrin SR: a nonnicotine oral medication for smoking cessation treatment
    - Chantix (varenicline): an oral medication. Use by pilots, bus drivers, and truck drivers is prohibited by the federal government

Good luck in your journey to a smoke-free life. Remember, if you have a relapse and start smoking again, you can quit again. Many people need to try several times before they are successful. If this happens to you, do not be too hard on yourself. Review the previous suggestions and begin again.

Stress or Urge Incontinence
(Loss of Urine)

Stress and urge incontinence are caused by relaxation of the muscles and ligaments of the pelvic floor, that is, the muscles and ligaments that support the bladder, uterus, urethra (tube leading from the bladder to the outside), lower bowel, and vagina. Because of this relaxation, which is commonly the result of stretching due to childbirth and normal loss of muscle elasticity with aging, any stress such as laughing, coughing, or sneezing can cause involuntary loss of urine or the need to urinate urgently, known as urge incontinence.

Urine can be irritating to the skin, so it is important to wash it off as soon as possible. The ammonia odor from urine leakage may also be distressing. Cotton underwear; the use of nondeodorized, unscented panty liners; and the use of wipes especially designed for the perineal area, such as baby wipes, will all help to prevent irritation, rashes, and cracking of skin. Skin cracking, irritation, and rashes will often increase the possibility of bacterial infection, especially in the warm, moist, genital area. Dusting with cornstarch will protect the skin from irritation. Only mild, unscented soaps should be used, and used sparingly, because soaps can be drying to skin. Perfumes (which are alcohol based) can also increase the drying effect and may cause an allergic reaction or chemical irritation to sensitive skin. Avoid bubble baths, vaginal hygiene products, and perfumed powders and talcum for the same reasons. Caffeine and smoking should also be avoided—both are bladder irritants (see Figure I.5). In addition, try to identify irritants that cause you to have urge incontinence and eliminate

Log of Times of Urine Loss, Circumstances of Loss, and Amount

	S	M	T	W	T	F	S
Week 1							
Week 2							
Week 3							
Week 4							

FIGURE I.5 Log of times of urine loss, circumstances of loss, and amount.

those. Some of these include citrus fruits and juices, caffeine (even the lesser amount in decaffeinated coffees, teas, and chocolate), and alcohol.

Diary of Incontinence

Code numbers for WHEN

1. Coughing/sneezing
2. Laughing/crying
3. Blowing nose
4. Climbing stairs

5. Bending over
6. Sitting or resting
7. Washing hands or dishes
8. Other times

Code letters for AMOUNT

a. A drop or two
b. A teaspoonful
c. A tablespoonful
d. More than a tablespoonful

Kegel (Pelvic Floor Muscle Strengthening) Exercises

Practice contracting, holding, and relaxing each time you urinate until you can stop the flow completely and start and stop at will. Then proceed to this exercise program.

Day 1: Repeated contracting, holding, and relaxing of pubococcygeus muscle (muscle band of perineal area) 4 times this day, 10 contractions and 10 relaxations each time.

Log for Pelvic Floor Exercise
(Place a checkmark in box for each exercise period each day)

	S	M	T	W	T	F	S
Week 1							
Week 2							
Week 3							
Week 4							

FIGURE I.6 Log for pelvic floor exercises.

Day 2: Increase to 20 contractions and 20 relaxations, 4 times this day.
Day 3: Increase to 30 contractions and 30 relaxations, 4 times this day.
Day 4: Increase to 40 contractions and 40 relaxations, 4 times this day.
Day 5: Increase to 70 contractions and 70 relaxations, 4 times this day.

Continue with Day 5 regimen, so you are now doing the exercise 4 times each day, contracting and relaxing 70 times at each of the four exercise periods (see Figure I.6).

You may want to ask your clinician about the vaginal cones or sphere to help you practice. Graduated weighted cones are available to assist in Kegel exercises; a cone is inserted in the vagina and Kegel exercises are performed using the cones' feedback; when weight of one cone can be maintained for 15 minutes when walking or standing, move to next weight. The sphere is inserted in the vagina to strengthen pelvic muscle tone. You can do Kegel exercises with the sphere in place as well.

1. Someone should accompany you to the facility where you are to have the abortion and wait there to take you home.
2. You may resume your normal physical activities according to the post-operative care instructions that will be given to you and as soon as you feel ready.
3. You may be given some medication (Methergine or Ergotrate, and/or an antibiotic) to take after your abortion. The first two medications will help your uterus return to its normal size and decrease bleeding. Antibiotics will help prevent infection. Follow the directions on how to take the pills. You may experience some uterine cramping (similar to menstrual cramps) with or without the Methergine or Ergotrate, because each of these medications causes the uterus to contract to help it to return to prepregnancy size. It is okay to take acetaminophen (Tylenol, Datril, Tempra, Valadol, Valorin, Acephen) for cramps, or ibuprofen (Motrin, Advil).
4. Because of the risk of infection, it is important not to have intercourse or to insert anything including fingers into your vagina for 2 to 3 weeks. Other forms of sexual activity or orgasm will not be harmful to your body. Do not douche at all and do not use tampons for 2 to 3 weeks after the procedure, or until you stop bleeding. You may also be given 3 to 5 days of antibiotics to help prevent infection. Be sure to complete this medication.
5. Bleeding will probably cease after 3 to 4 days, but may last up to 3 weeks. There may be no bleeding at all. If bleeding exceeds two sanitary pads an hour, if you have a fever, or are passing clots the size of a quarter or larger, call your clinician or the facility where the procedure was performed. If you continue to have bright red bleeding longer than 3 days, call your clinician. Bleeding should change from bright red to darker red and then to pink and then whitish mucousy discharge by the end of 3 weeks, and it should decrease in amount.
6. Menstruation (period) should resume in 4 to 6 weeks but may take as long as 8 weeks and as short as 2 weeks. You will probably ovulate (produce an egg) before you have a period, so protect yourself from pregnancy or abstain from vaginal-penile intercourse until you are using a contraceptive method.
7. You will be given an appointment with a clinician 2 to 3 weeks after your abortion. The clinician will check to see that your body is back to normal and will provide you with your desired form of contraception or schedule an appointment for a diaphragm or FemCap fitting 6 weeks after the abortion. An intrauterine device (IUD) can be inserted immediately after or within 3 weeks of a first-trimester miscarriage or abortion. Depo-Provera may be given the day of the abortion or within 5 days of the procedure. This appointment will also give you an opportunity to discuss your feelings. A friend or partner is welcome to see the clinician with you if you wish.

8. If you have chosen to use a hormonal contraceptive method, begin on the Sunday following the abortion procedure. If not, be sure to use another form of contraception such as spermicide and condoms when you resume sexual relations. Remember, you can become pregnant any time after your abortion if you are not using contraception. If you received Depo-Provera after your abortion, it is still important to return for your postabortion checkup 2 to 3 weeks after the procedure. You can then schedule your next Depo-Provera shot. If you choose to use the contraceptive implant, you can schedule an appointment for its insertion at the time of your postoperative visit.

9. If you have a problem or concern, call the clinician's clinic or office at:

Website: http://teenadvice.about.com/cs/optionsabortion/a/exabortion_4.htm

I. DEFINITION

Syphilis is a sexually transmitted disease (STD) that can affect any organ in the body such as the bones, brain, and/or heart. It is spread by sexual contact and can also be passed on from the mother to her unborn baby. It is caused by the organism *Treponema pallidum*.

II. IMPORTANT INFORMATION

    A. Any sexually active person can get infected with syphilis. An untreated person can spread syphilis for 1 year after being infected.

    B. Symptoms can occur 10 to 90 days after sexual contact; the average is 21 days

III. USUAL SIGNS AND SYMPTOMS: WHAT YOU MAY EXPERIENCE

    A. *Primary syphilis.* The first sign of syphilis is a painless chancre (sore) at the site of entry of the syphilis organism in an average of about three weeks after infection has occurred. The chancre may occur on the vulva, labia, opening to vagina, clitoris, cervix, nipple, lip, roof of mouth, finger, bite area, opening to the urethra on the head of the penis, the shaft of the penis, the anal area, or the scrotum. You may notice painful and/or swollen glands in your groin area, on your neck, or under your arms. The chancre heals in 3 to 6 weeks and will go away even if not treated. If you are not diagnosed and treated, you will progress to secondary syphilis.

    B. *Secondary syphilis.* In 2 to 8 weeks or as long as 6 months after the chancre appears (average is 6 weeks), you will notice a rash on any part of your body. It can even appear on the palms of your hands or the soles of your feet. You may also have some hair loss so that your head has a moth-eaten look and you may lose part of your eyebrows. You may notice swollen glands in any part of your body, have a low-grade fever, a sore throat, headache, feel tired, have loss of appetite, and your joints may feel sore. This will last about 6 weeks and go away without treatment. If you are not diagnosed and treated, you will progress to latent syphilis.

    C. *Latent syphilis.* You will have no symptoms, although 25% of persons may have a chancre again. During primary and secondary syphilis and early latency, you are infectious to sexual partners. After 12 months have passed from the date of the initial infection, you are no longer infectious but the organism is in your blood. If you are not diagnosed and treated, you may remain in the latent stage for the rest of your life.

    D. *Tertiary syphilis.* One third of persons infected with syphilis and not treated will go into the tertiary stage. In this stage, your bones, skin, heart, or nervous system including your brain can be affected. Persons with tertiary syphilis can become unable to work or care for themselves and have a shortened life.

IV. DIAGNOSIS
A. History of sexual contact with a known infected person
B. Blood tests and examination of material from a chancre under a special microscope to see the syphilis organism

V. TREATMENT
The treatment of choice is penicillin given by injection. For those allergic to penicillin, other antibiotics can be used. The amount and treatment will depend on the stage of the syphilis.

VI. COMPLICATIONS
A. Progression of the disease to tertiary stage
B. Transmission of syphilis from a woman to her unborn baby, causing congenital syphilis in the baby. Congenital means present at birth. Congenital syphilis can cause permanent damage to the baby.

VII. PATIENT EDUCATION
A. Follow-up for second dose of medications as instructed by health care provider
B. Use barrier contraception (condom) each time you have sexual intercourse
C. Look for signs on your partner before having sex. If you see a sore (chancre), rash, swelling, or discharge, consider a checkup for both of you before having sex.
D. If you think you may have contracted syphilis or any other STD, avoid having sex and visit a local STD clinic
E. If you are diagnosed with syphilis, report any sexual partners to your clinician so they can be notified and treated, or notify them to seek treatment
F. Return for testing after treatment for primary or secondary syphilis at 6 and 12 months; for latent syphilis, return for testing at 6, 12, and 24 months
G. There is no immunity to syphilis, so you can be reinfected by an infected partner

Return for treatment if you believe you have been infected again.

Special Notes:_____

Clinician:_____

For more information call the Centers for Disease Control and Prevention (CDC) STD hotline at 1-800-CDC-INFO. Phone numbers of free (or almost free) STD clinics are listed in the Community Service Numbers in the government pages of your local phone book.
Website: http://www.cdc.gov/std/syphilis/default.htm

I. DEFINITION
Trichomoniasis is a parasitic infection occurring in the female vagina or urethra, or male urethra and prostate. The infection is usually sexually transmitted, although it has been identified in nonsexually active women.

II. SIGNS AND SYMPTOMS
A. May appear 5 to 30 days after contact
B. In female, symptoms include:
  1. Foul-smelling, greenish yellow, frothy vaginal discharge (often fishy)
  2. Painful intercourse or urination
  3. Discomfort on tampon insertion
  4. Itchiness of the perineal area and vagina
  5. Redness and irritation of the vulva and upper thigh
  6. Pap smear may be abnormal
  7. Some patients may not have any symptoms
C. In male, symptoms include:
  1. Mild itch or discomfort in penis
  2. Moisture at tip of penis disappearing spontaneously
  3. Slight early morning discharge from penis before first urination
D. Untreated symptoms in female or male can progress to infection of neighboring urinary and reproductive organs

III. DIAGNOSIS
A. Female evaluation may include:
  1. Vaginal examination to check for trichomoniasis and to rule out yeast infections and bacterial infections such as gonorrhea or bacterial vaginosis
  2. Blood test to rule out syphilis
B. Male evaluation may include:
  1. Examination for gonorrhea or urinary tract infection
  2. Blood test for syphilis

IV. TREATMENT
The male should seek treatment after exposure to a partner with the infection. He may have no symptoms but could harbor the parasite in his urethra or prostate.

It is very important to report any medical conditions you have (especially seizure disorder) or any medication you take regularly before taking any treatment.

V. PATIENT EDUCATION
A. Take no alcohol during the 48 hours after treatment (medication) per instructions from your clinician

B. For minor side effects of medication (nausea, dizziness, or metallic taste), take medication with some food or milk
C. Advise sexual contact(s) to seek simultaneous treatment
D. Use condoms until all partners are treated

VI. FOLLOW-UP

Return to your clinician if symptoms persist or if new symptoms occur

Special notes: _____

Clinician: _____

For more information call Centers for Disease Control and Prevention (CDC) Sexually Transmitted Disease (STD) hotline at 1-800-CDC-INFO. Phone numbers of free (or almost free) STD clinics are listed in the Community Service Numbers in the government pages of your local phone book.

Websites: http://www.cdc.gov; http://www.cdc.gov/NCIDOD/dpd/parasites/trichomonas/default.htm

I. DEFINITION/MECHANISM OF ACTION

The vaginal contraceptive sponge looks like a small doughnut with a hollow in the center. The hollow area fits over the cervix. The sponge measures about one and three fourths of an inch in diameter. Across the bottom is a string loop to provide for easy removal. The sponge is polyurethane and contains the spermicide nonoxynol-9. It provides a barrier between the sperm and the cervix, traps sperm within the sponge, and releases spermicide to inactivate sperm over 24 hours.

II. EFFECTIVENESS AND BENEFITS
   A. 89% to 90.8% effectiveness
   B. May be inserted before intercourse and left in place for up to 24 hours
   C. Latex-free
   D. Over the counter—no prescription needed
   E. No need to add extra spermicide within 24 hours

III. SIDE EFFECTS AND DISADVANTAGES
   A. Vaginal irritation from the sponge
   B. Vaginal irritation from the spermicide in the sponge
   C. Sensation of something in the vagina
   D. Difficulty in inserting or removing the sponge
   E. Some concern about sponge using increasing the risk of toxic shock syndrome if not used as directed. Use with care or do not use during menses.
   F. Frequent use of nonoxynol-9 can cause genital irritation and increase the risk of HIV and other sexually transmitted diseases

IV. EXPLANATION OF METHOD
   A. How to insert
     1. Read instructions carefully before using
     2. Wash your hands before opening the package
     3. Open package carefully to avoid tearing the sponge
     4. Wet the sponge with water
     5. Insert in vagina as you would a tampon
     6. The sponge can be inserted any time up to 24 hours before sexual intercourse. There is no need to add spermicide once the sponge has been moistened with water and inserted.
     7. The sponge can be left in place for up to 24 hours from the time you inserted it and offers protection for each act of intercourse
   B. How to remove
     1. Read printed instructions carefully
     2. Wash your hands with soap and water
     3. Remember to remove sponge slowly to avoid tearing it
     4. Do not flush the sponge down the toilet

5. Special removal instructions
   a. If the sponge appears to be stuck, relax your vaginal muscles and bear down, and you should be able to remove it without difficulty
   b. The sponge may turn upside down in the vagina, making the string more difficult to find. To find the string, run your finger around the edge on the back side of the sponge until you feel the string. If you cannot find the loop, grasp the sponge between your thumb and forefinger and remove it slowly.
C. Remember that the sponge cannot get lost in the vagina

V. ADDITIONAL INFORMATION
A. It is okay to use the sponge while swimming or bathing
B. The sponge should be used only once and then discarded

VI. DANGER SIGNS OF TOXIC SHOCK SYNDROME
A. Fever (temperature higher than 101°F)
B. Diarrhea
C. Vomiting
D. Muscle aches
E. Rash (sunburn-like)

Yearly physical examination including Pap smear is recommended

Website: http://www.todaysponge.com

All women have a normal discharge called leukorrhea; the amount and consistency vary with each individual. This discharge is generally of a mucus-like consistency and tends to increase during the menstrual cycle up to 2 weeks before menstruation. A normal vaginal discharge may vary slightly in color, although it is usually clear or white, has no unpleasant odor, and is not itchy or irritating to the skin. Occasionally, a woman may notice a fishy or musty-smelling discharge if she has recently had vaginal inter-course. This may be caused by dead sperm being cleansed from the vagina. If this occurs persistently, do not confuse it with a bacterial infection or overgrowth called vaginosis. Have it checked by a clinician. Some methods of birth control may affect the amount of normal vaginal discharge.

Hints for Prevention of Vaginal Infection

1. Even under the best conditions, vaginal infections sometimes occur. Do not panic if you discover that you have such an infection. Treat it with common sense: cleanliness, pelvic rest (no intercourse), prescribed medications, and wear sensible clothing (cotton panties, cotton crotch panties, no panty hose under slacks, no underwear to bed).
2. Cleanliness and personal hygiene are very important. Keep clean by bathing (shower or tub, but be sure you disinfect the tub before and after use) with soap and water. Vaginal deodorants can be irritating and are worthless in treating or preventing an infection. Avoid all use of feminine hygiene sprays and deodorants as well as deodorant or scented tampons, pads, panty liners, and toilet papers because these products tend to alter the natural environment of the vagina and make it more susceptible to irritation and/or infection.
3. *Routine douching is never recommended.* It can be harmful if done when an infection is already present. For example, the pressure of the douche solution may cause the infection to spread into the womb (uterus) and become even worse. In addition, the douche solution removes the natural cleansing secretions of the vagina that normally help to maintain an environment that prevents infections. Indiscriminate douching with various commercial products may aggravate existing conditions, set up a chemical vaginitis (inflammation, irritation of the vagina), or contribute to a pelvic infection. Only douche under the direction of a clinician, following directions carefully.
4. To prevent both vaginal and bladder infections from occurring, wear cotton underwear or underwear and panty hose with a cotton crotch and no underwear while sleeping; change tampons or sanitary napkins after each urination or bowel movement; wipe yourself in the front first and then the back after going to the bathroom; urinate after intercourse and/or genital stimulation; and drink plenty of fluids (at least 6 glasses of water a day); cranberry juice or cranberry tablets may be helpful in avoiding infection.

Rules to Follow if You Have a Vaginal Infection (Vaginitis) or a Vaginosis

1. Take the entire course of medication exactly as prescribed. If you do not, the infection may go underground temporarily and then return and be more troublesome than before.
2. If you are treating an infection with vaginal cream or suppositories, remain lying down in bed for at least 15 minutes after insertion to allow the medication to spread deeply around the cervix, where it is needed. Standing up may cause the medicine to seep outward toward the vaginal opening.
3. Do not use tampons for protection because they will absorb the medication and reduce its effectiveness. Instead, use unscented external pads or small minipads to prevent staining underwear.
4. If you have a vaginal infection and use a diaphragm, soak diaphragm for 30 minutes with Betadine scrub (not solution) or 70% rubbing alcohol after using prescribed medication for 2 days and again when medication is completed. Use alcohol for your FemCap or Lea's Shield.
5. Sexual relations should be avoided for at least 1 week, and preferably throughout the entire course of treatment. Intercourse can be very irritating to the inflamed vagina and cervix during an infection and can slow down the healing process. In addition, the bacteria or other organisms that cause your infection might spread to your partner; if the partner is male, he should use a condom during the entire treatment period. Note that females can share vaginal infections with their female partners.
6. Insufficient lubrication prior to intercourse may contribute significantly to vaginal infections (and bladder infections). Water-soluble jelly can be used for lubrication. There are also vaginal lubricants and moisturizers especially for perimenopausal and postmenopausal women.

Bibliographies

ABDOMINAL AND PELVIC PAIN

Ahonen, K. A. (2009). Ovarian cancer: Clinical and genetic considerations. *Advance for Nurse Practitioners, 17*(1), 47–49.

Flowers, J. (2008). Uterine fibroids: Brief overview of presentation, diagnosis and treatment. *Advance for Nurse Practitioners, 16*(10), 36–40.

Hornick, L., & Slocumb, J. C. (2008). Treating chronic pelvic pain: Focus on pain triggers and neurogenic inflammation. *Advance for Nurse Practitioners, 16*(2), 44–53.

Lippert, J., Wilkins, G., & Hornick, L. (2008). Endometriosis: Toward more timely treatment. *The Clinical Advisor, 11*(2), 28–32.

Menon, S., Sammel, M. D., Vichnin, M., & Barnhart, K. T. (2007). Risk factors for ectopic pregnancy. *Journal of Pediatric and Adolescent Gynecology, 20*(3), 181–185.

Witt, C. M., Reinhold, T., Brinkhaus, B., Roll, S., Jena, S., & Willich, S. N. (2008). Acupuncture in patients with dysmenorrhea: A randomized study on clinical effectiveness and cost effectiveness in usual care. *American Journal of Obstetrics and Gynecology, 198*(2), 166e1–166e8.

Zitkus, B. S. (2009). Evaluation of the acute abdomen. *Advance for Nurse Practitioners, 17*(2), 28–35.

ABNORMAL VAGINAL BLEEDING

Chapa, H. O., Venegas, G., Antonetti, A. G., Van Duyne, C. P., Sandate J., & Bakker, K. (2009). In-office endometrial ablation using a third-generation uterine balloon therapy system: 12-month prospective follow-up on menstrual patterns and dysmenorrhea impact. *The Journal of Reproductive Medicine, 54*(11–12), 678–684.

Food and Drug Administration. (2009, Nov 13). *FDA approves Lysteda to treat heavy menstrual bleeding* [Press release]. Retrieved from http://www.fda.gov/NewsEvents/Newsroom/PressAnnouncements/ucm190551.htm

Hale, G. E., Manconi, F., Luscombe, G., & Fraser, I. S. (2010). Quantitative measurements of menstrual blood loss in ovulatory and anovulatory cycles in middle- and late-reproductive age and the menopausal transition. *Obstetrics and Gynecology, 115*(2, Pt. 1), 249–256.

Hazard, D., & Harkins, G. (2009). Patient satisfaction with thermal balloon ablation for treatment of menorrhagia. *American Journal of Obstetrics and Gynecology, 200*(5), e21–e23.

James, A. H., Kouides, P. A., Abdul-Kadir, R., Edlund, M., Federici, A. B., Halimeh, S., . . . Winikoff, R. (2009). Von Willebrand disease and other bleeding disorders in women: Consensus on diagnosis and management from an international expert panel. *American Journal of Obstetrics and Gynecology, 201*(1), 12.e1–12.e8. Retrieved from http://dx.doi.org/10.1016/j.ajog.2009.04.024

Lopes, J. E., Jr., & Sherer, E. (2010). Managing menorrhagia: Evaluating and treating heavy menstrual bleeding. *Advance for NPs & PAs, 1*(2), 21–24.

Maggard, M. A., Yermilov, I., Li, Z., Maglione, M., Newberry, S., Suttorp, M., . . . Shekelle, P. G. (2008). Pregnancy and fertility following bariatric surgery: A systematic review. *The Journal of the American Medical Association, 300*(19), 2286–2296.

Metwally, M., Ong, K. J., Ledger, W. L., & Li, T. C. (2008). Does high body mass index increase the risk of miscarriage after spontaneous and assisted conception? A meta-analysis of the evidence. *Fertility and Sterility, 90*(3), 714–726.

Nejat, E. J., Polotsky, A. J., & Pal, L. (2010). Predictors of chronic disease at midlife and beyond—the health risks of obesity. *Maturitas, 65*(2), 106–111.

Peeters, A., Barendregt, J. J., Willekens, F., Mackenbach, J. P., Al Mamun, A., Bonneux, L., & the Netherlands Epidemiology and Demography Compression of Morbidity Research Group (NEDCOM). (2003). Obesity in adulthood and its consequences for life expectancy: A life-table analysis. *Annals of Internal Medicine, 138*(1), 24–32.

Penninx, J. P. M., Mol, B. W., & Bongers, M. Y. (2009). Endometrial ablation with paracervical block. *The Journal of Reproductive Medicine, 54*(10), 617–620.

Polotsky, A. J., Hailpern, S. M., Skurnick, J. H., Lo, J. C., Sternfeld, B., & Santoro, N. (2010). Association of adolescent obesity and lifetime nulliparity—the Study of Women's Health Across the Nation (SWAN). *Fertility and Sterility, 93*(6), 2004–2011.

ABORTION

Beal, M. W. (2007). Update on medication abortion. *Journal of Midwifery & Women's Health, 52*(5), 23–30.

Carbonell Esteve, J. L., Marí, J. M., Valero, F., Llorente, M., Salvador, I. Varela, L., . . . Muñoz, E. (2006). Sublingual versus vaginal misoprostol (400 μg) for cervical priming in first-trimester abortion: A randomized trial. *Contraception, 74*(4), 328–333.

Clark, W. H., Gold, M., Grossman, D., & Winikoff, B. (2007). Can mifepristone medical abortion be simplified? A review of the evidence and questions for future research. *Contraception, 75*(4), 245–250.

Davey, A. (2006). Mifepristone and prostaglandin for termination of pregnancy: Contraindications for use, reasons and rationale. *Contraception, 74*(1), 16–20.

Foster, A. M., Wynn, L., Rouhana, A., Diaz-Olavarrieta, C., Schaffer, K., & Trussell, J. (2006). Providing medication abortion information to diverse communities: Use patterns of a multilingual web site. *Contraception, 74*(3), 264–271.

Heikinheimo, O., Leminen, R., & Suhonen, S. (2007). Termination of early pregnancy using flexible, low-dose mifepristone-misoprostol regimens. *Contraception, 76*(6), 456–460.

Lohr, P. A., Reeves, M. F., Hayes, J. L., Harwood, B., & Creinin, M. D. (2007). Oral mifepristone and buccal misoprostol administered simultaneously for abortion: A pilot study. *Contraception, 76*(3), 215–220.

Marions, L. (2006). Mifepristone dose in the regimen with misoprostol for medical abortion. *Contraception, 74*(1), 21–25.

Moreau, C., Trussell, J., Desfreres, J., & Bajos, N. (2010). Patterns of contraceptive use before and after an abortion: Results from a nationally representative survey of women undergoing an abortion in France. *Contraception, 82*(4), 337–344.

ABUSE AND VIOLENCE

Campbell, J. C. (1995). *Assessing dangerousness.* Newbury Park, CA: Sage.

Chen, P. H., Rovi, S., Vega, M., Jacobs, A., & Johnson, M. S. (2005). Screening for domestic violence in a predominantly Hispanic clinical setting. *Family Practice, 22*(6), 617–623.

Chen, P. H., Rovi, S., Washington, J., Jacobs, A., Vega, M., Pan, K. Y., & Johnson, M. S. (2007). Randomized comparison of 3 methods to screen for domestic violence in family practice. *Annals of Family Medicine, 5*(5), 430–435.

Curry, M. A., Renker, P., Hughes, R. B., Robinson-Whelen, S., Oschwald, M., Swank, P. R., & Powers, L. E. (2009). Development of measures of abuse among women with disabilities and the characteristics of their perpetrators. *Violence Against Women, 15*(9), 1001–1025.

Family Violence Prevention Fund. (2009). *The facts on domestic, dating and sexual violence.* Retrieved from http://www.endabuse.org/content/action_center/detail/754

Hien, D., & Ruglass, L. (2009). Interpersonal partner violence and women in the United States: An overview of prevalence rates, psychiatric correlates and consequences and barriers to help seeking. *International Journal of Law and Psychiatry, 32*(1), 48–55.

Laughon, K., Renker, P., Glass, N., & Parker, B. (2008). Revision of the abuse assessment screen to address nonlethal strangulation. *Journal of Obstetric, Gynecologic, and Neonatal Nursing, 37*(4), 502–507.

MacMillan, H. L., Wathen, C. N., Jamieson, E., Boyle, M. H., Shannon, H. S., Ford-Gilboe, M., . . . McNutt, L. A. (2009). Screening for intimate partner violence in health care settings: A randomized trial. *The Journal of the American Medical Association, 302*(5), 493–501.

Wathen, C. N., Jamieson, E., MacMillan, H. L., & The McMaster Violence Against Women Research Group. (2008). Who is identified by screening for intimate partner violence? *Women's Health Issues, 18*(6), 423–432.

AMENORRHEA

Lee, S., Kil, W. J., Chun, M., Jung, Y. S., Kang, S. Y., Kang, S. H., Oh, Y. T. (2009). Chemotherapy-related amenorrhea in premenopausal women with breast cancer. *Menopause, 16*(1), 98–103.

Poyastro Pinheiro, A., Thornton L. M., Plotonicov, K. H., Tozzi, F., Klump, K. L., Berrettini, W. H., . . . Bulik, C. M. (2007). Patterns of menstrual disturbance in eating disorders. *The International Journal of Eating Disorders, 40*(5), 424–434.

Practice Committee of American Society for Reproductive Medicine. (2008). Current evaluation of amenorrhea. *Fertility and Sterility, 90*(Suppl. 2), S219–S225.

Taffe, J. R., Cain, K. C., Mitchell, E. S., Woods, N. F., Crawford, S. L, & Harlow, S. D. (2010). "Persistence" improves the 60-day amenorrhea marker of entry to late-stage menopausal transition for women aged 40 to 44 years old. *Menopause, 17*(1), 191–193.

Tavasoli, F., Hafizi, L., & Aalami, M. (2009). Pelvic endometriosis in a patient with primary amenorrhea. *Medical Journal of Reproduction and Infertility, 10*(2), 151.

Thompson, S. H. (2007). Characteristics of the female athlete triad in collegiate cross-country runners. *Journal of American College Health, 56*(2), 129–136.

BREAST CONDITIONS

Dietrich, J. E., & Brandt, M. L. (2009). Disorders of the adolescent breast. *The Female Patient, 34*, 22–26.

Duffy, C., Perez, K., & Partridge, A. (2007). Implications of phytoestrogen intake for breast cancer. *A Cancer Journal for Clinicians, 57*(5), 260–277.

Edwards, Q. T., Seibert, D., Maradiegue, A., MacDonald, D., Jasperson, K., Lowstuter, K., & Weitzel, J. (2007). Breast cancer and the family tree: An issue for all practice settings. *Advance for Nurse Practitioners, 15*(5), 34–41.

Lee, E. (2009). Evidence-based management of benign breast diseases. *The American Journal for Nurse Practitioners, 13*(7–8), 22–31.

Saslow, D., Boetes, C., Burke, W., Harms, S., Leach, M.O. Lehman, C.D., . . . Russell, C. A. (2007). American Cancer Society guidelines for breast screening with an MRI as an adjunct to mammography. *A Cancer Journal for Clinicians, 57*, 75–89.

CERVIX, PAP SMEARS, HUMAN PAPILLOMAVIRUS

American Cancer Society. (2011). Cancer facts and figures 2009. Retrieved from http://www.cancer.org/research/cancerfactsfigures/cancerfactsfigures/cancer-facts-figures-2011

American College of Obstetricians and Gynecologists. (2009). Evaluation and management of abnormal cervical cytology and histology in adolescents. *Obstetrics and Gynecology, 113*(6), 1422–1425.

American College of Obstetricians and Gynecologists. (2009). Health care for undocumented immigrants. *Obstetrics and Gynecology, 113*(1), 251–254.

American Society for Colposcopy and Cervical Pathology. (2007). *Management of women with atypical squamous cells of undetermined significance (ASC-US)*. Retrieved from http://www.asccp.org/ Portals/9/docs/pdfs/Consensus%20Guidelines/algorithms_cyto_07.pdf

American Society for Colposcopy and Cervical Pathology. (2009). *Management of women with a histological diagnosis of cervical intraepithelial neoplasia grade 1 (CIN 1) preceeded by ASC-US,ASC-H,orLSILcytology*. Retrieved from http://www.asccp.org/pdfs/consensus/algorithms_hist_07.pdf

Cancer Research UK. (2009). Cervical cancer statistics: Key facts. Retrieved from http://info.cancerresearchuk.org/cancerstats/types/cervix/

Castle, P. E., Fetterman, B., Poitras, N., Lorey, T., Shaber, R., & Kinney, W. (2009). Five-year experience of human papillomavirus DNA and Papanicolaou test cotesting. *Obstetrics and Gynecology, 113*(3), 595–600.

Dillner, J., Rebolj, M., Birembaut, P., Petry, K. U., Szarewski, A., Munk, C., . . . Iftner, T. (2008). Long term predictive values of cytology and human papillomavirus testing in cervical cancer screening: Joint European cohort study. *British Medical Journal, 337*:a1754. doi:10.1136/bmj.a1754

Kaplan, J. E., Benson, C., Holmes, K. H., Brooks, J. T., Pau, A., & Masur, H. (2009). Guidelines for prevention and treatment of opportunistic infections in HIV-infected adults and adolescents: Recommendations from CDC, the National Institutes of Health, and the HIV Medicine Association of the Infectious Diseases Society of America. *Morbidity and MortalityWeekly Report, 58*(RR-4), 1–207. Retrieved from http://www.cdc.gov/mmwr/pdf/rr/rr58e324.pdf

National Health Service. (2009). *NHS Cervical cancer screening programme*. Retrieved from http://www.cancerscreening.nhs.uk/cervical/

Nationaal Programma Kankerbestrijding. (2009). *Monitor reference page: Cervical cancer screening*. Retrieved from http://www.npknet.nl/1521-p-1052

Naucler, P., Ryd, W., Törnberg, S., Strand, A., Wadell, G., Elfgren K., . . . Dillner, J. (2007). Human papillomavirus and Papanicolaou tests to screen for cervical cancer. *The New England Journal of Medicine, 357*(16), 1589–1597.

Ronco, G., Giorgi-Rossi, P., Carozzi, F., Confortini, M., Dalla Palma, P., Del Mistro, A., . . . Segnan, N. (2008). Results at recruitment from a randomized controlled trial comparing human papillomavirus testing alone with conventional cytology as the primary cervical cancer screening test. *Journal of the National Cancer Institute, 100*(7), 492–501.

Sawaya, G. F., Iwaoka-Scott, A. Y., Kim, S., Wong, S. T., Huang, A. J., Washington, A. E. & Pérez-Stable, E. J. (2009). Ending cervical cancer screening: Attitudes and beliefs from ethnically diverse older women. *American Journal of Obstetrics and Gynecology, 200*(1), 40.e1–40.e7.

Smith, R. A., Cokkinides, V., Brooks, D., Saslow, D., & Brawley O. W. (2009). Cancer screening in the United States, 2010: A review of current American Cancer Society guidelines and issues in cancer screening. *A Cancer Journal for Clinicians, 60*(2), 99–119.

Solomon, D., Davey, D., Kurman, R., Moriarty, A., O'Connor, D., Prey, M., . . . Young, N. for the Forum Group Members and the Bethesda 2001 workshop. (2002). The 2001 Bethesda system. *Journal of the American Medical Association, 287*(16), 2114–2119.

Stoler, M. H. (2002). New Bethesda terminology and evidence-based management guidelines for cervical cytology findings. *The Journal of the American Medical Association, 287*(16), 2140–2141.

U.S. Census Bureau. (2004). *U.S. interim projections by age, sex, race, and Hispanic origin: 2000–2050*. Retrieved from http://www.census.gov/population/www/projections/usinterimproj

U.S. Preventive Services Task Force. (2011). *Screening for cervical cancer*. Retrieved from http://www.ahrq.gov/clinic/pocketgd1011/gcp10s2.htm

Wright, T. C., Jr., Massad, L. S., Dunton, C. J., Spitzer, M., Wilkinson, E. J., & Solomon, D. for the 2006 American Society for Colposcopy and Cervical Pathology-sponsored Consensus Conference. (2007). *American Journal of Obstetrics & Gynecology, 197*(4), 340–345. doi:10.1016/j.ajog.2007.07.050

COMPLEMENTARY AND ALTERNATIVE THERAPIES

Alraek, T., Borud, E., & White, A. (2011). Selecting acupuncture treatment for hot flashes: A Delphi consensus compared with a clinical trial. *Journal of Alternative Complementary Medicine, 17*(1), 33–38. doi:10.1089/acm.2010.0070

Anastasi, J. K., Chang, M., & Capili, B. (2011). Herbal supplements: Talking with your patients. *Journal for Nurse Practitioners, 7*(1), 29–35.

Barnard, K., & Colón-Emeric, C. (2010). Extraskeletal effects of vitamin D in older adults: Cardiovascular disease, mortality, mood, and cognition. *The American Journal of Geriatric Pharmacotherapy, 8*(1), 4–33.

Bercaw, J., Maheshwari, B., & Sangi-Haghpeykar, H. (2010). The use during pregnancy of prescription, over-the-counter, and alternative medications among Hispanic women. *Birth, 37*(3), 211–218.

Bosage, P. M., & Freeman, S. (2009). Bioidentical hormones, compounding and evidence-based medicine: What women's health practitioners need to know. *Journal for Nurse Practitioners, 5*(6), 421–427.

Gossler, S. M. (2010). Use of complementary and alternative therapies during pregnancy, postpartum, and lactation. *Journal of Psychosocial Nursing and Mental Health Services, 48*(11), 30–36.

Green, A. K., Hankison, S. E., Bertone-Johnson, E. R., & Tamimi, R. M. (2009). Mammographic density, plasma vitamin D levels and risk of breast cancer in postmenopausal women. *International Journal of Cancer, 127*(3), 667–674. doi:10.1002/ijc.25075

Griffith, R., & Tengnah, C. (2010). Regulation of herbal medicines. *British Journal of Community Nursing, 15*(9), 445–448.

Kelley, K. W., & Carroll, D. G. (2010). Evaluating the evidence for over-the-counter alternatives for relief of hot flashes in menopausal women. *Journal of the American Pharmacists Association, 50*(5), e106–e115.

Knight, J. A., Wong, J., Blackmore, K. M., Raboud, J. M., & Vieth, R. (2010). Vitamin D association with estradiol and progesterone in young women. *Cancer Causes & Control, 21*(3), 479–483.

Lakhan, S. E., & Vieira, K. F. (2010). Nutritional and herbal supplements for anxiety and anxiety-related disorders: Systematic review. *Nutrition Journal, 9*(1), 42.

Lloyd, K. B., & Hornsby, L. B. (2009). Complementary and alternative medications for women's health issues. *Nutrition in Clinical Practice, 24*(5), 589–608.

Lunny, C. A., & Fraser, S. N. (2010). The use of complementary and alternative medicines among a sample of Canadian menopausal-aged women. *Journal of Midwifery & Women's Health, 55*(4), 335–343.

McKenzie, S. C., & Rahman, A. (2010). Bradycardia in a patient taking black cohosh. *The Medical Journal of Australia, 193*(8), 479–481.

Meier, B., & Spriano, D. (2010). Modern HPTLC—a perfect tool for quality control of herbals and their preparations. *Journal of AOAC International, 93*(5), 1399–1409.

Micozzi, M. S., & Pribitkin, E. A. (2010). Common herbal remedies, adverse reactions, and dermatologic effects. *Skinmed, 8*(1), 30–36.

Millen, A. E., Wactawski-Wende, J., Pettinger, M., Melamed, M. L., Tylavsky, F. A., Liu, S., . . . Jackson, R. D. (2010). Predictors of serum 25-hydroxyvitamin D concentrations among postmenopausal women: The women's health initiative calcium plus vitamin D clinical trial. *The American Journal of Clinical Nutrition, 91*(5), 1324–1335.

Morgan, L. M., Major, J. L., Meyer, R. E., & Mullenix, A. (2009). Multivitamin use among non-pregnant females of childbearing age in the Western North Carolina multivitamin distribution program. *North Carolina Medical Journal, 70*(5), 386–390.

Ross, A. C., Manson, J. E., Abrams, S. A., Aloia, J. F., Brannon, P. M., Clinton, S. K., . . . Shapses, S. A. (2010). The 2011 report on dietary reference intakes for calcium and vitamin D from the Institute of Medicine: What clinicians need to know. *The Journal of Clinical Endocrinology and Metabolism, 96*(1), 69–71. doi:10.1210/jc.2010–2704

Sarris, J., & Kavanagh, D. J. (2009). Kava and St. John's wort: Current evidence for use in mood and anxiety disorders. *Journal of Alternative and Complementary Medicine, 15*(8), 827–836.

Sassarini, J., & Lumsden, M. A. (2010). Hot flashes: Are there effective alternatives to estrogen? *Menopause International, 16*(2), 81–88.

Schonberg, M. A., & Wee, C. C. (2005). Menopausal symptom management and prevention counseling after the Women's Health Initiative among women seen in an internal medicine practice. *Journal of Women's Health, 14*(6), 507–514.

Serby, M. J., Yhap, C., & Landron, E. Y. (2010). A study of herbal remedies for memory complaints. *The Journal of Neuropsychiatry and Clinical Neurosciences, 22*(3), 345–347.

Shams, T., Setia, M. S., Hemmings, R., McCusker, J., Sewitch, M., & Ciampi, A. (2010). Efficacy of black cohosh-containing preparations on menopausal symptoms: A meta-analysis. *Alternative Therapies in Health and Medicine, 16*(1), 36–44.

Sharan, C., Halder, S. K., Thota, C., Jaleel, T., Nair, S., & Al-Hendy, A. (2011). Vitamin D inhibits proliferation of human uterine leiomyoma cells via catechol-O-methyltransferase. *Fertility and Sterility, 95*(1), 247–253.

Staud, R. (2011). Effectiveness of CAM therapy: Understanding the evidence. *Rheumatic Diseases Clinics of North America, 37*(1), 9–17.

Whelan, A. M., Jurgens, T. M., & Naylor, H. (2009, Fall). Herbs, vitamins and minerals in the treatment of premenstrual syndrome: A systematic review. *The Canadian Journal of Clinical Pharmacology, 16*(3), e407–e429.

CONTRACEPTION AND EMERGENCY CONTRACEPTION

Ahern, R., Frattarelli, L. A., Delto, J., & Kaneshiro, B. (2010). Knowledge and awareness of emergency contraception in adolescents. *Journal of Pediatric and Adolescent Gynecology, 23*(5), 273–278. doi:10.1016/j.jpag.2010.02.010

Bonny, A. E., Secic, M., & Cromer, B. A. (2011). Relationship between weight and bone mineral density in adolescents on hormonal contraception. *Journal of Pediatric and Adolescent Gynecology, 24*(1), 35–38.

Brache, V., & Faundes, A. (2010). Contraceptive vaginal rings: A review. *Contraception, 82*(5), 418–427.

Burkman, R. T., & Carson, S. A. (2008). Noncontraceptive health benefits of progestin-only contraceptive agents. *The Female Patient, 33*(8), 47–52.

Curtis, K. M., Jamieson, D. J., Peterson, H. B., & Marchbanks, P. A. (2010). Adaptation of the World Health Organization's Medical Eligibility Criteria for Contraceptive Use for use in the United States. *Contraception, 82*(1), 3–9. doi:10.1016/j.contraception.2010.02.014

Durand, M., Koistinen, R., Chirinos, M., Rodríguez, J. L., Zambrano, E., Seppälä, M., & Larrea, F. (2010). Hormonal evaluation and midcycle detection of intrauterine glycodelin in women treated with levonorgestrel as in emergency contraception. *Contraception, 82*(6), 526–533. doi:10.1016/j.contraception.2010.05.015

Farr, S. L. Curtis, K. M., Robbins, C. L, Zapata, L. B., & Dietz, P. M. (2011). Use of contraception among US women with frequent mental distress. *Contraception, 77*, 230–233. doi:10.1016/j.contraception.2010.07.005

Fehring, R. J., & Schneider, M. (2008). Variability in the hormonally estimated fertile phase of the menstrual cycle. *Fertility and Sterility, 90*(4), 1232–1235. doi:10.1016/j.fertnstert.2007.10.050

Fehring, R. J., Schneider, M., & Barron, M. L. (2008). Efficacy of the Marquette method of natural family planning. *The American Journal of Maternal Child Nursing, 33*(6), 348–354. Retrieved from http://www.mcnjournal.com/

Fine, P. M. (2011, February). A new option in emergency contraception. *The Female Patient, 36*, 41–44.

Fox, M. C., Oat-Judge, J., Severson, K., Jamshidi, R. M., Singh, R. H., McDonald-Mosley, R., & Burke, A. E. (2011). Immediate placement of intrauterine devices after first and second trimester pregnancy termination. *Contraception, 83*(1), 34–40. doi:10.1016/j.contraception.2010.06.018

Fraser, I. S. (2010). Non-contraceptive health benefits of intrauterine hormonal systems. *Contraception, 82*(5), 396–403. doi:10.1016/j.contraception.2010.05.005

Gaffield, M. E., & Culwell, K. R. (2010, March). New recommendations on the safety of contraceptive methods for women with medical conditions: World Health Organization's Medical eligibility criteria for contraceptive use, fourth edition. *IPPF Medical Bulletin, 44*(1), 1–5.

Gemzell-Danielsson, K. (2010). Mechanism of action of emergency contraception. *Contraception, 82*(5), 404–409. doi:10.1016/j.contraception.2010.05.004

Grimes, D. A., Jensen, J. T., Atlas, R. O., Nelson, A. L., & Kaunitz, A. M. (2008). Intrauterine contraception: A new perspective. *Supplement to the Female Patient*, 1–24.

Harper, C. C., Weiss, D. C., Speidel, J. J., & Raine-Bennett, T. (2008). Over-the-counter access to emergency contraception for teens. *Contraception, 77*(4), 230–233.

Hatcher, R. A., Cates, W., Kowal, D., Nelson, A. L., & Trussell, J. (2011). *Contraceptive technology* (20th ed.). New York, NY: Ardent Media.

Heikinheimo, O., Lehtovirta, P., Aho, I., Ristola, M., & Paavonen, J. (2011). The levonorgestrel-releasing intrauterine system in human immunodeficiency virus-infected women: A 5-year follow-up study. *American Journal of Obstetrics and Gynecology, 204*(2), 126.e1–e4. doi: 10.1016/j.ajog.2010.09.002

Heikinheimo, O., Leminen, R., & Suhonen, S. (2007). Termination of early pregnancy using flexible, low-dose mifepristone-misoprostol regimens. *Contraception, 76*(6), 456–460. doi:10.1016/j.contraception.2007.08.012

Helmerhorst, F. M., Belfield, T., Kulier, R., Maitra, N., O'Brien, P., & Grimes, D. A. (2006). The Cochrane fertility regulation group: Synthesizing the best evidence about family planning. *Contraception, 74*(4), 280–286.

Johnson, C. C., Burkman, R. T., Gold, M. A., Brown, R. T., Harel, Z., Bruner, A., . . . Bone, H. G. (2008). Longitudinal study of depot medroxyprogesterone acetate (Depo-Provera®) effects on bone health in adolescents: Study design, population characteristics and baseline bone mineral density. *Contraception, 77*(4), 239–248.

Kaskowitz, A. P., Carlson, N., Nichols, M., Edelman, A., & Jensen, J. (2007). Online availability of hormonal contraceptives without a health care examination: Effect of knowledge and health care screening. *Contraception, 76*(4), 273–277. doi:10.1016/j.contraception.2007.06.009

Kinsella, E. O., Crane, L. A., Ogden, L. G., & Stevens-Simon, C. (2007). Characteristics of adolescent women who stop using contraception after use at first sexual intercourse. *Journal of Pediatric and Adolescent Gynecology, 20*(2), 73–81. doi:10.1016.j.jpag.2007.01.004

Lewis, R. A., Taylor, D., Natavio, M. F., Melamed, A., Felix, J., & Mishell, D., Jr. (2010). Effects of the levonorgestrel-releasing intrauterine system on cervical mucus quality and sperm penetrability. *Contraception, 82*(6), 491–496. doi:10.1016/j.contraception.2010.06.006

Meyer, J. L., Gold, M. A., & Haggerty, C. L. (2011). Advance provision of emergency contraception among adolescent and young adult women: A systematic review of literature. *Journal of Pediatric and Adolescent Gynecology, 24*(1), 2–9. doi:10.1016/j.jpag.2010.06.002

Schwartz, J. (2009). Update on the female condom. *The Female Patient, 34*(6), 26–28.

Tepper, N. K., & Curtis, K. M. (2010). Contraceptive safety: US medical eligibility criteria. *The Female Patient, 35*(10), 55–58.

Westhoff, C., Jain, J. K., Milsom, I., & Ray, A. (2007). Changes in weight with depot medroxyprogesterone acetate subcutaneous injection 104 mg/0.65 mL. *Contraception, 75*(4), 261–267.

World Health Organization. (2004). *Medical eligibility criteria for contraceptive use.* (3rd ed.). Geneva, Switzerland: World Health Organization.

World Health Organization. (2009). *Medical eligibility criteria for contraceptive use* (4th ed.). Geneva, Switzerland: World Health Organization. Retrieved from http://whqlibdoc.who.int/publications/2010/9789241563888_eng.pdf

Wysocki, S., Deal, M., & Levine, J. P. (2010). Exploring the benefits of non-daily hormonal contraception. *Current Medical Evidence, 3*(8), 1–11.
Zapata, L. B., Whiteman, M. K., Tepper, N. K., Jamieson, D. J., Marchbanks, P. A., & Curtis, K. M. (2010). *Contraception, 82*(1), 41–55. doi:10.1016/j.contraception.2010.02.011
Zieman, M., Hatcher, R. A., Cwiak, C., Darney, P. D., Creinin, M. D., & Stosur, H. R. (2010). *2010–2012 Managing Contraception for your pocket*. Atlanta, GA: Bridging the Gap Communications.

HIV/AIDS

Campsmith, M. L., Rhodes, P. H., Hall, H. I., & Green, T. A. (2010). Undiagnosed HIV prevalence among adults and adolescents in the United States at the end of 2006. *Journal of Acquired Immune Deficiency Syndromes, 53*(5), 619–624. doi:10.1097/QAI.0b013e3181bf1c45
Colbert, A. M., Kim, K. H., Sereika, S. M., & Erlen, J. A. (2010). An examination of the relationships among gender, health status, social support, and HIV-related stigma. *The Journal of the Association of Nurses in AIDS Care, 21*(4), 302–313. doi:10.1016/j.jana.2009.11.0004
Crepaz, N., Marshall, K. J., Aupont, L. W., Jacobs, E. D., Mizuno, Y., Kay, L. S., . . . O'Leary, A. (2009). The efficacy of HIV/STI behavioral interventions for African American females in the United States: A meta-analysis. *American Journal of Public Health, 99*(11), 2069–2078. doi: 10.2105/AJPH.2008.139519
DeMarco, R. F. (2010). Palliative care and African American women living with HIV: Graduate students learn to create tailored quality improvement projects. *The Journal of Nursing Education, 49*(8), 462–465.
DeMarco, R. F., Kendricks, M., Dolmo, Y., Looby, S., & Rinne, K. (2009). The effect of prevention messages and self-efficacy skill building with inner-city women at risk for HIV infection. *The Journal of the Association of Nurses in AIDS Care, 20*(4), 283–292.
DeMarco, R. F., & Stokes, C. (2010). Midlife black women living with HIV/AIDS in the United States: A treatment strategy using peer-led, structured writing in a group with global possibilities. Online publication of treatment strategies-AIDS.
Dieffenbach, C. W., & Fauci, A. S. (2009). Universal voluntary testing and treatment for prevention of HIV transmission. *The Journal of the American Medical Association, 301*(22), 2380–2382.
Doherty, I. A., Schoenbach, V. J., & Adimora, A. A. (2009). Sexual mixing patterns and heterosexual HIV transmission among African Americans in the southeastern United States. *Journal of Acquired Immune Deficiency Syndromes, 52*(1), 114–120. doi:10.1097/QAI.0b013e3181ab5e10
El-Bassel, N., Caldeira, N. A., Ruglass, L. M., & Gilbert, L. (2009). Addressing the unique needs of African American women in HIV prevention. *American Journal of Public Health, 99*(6), 996–1001. doi:10.2105/AJPH.2008.140541
El-Sadr, W. M., Mayer, K. H., & Hodder, S. L. (2010). AIDS in America—forgotten but not gone. *The New England Journal of Medicine, 362*(11), 967–970.
Hall, H. I., Song, R., Rhodes, P., Prejean, J., An, Q., Lee, L. M., . . . Janssen, R. S. for the HIV Incidence Surveillance Group. (2008). Estimation of HIV incidence in the United States. *The Journal of the American Medical Association, 300*(5), 520–529. doi:10.1001/jama.300.5.520
Jacobs, R. J., & Thomlison, B. (2009). Self-silencing and age as risk factors for sexually acquired HIV in midlife and older women. *Journal of Aging and Health, 21*(1), 102–128.
Jemmott, L. S., Jemmott, J. B., III, & O'Leary, A. (2007). Effects on sexual risk behavior and STD rate of brief HIV/STD prevention interventions for African American women in primary care settings. *American Journal of Public Health, 97*(6), 1034–1040. doi:10.2105/AJPH.2003.020271
Myers, H. F., Sumner, L. A., Ullman, J. B., Loeb, T. B., Carmona, J. V., & Wyatt, G. E. (2009). Trauma and psychosocial predictors of substance abuse in women impacted by HIV/AIDS. *The Journal of Behavioral Health Services & Research, 36*(2), 233–246.

INFERTILITY

Bartlett, J. G., Auwaerter, P. G., & Pham, P. (2008). Carrier tests among infertile women. *Journal of Genetic Counseling, 17*, 84–91.

Das, A., Borah, T., & Panda, S. (2010). Spontaneous pregnancy in primary amenorrhea: A case report [Farsi]. *Journal of Reproduction and Infertility, 11*(1), 59–60.

Duffy, C., & Allen, S. (2009). Medical and psychosocial aspects of fertility after cancer. *Cancer Journal, 15*(1), 27–33.

Ganie, M. A., Laway, B. A., Qazi, S., Jehangir, M., Butt, T. P., & Koul, S. (2010). Spontaneous successful pregnancy in post-surgical hypopituitarism: A case report. *Turkish Journal of Endocrinology and Metabolism, 14*(1), 23–25.

Hodgson, D. C., Pintilie, M., Gitterman, L., DeWitt, B., Buckley, C. A., Ahmed, S., . . . Gospodarowicz, M. K. (2007). Fertility among female hodgkin lymphoma survivors attempting pregnancy following ABVD chemotherapy. *Hematological Oncology, 25*(1), 11–15.

Janse, F., Knauff, E. A., Niermeijer, M. F., Eijkemans, M. J., Laven, J. S., Lambalk, C. B., . . . Goverde, A. J. (2010). Similar phenotype characteristics comparing familial and sporadic premature ovarian failure. *Menopause, 17*(4), 758–765.

Legro, R. S., Barnhart, H. X., Schlaff, W. D., Carr, B. R., Diamond, M. P., Carson, S. A., . . . Myers, E. R. (2007). Clomiphene, metformin, or both for infertility in the polycystic ovary syndrome. *The New England Journal of Medicine, 356*, 551–566.

Pastore, L. M., Morris, W. L., & Karns, L. B. (2008). Emotional reaction to fragile X premutation carrier tests among infertile women. Johns Hopkins POC-IT Center. ABX Guide. *Journal of Genetic Counseling, 17*(1), 84–91. Retrieved from hopkins-abxguide.org

Practice Committee of the American Society for Reproductive Medicine. (2008). Progesterone supplementation during the luteal phase and in early pregnancy in the treatment of infertility: An educational bulletin. *Fertility and Sterility, 89*(4), 789–792.

Soni, S., & Badawy, S. Z. (2010). Celiac disease and its effect on human reproduction: A review. *The Journal of Reproductive Medicine, 55*(1–2), 3–8.

Yanushpolsky, E., Hurwitz, S., Greenberg, L., Racowsky, C., & Hornstein, M. D. (2008). Comparison of Crinone 8% intravaginal gel and intramuscular progesterone supplementation for in vitro fertilization/embryo transfer in women under age 40: Interim analysis of a prospective randomized trial. *Fertility and Sterility, 89*(2), 485–487.

INTERSTITIAL CYSTITIS

El Khoudary, S. R., Talbott, E. O., Bromberger, J. T., Chang, C. C., Songer, T. J., & Davis, E. L. (2009). Severity of interstitial cystitis symptoms and quality of life in female patients. *Journal of Women's Health, 18*(9), 1361–1368. doi:10.1089/jwh.2008.1270

Hsieh, C. H., Chang, S. T., Hsieh, C. J., Hsu, C. S., Kuo, T. C., Chang, H. C., & Lin, Y. H. (2008). Treatment of interstitial cystitis with hydrodistention and bladder training. *International Urogynecology Journal andPelvic Floor Function, 19*(10), 1379–1384. doi:10.1007/s00192-008-0640-9

Kilpatrick, L. A., Ornitz, E., Ibrahimovic, H., Hubbard, C. S., Rodríguez, L. V., Mayer, E. A., & Naliboff, B. D. (2010). Gating of sensory information differs in patients with interstitial cystitis/painful bladder syndrome. *The Journal of Urology, 184*(3), 958–963. doi:10.1016/j.juro.2010.04.083

Mayo Clinic.(n.d.). *Interstitial cystitis.* Retrieved from http://www.mayoclinic.com/health/interstitial-cystitis/DS00497

National Kidney and Urologic Diseases Information Clearinghouse. (n.d.). *Interstitial cystitis/painful bladder syndrome.* Retrieved from http://kidney.niddk.nih.gov/kudiseases/pubs/interstitialcystitis/

Nickel, J. C., Tripp, D. A., Pontari, M., Moldwin, R., Mayer, R., Carr, L. K., . . . Nordling, J. (2010). Interstitial cystitis/painful bladder syndrome and associated medical conditions with an emphasis on irritable bowel syndrome, fibromyalgia and chronic fatigue syndrome. *The Journal of Urology*, *184*(4), 1358–1363. doi:10.1016/j.juro.2010.06.005

Terris, M. K., & Sajadi, K. P. Urethritis. *WebMD*. Retrieved from http://www.emedicine.com/med/topic2342.htm

Warren, J. W., Brown, J., Tracy, J. K., Langenberg, P., Wesselmann, U., & Greenberg, P. (2008). Evidence-based criteria for pain of interstitial cystitis/painful bladder syndrome in women. *Urology*, *71*(3), 444–448. doi:10.1016/j.urology.2007.10.062

MENOPAUSE, HORMONE THERAPY

Altman, A. M., Moore, A., Speroff, L., & Wysocki, S. (2009). Tackling the tricky issue of bioidentical hormones. *Women's Health Care: A Practical Journal for Nurse Practitioners*, *8*(7), 7–15.

Banks, E., & Canfell, K. (2009). Invited commentary: Hormone therapy risks and benefits—The Women's Health Initiative findings and the postmenopausal estrogen timing hypothesis. *American Journal of Epidemiology*, *170*(1), 24–28.

Bjørge, T., Engeland, A., Tretli, S., & Weiderpass, E. (2008). Body size in relation to cancer of the uterine corpus in 1 million Norwegian women. *International Journal of Cancer*, *120*(2), 378–383.

Brown, L. (2008). Pathology of uterine malignancies. *Clinical Oncology (Royal College of Radiologists)*, *20*, 433–437.

Burdette, L., Moore, A., Speroff, L., & Wysocki, S. (2009). Hormone therapy in menopause: Applying research findings to optimal patient care and education. *Women's Health Care: A Practical Journal for Nurse Practitioners*, *8*(5), 10–21.

Chollet, J. A. (2010, December). Progress in vulvovaginal atrophy treatments. *The Female Patient*, *35*, 29–31.

Crosbie, E. J., Zwahlen, M., Kitchener, H. C., Egger, M., & Renehan, A. G. (2010). Body mass index, hormone replacement therapy, and endometrial cancer risk: A meta-analysis. *Cancer Epidemiology, Biomarkers & Prevention*, *19*(12), 3119–3130. doi:10.1158/1055-9965.EPI-10-0832

Fournier, A., Berrino, F., & Clavel-Chapelon, F. (2008). Unequal risks for breast cancer associated with different hormone replacement therapies: Results from the E3N cohort study. *Breast Cancer Research and Treatment*, *107*(1), 103–111.

Freeman, S. B. (2009). Micronized progesterone: An important option for oral hormone therapy. *Women's Health Care: A Practical Journal for Nurse Practitioners*, *8*(12), 7–14.

Haumschild, M. S., & Haumschild, R. J. (2010). Postmenopausal females and the link between oral bisphosphonates and osteonecrosis of the jaw: A clinical review. *Journal of the American Academy of Nurse Practitioners*, *22*(10), 534–539.

Kellogg-Spadt, S. (2010, April). Vulvovaginal atrophy. *Advance for Nurse Practitioners*, *18*(4), 31–34, 55.

Lyytinen, H., Pukkala, E., & Ylikorkala, O. (2009). Breast cancer risk in postmenopausal women using estradiol-progestogen therapy. *Obstetrics and Gynecology*, *113*(1), 65–73.

Margolis, M. B. (2010, May). How drug delivery and pharmacokinetics impact estrogen therapy. *The Female Patient (Supplement)*, 1–8.

Moore, A. (2010). Bioidentical hormone therapy: What practitioners need to know now. *Women's Health Care: A Practical Journal for Nurse Practitioners*, *9*(5), 10–17.

Mørch, L. S., Lökkegaard, E., Kierkegaardm, E., Andreasen, A. H., Krüger-Kjaer, S., & Lidegaard, O. (2009). Hormone therapy and ovarian cancer. *Journal of the American Medical Association*, *302*(3), 298–305. doi:10.1001/jama.2009.1052

Prentice, R. L., Manson, J. E., Langer, R. D., Anderson, G. L., Pettinger, M., Jackson, R. D., . . . Rossouw, J. E. (2009). Benefits and risks of postmenopausal hormone therapy when it is initiated soon after menopause. *American Journal of Epidemiology*, *170*(1), 12–23.

Roberts, H. (2010). Long-term hormone therapy—a Cochrane Summary. *The Female Patient*, *35*(12), 50–53.

Schmidt, C. A. B. (2010). HRT/ERT: Best practice recommendations. *Clinician Reviews*, *20*(12), 32–38.

Theroux, R. (2010). Women's decision making during the menopausal transition. *Journal of the American Academy of Nurse Practitioners, 22*(11), 612–621.

Wysocki, S. (2009). Local estrogen therapy—preferred treatment for symptoms of menopausal vulvovaginal atrophy. *Women's Health Care: A Practical Journal for Nurse Practitioners, 8*(11), 8–16.

MENSTRUAL CYCLE: DYSMENORRHEA, PREMENSTRUAL SYNDROME, AMENORRHEA

Ballagh, S. A., & Heyl, A. (2008). Communicating with women about menstrual cycle symptoms. *The Journal of Reproductive Medicine, 53*(11), 837–846.

Bertone-Johnson, E. R., Hankinson, S. E., Johnson, S. R., & Manson, J. E. (2008). Cigarette smoking and the development of premenstrual syndrome. *American Journal of Epidemiology, 168*(8), 938–945.

Bertone-Johnson, E. R., Hankinson, S. E., Johnson, S. R., & Manson, J. E. (2009). Timing of alcohol use and the incidence of premenstrual syndrome and probable premenstrual dysphoric disorder. *Journal of Women's Health, 18*(12), 1945–1953.

Bertone-Johnson, E. R., Hankinson, S. E., Willett, W. C., Johnson, S. R., & Manson, J. E. (2010). Adiposity and the development of premenstrual syndrome. *Journal of Women's Health, 19*(11), 1955–1962.

Brown, J., O'Brien, P., Marjoribanks, J., & Wyatt, K. (2009). Selective serotonin reuptake inhibitors for premenstrual syndrome. *Cochrane Database of Systemic Reviews.*

Canning, S., Waterman, M., Orsi, N., Ayres, J., Simpson, N., & Dye, L. (2010). The efficacy of Hypericum perforatum (St. John's wort) for the treatment of premenstrual syndrome: A randomized, double-blind, placebo-controlled trial. *CNS Drugs, 24*(3), 207–225.

Daley, A. (2009). Exercise and premenstrual symptomatology: A comprehensive review. *Journal of Women's Health, 18*(6), 895–899.

Doubova, S. V., Morales, H. R., Hernández, S. F., del Carmen Martínez-García, M., deCossío Ortiz, M. G., Soto, M. A., . . . Lozoya, X. (2007). Effect of a Psidii guajavae folium extract in the treatment of primary dysmenorrhea: A randomized clinical trial. *Journal of Ethnopharmacology, 110*(2), 305–310. doi:10.1016/j.jep.2006.09.033

Ford, O., Lethaby, A., Roberts, H., & Mol, B. W. J. (2009). Progesterone for premenstrual syndrome. *Cochrane Database of Systemic Reviews.*

French, L. (2008). Dysmenorrhea in adolescents: Diagnosis and treatment. *Paediatric Drugs, 10*(1), 1–7.

Halbreich, U. (2008). Selective serotonin reuptake inhibitors and initial oral contraceptives for the treatment of PMDD: Effective but not enough. *CNS Spectrums, 13*(7), 566–572.

Lemmens-Gruber, R., & Kamyar, M. (2008). Pharmacology and clinical relevance of vasopressin antagonists. *Internist (Berl), 49*(5), 628–30, 632–634. doi:10.1007/s00108-008-2017-z

Ozgoli, G., Selselei, E. A., Mojab, F., & Majd, H. A. (2009). A randomized, placebo-controlled trial of Gingko biloba in treatment of premenstrual syndrome. *Journal of Alternative and Complementary Medicine, 15*(8), 845–851.

Panay, N. (2008). Understanding the pain: Managing severe PMS. *The Practicing Midwife, 11*(8), 26–29.

Proctor, M. L., Murphy, P. A., Pattison, H. M., Suckling, J., & Farquhar, C. M. (2007). Behavioral interventions for primary and secondary dysmenorrhea. *Cochrane Database Systemic Reviews*, (3) CD002248. doi:10.1002/14651858.CD002248.pub3

Rapkin, A. J., & Mikacich, J. A. (2008). Premenstrual syndrome and premenstrual dysphoric disorder in adolescents. *Current Opinion in Obstetrics and Gynecology, 20*(5), 455–463.

Schiøtz, H. A., Jettestad, M., & Al-Heeti, D. (2007). Treatment of dysmenorrhea with a new TENS device (OVA). *Journal of Obstetrics and Gynaecology, 27*(7), 726–728. doi:10.1080/01443610701612805

Sharma, P., Malhotra, C., Taneja, D. K., & Saha, R. (2008). Problems related to menstruation amongst adolescent girls. *Indian Journal of Pediatrics, 75*(2), 125–129. doi:10.1007/s12098-008-0018-5

Tschudin, S., Bertea, P. C., & Zemp, E. (2010). Prevalence and predictors of premenstrual syndrome and premenstrual dysphoric disorder in a population-based sample. *Archives of Women's Mental Health, 13*(6), 485–494.

van Die, M. D., Bone, K. M., Burger, H. G., Reece, J. E., & Teede, H. J. (2009). Effects of a combination of Hypericum perforatum and Vitex agnus-castus on PMS-like symptoms in late-perimenopausal women: Findings from a subpopulation analysis. *Journal of Alternative and Complementary Medicine, 15*(9), 1045–1048.

Wallenstein, G. V., Blaisdell-Gross, B., Gajria, K., Guo, A., Hagan, M., Kornstein, S. G., & Yonkers, K. (2008). Development and validation of the Premenstrual Symptoms Impact Survey (PMSIS): A disease-specific quality of life assessment tool. *Journal of Women's Health, 17*, 439–450.

Witt, C. M., Reinhold, T., Brinkhaus, B., Roll, S., Jena, S., & Willich, S. N. (2008). Acupuncture in patients with dysmenorrhea: A randomized study on clinical effectiveness and cost-effectiveness in usual care. *American Journal of Obstetrics and Gynecology, 198*, 1–8. doi:10.1016/j.ajog.2007.07.041

Yang, M., Gricar, J. A., Maruish, M. E., Hagan, M. A., Kornstein, S. G., & Wallenstein, G. V. (2010). Interpreting premenstrual symptoms impact survey scores using outcomes in health-related quality of life and sexual drive impact. *Journal of Reproductive Medicine, 55*(1–2), 41–48.

Zhu, X., Proctor, M., Bensoussan, A., Wu, E., & Smith, C. A. (2008). Chinese herbal medicine for primary dysmenorrhea. *Cochrane Database Systemic Reviews*, (2): CD005288. doi:10.1002/14651858.CD005288.pub3.

MENTAL HEALTH AND EMOTIONAL ISSUES

Alschuler, K. N., Hoodin, F., & Byrd, M. R. (2009). Rapid assessment for psychopathology in a college health clinic: Utility of college student specific questions. *Journal of American College Health, 58*(2), 177–179.

Blier, P., Ward, H. E., Tremblay, P., Laberge, L., Hébert, C., & Bergeron, R. (2009). Combination of antidepressant medications from treatment initiation for major depressive disorder: A double-blind randomized study. *The American Journal of Psychiatry, 166*, 1–8. doi:10.1176/appi.ajp.2009.09020186

Bostwick, J. M. (2010, April 29). A generalist's guide to treating patients with depression with an emphasis on using side effects to tailor antidepressant therapy. *Mayo Clinic Proceedings, 85*(6), 538–550. doi:10.4065/mcp.2009.0565

Druss, B. G., von Esenwein, S. A., Compton, M. T., Rask, K. J., Zhao, L., & Parker, R. M. (2010). A randomized trial of medical care management for community mental health settings: The primary care access, referral, and evaluation (PCARE) study. *The American Journal of Psychiatry, 167*(2), 151–159. doi:10.1176/appi.ajp.2009.09050691

Gill, J. M., Klinkman, M. S., & Chen, Y. X. (2010). Antidepressant medication use for primary care patients with and without medical comorbidities: A national electronic health record (EHR) network study. *Journal of the American Board of Family Medicine, 23*(4), 499–508.

Hackley, B. (2010). Antidepressant medication use in pregnancy. *Journal of Midwifery and Women's Health, 55*(2), 90–100.

Hackley, B., Sharma, C., Kedzior, A., & Sreenivasan, S. (2010). Managing mental health conditions in primary settings. *Journal of Midwifery & Women's Health, 55*(1), 9–19.

Ladabaum, U., Sharabidze, A., Levin, T. R., Zhao, W. K., Chung, E., Bacchetti, P., . . . Pepin, C. J. (2010). Citalopram provides little or no benefit in nondepressed patients with irritable bowel syndrome. *Clinical Gastroenterology and Hepatology, 8*(1), 42–48.e1

Mansfield, A. J., Kaufman, J. S., Marshall, S. W., Gaynes, B. N., Morrissey, J. P., & Engel, C. C. (2010). Deployment and the use of mental health services among U.S. Army wives. *The New England Journal of Medicine, 362*(2), 101–109.

Mark, T. L. (2010). For what diagnoses are psychotropic medications being prescribed? A nationally representative survey of physicians. *CNS Drugs, 24*(4), 319–326.

McMullen, L. M., & Herman, J. (2009). Women's accounts of their decision to quit taking antidepressants. *Qualitative Health Research, 19*(11), 1569–1579.

O'Connor, E. A., Whitlock, E. P., Beil, T. L., & Gaynes, B. N. (2009). Screening for depression in adult patients in primary care settings: A systematic evidence review. *Annals of Internal Medicine, 151*(11), 793–803.

Ostacher, M. J., Perlis, R. H., Nierenberg, A. A., Calabrese, J., Stange, J. P., Salloum, I., . . . Sachs, G. S. for the STEP-BD Investigators. (2010). Impact of substance use disorders on recovery from episodes of depression in bipolar disorder patients: Prospective data from the Systemic Treatment Enhancement Program for Bipolar Disorder (STEP-BD). *The American Journal of Psychiatry, 167*(3), 289–297. doi:org/10.1176/appi.ajp.2009.09020299

Pizzi, C., Mancini, S., Angeloni, L., Fontana, F., Manzoli, L., & Costa, G. M. (2009). Effects of selective serotonin reuptake inhibitor therapy on endothelial function and inflammatory markers in patients with coronary heart disease. *Clinical Pharmacology and Therapeutics, 86*(5), 527–532.

Sansone, R. A., & Sansone, L. A. (2010). Emotional hyper-reactivity in borderline personality disorder. *Psychiatry (Edgmont), 7*(9), 16–20. doi:10.1038/clpt.2009.121

Sassarini, J., & Lumsden, M. A. (2010). Hot flushes: Are there effective alternatives to estrogen? *Menopause International, 16*(2), 81–88.

OSTEOPOROSIS

Barrett-Connor, E., Cox, D. A., Song, J., Mitlak, B., Mosca, L., & Grady, D. (2009). Raloxifene risk for stroke based on the Framingham stroke risk score. *The American Journal of Medicine, 122*(8), 754–761.

Becker, C. (2010). Another selective estrogen-receptor modulator for osteoporosis. *New England Journal of Medicine, 362*, 752–754.

Bell, K. J. L., Hayen, A., Macaskill, P., Irwig, L., Craig, J. C., Ensrud, K., & Bauer, D. C. (2009). Value of routine monitoring of bone mineral density after starting bisphosphonate treatment: Secondary analysis of trial data. *British Medical Journal, 338*, b2266. doi:10.1136/bmj.b2266

Black, D. M., Kelly, M. P., Genant, H. K., Palermo, L., Eastell, R., Bucci-Rechtweg, C., . . . Bauer, D. C. (2010). Bisphosphonates and fractures of the subtrochanteric or diaphyseal femur. *New England Journal of Medicine, 362*(19), 1761–1771.

Capeci, C. M., & Tejwani, N. C. (2009). Bilateral low-energy simultaneous or sequential femoral fractures in patients on long-term alendronate therapy. *The Journal of Bone and Joint Surgery (American), 91*(11), 2556–2561. doi:10.2106/JBJS.H.01774

Cardwell, C. R., Abnet, C. C., Cantwell, M. M., & Murray, L. J. (2010). Exposure to oral bisphosphonates and risk of esophageal cancer. *The Journal of the American Medical Association, 304*(6), 657–663. doi:10.1001/jama.2010.1098

Cummings, S. R., Ensrud, K., Delmas, P. D., LaCroix, A. Z., Vukicevic, S., Reid, D. M., . . . Eastell, R. (2010). Lasofoxifene in postmenopausal women with osteoporosis. *The New England Journal of Medicine, 362*(8), 686–696.

Delmas, P. D., Munoz, F., Black, D. M., Cosman, F., Boonen, S., Watts, N. B., . . . Eastell, R. (2009). Effects of yearly zoledronic acid 5 mg on bone turnover markers and relation of PINP with fracture reduction in postmenopausal women with osteoporosis. *Journal of Bone and Mineral Research, 24*(9), 1544–1551. doi:10.1359/jbmr.090310

Favia, G., Pilolli, G. P., & Maiorano, E. (2009). Osteonecrosis of the jaw correlated to bisphosphonate therapy in non-oncologic patients: Clinicopathological features of 24 patients. *The Journal of Rheumatology, 36*(12), 2780–2787. doi:10.3899/jrheum.090455

Green, J., Czanner, G., Reeves, G., Watson, J., Wise, L., & Beral, V. (2010). Oral bisphosphonates and risk of cancer of oesophagus, stomach, and colorectum: Case-control analysis within a UK primary care cohort. *British Medical Journal, 341*, 4444. doi:10.1136/bmj.c4444

Higgs, D., & Kessenich, C. (2010). Complementary therapies in osteoporosis. *Journal for Nurse Practitioners, 6*(3), 193–198.

Ing-Lorenzini, K., Desmeules, J., Plachta, O., Suva, D., Dayer, P., & Peter, R. (2009). Low-energy femoral fractures associated with the long-term use of bisphosphonates: A case series from a Swiss university hospital. *Drug Safety, 32*(9), 775–785.

Jamal, S. A. (2009). Themes—New treatment modalities for osteoporosis. *Canadian Orthopaedic Association*. Retrieved from http://www.coa-aco.org/coa_bulletin/issue_73/themes-new-treatment-modalities-for-osteoporosis.html

Lenart, B. A., Neviaser, A. S., Lyman, S., Chang, C. C., Edobor-Osula, F., Steele, B., . . . Lane, J. M. (2009). Association of low-energy femoral fractures with prolonged bisphosphonate use: A case control study. *Osteoporosis International, 20*(8), 1353–1362.

Liu, J., Ho, S. C., Su, Y. X., Chen, W. Q., Zhang, C. X., & Chen, Y. M. (2009). Effect of long-term intervention of soy isoflavones on bone mineral density in women: A meta-analysis of randomized controlled trials. *Bone, 44*(5), 948–953.

Loke, Y. K., Jeevanantham, V., & Singh, S. (2009). Bisphosphonates and atrial fibrillation: Systematic review and meta-analysis. *Drug Safety, 32*(3), 219–228. doi:10.2165/00002018-200932030-00004

Mosca, L., Grady, D., Barrett-Connor, E., Collins, P., Wenger, N., Abramson, B. L., . . . Kornitzer, M. (2009). Effect of raloxifene on stroke and venous thromboembolism according to subgroups in postmenopausal women at increased risk of coronary heart disease. *Stroke, 40*(1), 147–155.

National Osteoporosis Foundation. (2009). *Clinicians guide to prevention and treatment of osteoporosis*. Retrieved from http://www.nof.org/professionals/clinical-guidelines

O'Donnell, S., Cranney, A., Wells, G. A., Adachi, J. D., & Reginster, J. Y. (2008). Strontium ranelate for preventing and treating postmenopausal osteoporosis (review). *Cochrane Database of Systematic Reviews*. Retrieved from http://www2.cochrane.org/reviews/en/ab005326.html

Recker, R. R., Ste-Marie, L. G., Langdahl, B., Czerwinski, E., Bonvoisin, B., Masanauskaite, D., . . . Felsenberg, D. (2009). Effects of intermittent intravenous ibandronate injections on bone quality and micro-architecture in women with postmenopausal osteoporosis: The DIVA study. *Bone, 46*(3), 660–665.

Sørensen, H. T., Christensen, S., Mehnert, F., Pedersen, L., Chapuriat, R. D., Cummings, S. R., & Baron, J. A. (2008). Population based case-control study. *British Medical Journal, 336*(7648), 813–816. doi:10.1136/bmj.39507.551644.BE

Thorpe, B. M. (2009). Advances in the treatment of postmenopausal osteoporosis. *Journal for Nurse Practitioners, 5*(6, Suppl. 1), s3–s33.

Tucker, K. L., Jugdaohsingh, R., Powell, J. J., Qiao, N., Hannan, M. T., Sripanyakorn, S., . . . Kiel, D. P. (2009). Effects of beer, wine and liquor intakes on bone mineral density in older men and women. *The American Journal of Clinical Nutrition, 89*(4), 1188–1196. doi:10.3945/ajcn.2008.26765

World Health Organization Collaborating Centre for Metabolic Bone Diseases, University of Sheffield, UK.FRAX®: WHO Fracture Risk Assessment Tool. (2009). Retrieved from http://www.shef.ac.uk/FRAX

POLYCYSTIC OVARY SYNDROME

Azziz, R., Carmina, E., Dewailly, D., Diamanti-Kandarakis, E., Escobar-Morreale, H. F., Futterweit, W., . . . Witchel, S. F. (2009). The Androgen Excess and PCOS Society criteria for the polycystic ovary syndrome: The complete task force report. *Fertility and Sterility, 91*(2), 456–488.

Berrino, F., Bellati, C., Secreto, G., Camerini, E., Pala, V., Panico, S., . . . Kaaks, R. (2001). Reducing bioavailable sex hormones through a comprehensive change in diet: The diet and androgens (DIANA) randomized trial. *Cancer Epidemiology, Biomarkers & Prevention, 10*(1), 25–33.

Dunaif, A., Chang, J., & Franks, S. (2008). *Polycystic ovary syndrome: Current controversies, from the ovary to the pancreas.* Totowa, NJ: Humana Press.

Hart, R., & Norman, R. (2006). Polycystic ovarian syndrome—prognosis and outcomes. *Best Practice & Research Clinical Obstetrics & Gynaecology, 20*(5), 751–778.

Mayo Clinic Staff. (2011). *Clinical manifestations of polycystic ovary syndrome in adults.* Retrieved from http://www.uptodate.com/home/index.html

Mayo Clinic Staff. (2011). *Treatment of polycystic ovary syndrome in adults.* Retrieved from http://www.mayoclinic.com/health/polycystic-ovary-syndrome/DS00423/DSECTION=treatments-and-drugs

Purdue, G. L. (2010). Polycystic ovary syndrome: A threat to appearance, menstruation, and fertility. *American Nurse Today, 5*(9), 65–67.

Radosh, L. (2009). Drug treatments for polycystic ovary syndrome. *American Family Physician, 79,* 671.

Segars, J. H., & DeCherney, A. H. (2010). Is there a genetic basis for polycystic ovary syndrome? *The Journal of Clinical Endocrinology and Metabolism, 95,* 2058–2060.

U.S. Department of Health and Human Services Office on Women's Health. *Polycystic ovary syndrome: Frequently asked questions.* Retrieved from www.womenshealth.gov/faq/polycystic-ovary-syndrome.cfm

PRECONCEPTION CARE

Berghella, V., Buchanan, E., Pereira, L., & Baxter, J. K. (2010). Preconception care. *Obstetrical & Gynecological Survey, 65*(2), 119–131.

Canady, R. B., Tiedje, L. B., & Lauber, C. (2008). Preconception care & pregnancy planning: Voices of African American women. *Maternal & Child Health Journal, 33*(2), 90–97.

Cartwright, A., Wallymahmed, M., Macfarlane, I., & Casson, I. (2009). What do women with diabetes know about pregnancy and contraception? *Practical Diabetes International, 26*(6), 238–242.

Centers for Disease Control and Prevention. (2008). Update on overall prevalence of major birth defects—Atlanta, Georgia, 1978–2005. *Morbidity & Mortality Weekly Report,57*(1), 1–5.

Chuang, C. H., Velott, D. L., & Weisman, C. S. (2010). Exploring knowledge and attitudes related to pregnancy and preconception health in women with chronic medical conditions. *Maternal & Child Health Journal, 14,* 713–719.

Coonrod, D. V., Bruce, N. C., Malcolm, T. D., Drachman, D., & Frey, K. A. (2009). Knowledge and attitudes regarding preconception care in a predominantly low-income Mexican American population. *American Journal of Obstetrics & Gynecology, 200*(6), 686.e1–e7.

Coulthard, T., & Hawthorne, G. (2008). Type 2 diabetes in pregnancy: More to come? *Practical Diabetes International, 25*(9), 359–361.

Curtis, M. G. (2010). Preconception care: Clinical and policy implications of the preconception agenda. *Journal of Clinical Outcomes Management, 17*(4), 167–172.

Dunlop, A. L., Jack, B. W., Bottalico, J. N., Lu, M. C., James, A., Shellhaas, C. S., . . . Prasad, M. R.(2008). The clinical content of preconception care: Women with chronic medical conditions. *American Journal of Obstetrics and Gynecology, 199*(6 Suppl. 2), S310–S327.

Floyd, R. L., Jack, B. W., Cefalo, R., Atrash, H., Mahoney, J., Herron, A., . . . Sokol, R. J. (2008). The clinical content of preconception care: Alcohol, tobacco, and illicit drug exposures. *American Journal of Obstetrics and Gynecology, 199*(6 Suppl. 2), S333–S339.

Frey, K. A., Navarro, S. M., Kotelchuck, M., & Lu, M. C. (2008). The clinical content of preconception care: Preconception care for men. *American Journal of Obstetrics and Gynecology, 199*(6 Suppl. 2), S389–S395.

Frieder, A., Dunlop, A. L., Culpepper, L., & Bernstein, P. S. (2008). The clinical content of preconception care: Women with psychiatric conditions. *American Journal of Obstetrics and Gynecology, 199*(6 Suppl. 2), S328–S332.

Grivell, R., Dodd, J., & Robinson, J. (2009). The prevention and treatment of intrauterine growth restriction. *Best Practice & Research, Clinical Obstetrics & Gynaecology, 23*(6), 795–807.

Heavey, E. (2010). Don't miss preconception care opportunities for adolescents. *The American Journal of Maternal Child Nursing, 35*(4), 213–219.

Hughes, C., Spence, D., Holmes, V. A., & McCorry, N. K. (2010). Preconception care for women with diabetes: The midwife's role. *British Journal of Midwifery, 18*, 144, 146–149.

Karakantza, M., Androutsopoulos, G., Mougiou, A., Sakellaropoulos, G., Kourounis, G., & Decavalas, G. (2008). Inheritance and perinatal consequences of inherited thrombophilia in Greece. *International Journal of Gynaecology and Obstetrics, 100*(2), 124–129.

Kerrigan, A. M., & Kingdon, C. (2010). Maternal obesity and pregnancy: A retrospective study. *Midwifery, 26*(1), 138–146.

Klerman, L.V., Jack, B. W., Coonrod, D. V., Lu, M. C., Fry-Johnson, Y. W., & Johnson, K. (2008). The clinical content of preconception care: Care of psychosocial stressors. *American Journal of Obstetrics & Gynecology, 199*(6 Suppl. 2), S362–S366.

Mortagy, I., Kielmann, K., Baldeweg, S. E., Modder, J., & Pierce, M. B. (2010). Integrating preconception care for women with diabetes into primary care: A qualitative study. *The British Journal of General Practice, 60*(580), 815–821.

Sanders, L. B. (2009). Reproductive life plans: Initiating the dialogue with women. *The American Journal of Maternal Child Nursing, 34*(6), 342–347.

Thompson, B. K., Peck, M., & Brandert, K. T. (2008). Integrating preconception health into public health practice: A tale of three cities. *Journal of Women's Health, 17*(5), 723–727.

Valika, B. K., & Urban, R. J. (2009). Preconception care for the type 2 diabetic mother: A review on current care guidelines. *Current Women's Health Reviews, 5*, 109–116.

Whitty, J. E. (2010). Cystic fibrosis in pregnancy. *Clinical Obstetrics and Gynecology, 53*(2), 369–376.

SEXUALITY AND SEXUAL DYSFUNCTION

Abdo, C. H. N., Valadares, A. L. R., Oliveira, W. M., Scanavino, M. T., & Afif-Abdo, J. (2010). Hypoactive sexual desire disorder (HSDD) in a population-based study of Brazilian women: Associated factors classified according to their importance. *Menopause, 17*, 1114–1121.

Abu Ali, R. M., Al Hajeri, R. M., Khader, Y. S., Shegem, N. S., & Ajlouni, K. M. (2008). Sexual dysfunction in Jordanian diabetic women. *Diabetes Care, 31*(8), 1580–1581.

Adler, J., Zanetti, R., Wight, E., Urech, C., Fink, N., & Bitzer, J. (2008). Sexual dysfunction after premenopausal stage I and II breast cancer: Do androgens play a role? *The Journal of Sexual Medicine, 5*(8), 1898–1906.

Brotto, L. A., Bitzer, J., Laan, E., Leiblum, S., & Luria, M. (2010). Women's sexual desire and arousal disorders. *The Journal of Sexual Medicine, 7*(1, Pt. 2), 586–614.

Carvalheira, A. A., Brotto, L. A., & Leal, I. (2010). Women's motivations for sex: Exploring the diagnostic and statistical manual, fourth edition, text revision criteria for hypoactive sexual desire and female sexual arousal disorders. *The Journal of Sexual Medicine, 7*(4, Pt. 1), 1454–1463.

Carvalho, J., & Nobre, P. (2010). Sexual desire in women: An integrative approach regarding psychological, medical, and relationship dimensions. *The Journal of Sexual Medicine, 7*(5), 1807–1815.

Castelo-Branco, C., Palacios, S., Combalia, J., Ferrer, M., & Traveria, G. (2009). Risk of hypoactive sexual desire disorder and associated factors in a cohort of oophorectomized women. *Climacteric, 46*, 168–193.

Dennerstein, L., Hayes, R., Sand, M., & Lehert, P. (2009). Attitudes toward and frequency of partner interactions among women reporting decreased sexual desire. *The Journal of Sexual Medicine, 6*(6), 1668–1673.

Graziottin, A., Koochaki, P. E., Rodenberg, C. A., & Dennerstein, L. (2009). The prevalence of hypoactive sexual desire disorder in surgically menopausal women: An epidemiological study of women in four European countries. *The Journal of Sexual Medicine, 6*(8), 2143–2153.

Janssen, E., McBride, K. R., Yarber, W., Hill, B. J., & Butler, S. M. (2008). Factors that influence sexual arousal in men: A focus group study. *Archives of Sexual Behavior, 37*(2), 252–265.

McCabe, M., Althof, S. E., Assalian, P., Chevret-Measson, M., Leiblum, S. R., Simonelli, C., & Wylie, K. (2010). Psychological and interpersonal dimensions of sexual function and dysfunction. *The Journal of Sexual Medicine, 7*(1, Pt. 2), 327–336.

Nygaard, I. (2008). Sexual dysfunction prevalence rates: Marketing or real? *Obstetrics and Gynecology, 112*(5), 968–969.

Shifren, J. L., Monz, B. U., Russo, P. A., Segreti, A., & Johannes, C. B. (2008). Sexual problems and distress in United States women: Prevalence and correlates. *Obstetrics and Gynecology, 112*(5), 970–978. doi:10.1097/AOG.0b013e3181898cdb

Sidi, H., Naing, L., Midin, M., & Nick Jaafar, N. R. (2008). The female sexual response cycle: Do Malaysian women conform to the circular model? *The Journal of Sexual Medicine, 5*(10), 2359–2366.

Toates, F. (2009). An integrative theoretical framework for understanding sexual motivation, arousal, and behavior. *Journal of Sex Research, 46*(2–3), 168–193.

Valadares, A. L., Pinto-Neto, A. M., Osis, M. J., Conde, D. M., Sousa, M. H., & Costa-Paiva, L. (2008). The sexuality of middle-aged women with a sexual partner: A population-based study. *Menopause, 15*, 706–713.

SEXUALLY TRANSMITTED DISEASES, VAGINITIS, VAGINOSIS

Alicea-Alvarez, N., Hellier, S. D., Jack, L. W., & Lundberg, G. G. (2011). A pilot study of Chlamydia screening among high school girls. *Journal for Nurse Practitioners, 7*(1), 25–28.

Bavis, M. P., Smith, D. Y., & Siomos, M. Z. (2009). Genital herpes: Diagnosis, treatment, and counseling in the adolescent patient. *Journal for Nurse Practitioners, 5*(6), 415–420.

Bohbot, J. M., Vicaut, E., Fagnen, D., & Brauman, M. (2010). Treatment of bacterial vaginosis: A multicenter, double-blind, double-dummy, randomized phase III study comparing secnidazole and metronidazole. *Infectious Diseases in Obstetrics and Gynecology.* doi:10.1155/2010/705692

Brotman, R. M., Klebanoff, M. A., Nansel, T. R., Yu, K. F., Andrews, W. W., Zhang, J., & Schwebke, J. R. (2010). Bacterial vaginosis assessed by gram stain and diminished colonization resistance to incident gonococcal, chlamydial, and trichomonal genital infection. *The Journal of Infectious Diseases, 202*(12), 1907–1915.

Centers for Disease Control and Prevention. (2010, December 17). Sexually transmitted diseases treatment guidelines 2010. *Morbidity and Mortality Weekly Report, 59*, No. RR-12, 1–110.

Centers for Disease Control and Prevention. (2011). *Parasites: Lice.* Retrieved from http://www.cdc.gov/parasites/lice/

Coughlin, G., & Secor, M. (2010). Bacterial vaginosis: Update on evidence-based care. *Advance for Nurse Practitioners, 18*(1), 41–44, 53.

Donders, G., Bellen, G., Ausma, J., Verguts, L, Vaneldere, J., Hinoul, P., . . . Janssens, D. (2011). The effect of antifungal treatment on the vaginal flora of women with vulvo-vaginal yeast infection with or without bacterial vaginosis. *European Journal of Clinical Infectious Diseases, 30*, 59–63.

Ehrström, S., Daroczy, K., Rylander, E., Samuelsson, C., Johannesson, U., Anzén, B., & Påhlson, C. (2010). Lactic acid bacteria colonization and clinical outcome after probiotic supplementation in conventionally treated bacterial vaginosis and vulvovaginal candidiasis. *Microbes and Infection, 12*(10), 691–699.

Ford, J. (2008, August). Pesticide-resistant head lice. *Advance for Nurse Practitioners*, 53–55.

Giannini, C. M., Kim, H. K., Mortensen, J., Mortensen, J., Marsolo, K., & Huppert, J. (2010). Culture of non-genital sites increases the detection of gonorrhea in women. *Journal of Pediatric and Adolescent Gynecology, 23*(4), 246–252.

Holloway, D. (2010). Nursing considerations in patients with vaginitis. *British Journal of Nursing, 19*(16), 1040–1046.

Idso, C. (2009). Sexually transmitted infection prevention in newly single older women. *Journal for Nurse Practitioners, 5*(6), 440–453.

Javier, J. (2009, Winter). The treatment and prevention of head lice infestation. *Retail Clinician*, 1–8.

Johnson, S. R., Griffiths, H., & Humberstone, F. J. (2010). Attitudes and experience of women to common vaginal infections. *Journal of Lower Genital Tract Disease, 14*(4), 287–294.

Marrazzo, J. M., Thomas, K. K., Agnew, K., & Ringwood, K. (2010). Prevalence and risks for bacterial vaginosis in women who have sex with women. *Sexually Transmitted Diseases, 37*(5), 335–339.

Murphy, M. B., & Fitzpatrick, J. J. (2011). Illness intrusiveness of a Hepatitis C diagnosis: A pilot study and the implications of practice. *Journal for Nurse Practitioners, 7*(1), 46–50.

Payne, S. C., Cromer, P. R., Stanek, M. K., & Palmer, A. A. (2010). Evidence of African-American women's frustrations with chronic recurrent bacterial vaginosis. *Journal of the American Academy of Nurse Practitioners, 22*(2), 101–108.

Quan, M. (2010). Vaginitis: Diagnosis and management. *Postgraduate Medicine, 122*(6), 117–127.

Roth-Kaufmann, M. M. (2008). Hepatitis C infection. *Clinician Reviews, 18*(6), 18–23.

Ryan-Wenger, N. A., Neal, J. L., Jones, A. S., & Lowe, N. K. (2010). Accuracy of vaginal symptom self-diagnosis algorithms for deployed military women. *Nursing Research, 59*(1), 2–10.

Sherman, C. (2008, May). Staying up to date on managing hepatitis B. *The Clinical Advisor*, 17–20.

Tempera, G., & Furneri, P. M. (2010). Management of aerobic vaginitis. *Gynecologic and Obstetric Investigation, 70*(4), 244–249.

U.S. Preventive Services Task Force. (2005). *Screening for gonorrhea: Recommendation statement.* 1–11. AHRQ Publication No. 05-0579-A.

Van Der Pol, B. (2010). Diagnosing vaginal infections: It's time to join the 21st century. *Current Infectious Disease Reports, 12*(3), 225–230.

Ya, W., Reifer, C., & Miller, L. E. (2010). Efficacy of vaginal probiotic capsules for recurrent bacterial vaginosis: A double-blind, randomized, placebo-controlled study. *American Journal of Obstetrics and Gynecology, 203*(2), 120.e1–e6.

SMOKING CESSATION

Barnes, J., Dong, C. Y., McRobbie, H., Walker, N., Mehta, M., & Stead, L. F. (2010). Hypnotherapy for smoking cessation. *Cochrane Database of Systematic Reviews.* Retrieved from http://onlinelibrary.wiley.com/o/cochrane/clsysrev/articles/CD001008/frame.html

Boyle, R. G., Solberg, L. I., Asche, S. E., Boucher, J. L., Pronk, N. P., & Jensen, C. J. (2005). Offering telephone counseling to smokers using pharmacotherapy. *Nicotine & Tobacco Research, 7*(Suppl. 1), S19–S27.

Comer, L., & Grassley, J. S. (2010). A smoking cessation website for childbearing adolescents. *Journal of Obstetric, Gynecologic, and Neonatal Nursing, 39*(6), 695–702.

Ebbert, J. O., Yang, P., Vachon, C. M., Vierkant, R. A., Cerhan, J. R., Folsom, A. R., & Sellers, T. A. (2003). Lung cancer risk reduction after smoking cessation: Observations from a prospective cohort of women. *Journal of Clinical Oncology, 21*(5), 921–926.

Fairhurst, A. (2010). Developing a joined up approach to smoking cessation in primary and secondary care. *Nursing Times, 106*(37), 12–13.

Gangwisch, J. E., & Jacobson, C. M. (2009). New perspectives on assessment of suicide risk. *Current Treatment Options in Neurology, 11*(5), 371–376.

Guirguis, A. B., Ray, S. M., Zingone, M. M., Airee, A., Franks, A. S., & Keenum, A. J. (2010). Smoking cessation: Barriers to success and readiness to change. *Journal of the Tennessee Medical Association, 103*(9), 45–49.

Heatherton, T. F., Kozlowski, L. T., Frecker, R. C., & Fagerström, K. O. (1991). The Fagerström test for nicotine dependence: A revision of the Fagerström Tolerance Questionnaire. *British Journal of Addiction, 86*(9), 1119–1127.

Johnson, T. S. (2010). A brief review of pharmacotherapeutic treatment options in smoking cessation: Bupropion versus varenicline. *Journal of the American Academy of Nurse Practitioners, 22*(10), 557–563.

Langley, T. E., Szatkowski, L., Gibson, J., Huang, Y., McNeill, A. J., Coleman, T., & Lewis, S. (2010). Validation of The Health Improvement Network (THIN) primary care database for monitoring prescriptions for smoking cessation medications. *Pharmacoepidemiology and Drug Safety, 19*(6), 586–590.

Malucky, A. (2010). Brief evidence-based interventions for nurse practitioners to aid patients in smoking cessation. *Journal for Nurse Practitioners, 6*(2), 126–131.

Oncken, C., Dornelas, E., Greene, J., Sankey, H., Glasmann, A., Feinn, R., & Kranzler, H. R. (2008). Nicotine gum for pregnant smokers: A randomized controlled trial. *Obstetrics and Gynecology, 112*(4), 859–867.

Parsons, A., Daley, A., Begh, R., & Aveyard, P. (2010). Influence of smoking cessation after diagnosis of early stage lung cancer on prognosis: Systematic review of observational studies with meta-analysis. *British Medical Journal, 340*:b5569. doi:10.1136/bmj.b5569

Prokhorov, A. V., Hudmon, K. S., Marani, S., Foxhall, L., Ford, K. H., Luca, N.S., . . . Gritz, E. R. (2010). Engaging physicians and pharmacists in providing smoking cessation counseling. *Archives of Internal Medicine, 170*(18), 1640–1646.

Rodriguez, J., Jiang, R., Johnson, W. C., MacKenzie, B. A., Smith, L. J., & Barr, R. G. (2010). The association of pipe and cigar use with cotinine levels, lung function, and airflow obstruction: A cross-sectional study. *Annals of Internal Medicine, 152*(4), 201–210.

Sreedharan, J., Muttappallymyalil, J., & Venkatramana, M. (2010). Nurses' attitude and practice in providing tobacco cessation care to patients. *Journal of Preventative Medicine and Hygiene, 51*(2), 57–61.

URINARY TRACT INFECTIONS AND URINARY INCONTINENCE

Barclay, L. (2008). Best practices to treat urinary tract infections. *Urologic Nursing, 28*(5), 333–341.

Barclay, L. (2008). New guidelines for management of urinary tract infection in nonpregnant women. *Obstetrics & Gynecology, 111*(3), 785–794.

Bennett, G. L., Hecht, E. M., Tanpitukpongse, T. P., Babb, J. S., Taouli, B., Wong, S., . . . Lee, V. S. (2009). MRI of the urethra in women with lower urinary tract symptoms: Spectrum of findings at static and dynamic imaging. *American Journal of Roentgenology, 193*(6), 1708–1715. doi:10.2214/AJR.08.1547AJR

Borello-France, D. F., Handa, V. L., Brown, M. B., Goode, P., Kreder, K., Scheufele, L. L., . . . Weber, A. M. (2007). Pelvic-floor muscle function in women with pelvic organ prolapse. *Physical Therapy, 87*(4), 399–407. doi:10.2522/ptj.20060160

Chen, S. L., Jackson, S. L., & Boyko, E. J. (2009). Diabetes mellitus and urinary tract infection: Epidemiology, pathogenesis and proposed studies in animal models. *The Journal of Urology, 182*(Suppl. 6), S51–S56.

Gopal, M., Sammel, M. D., Arya, L. A., Freeman, E. W., Lin, H., & Gracia, C. (2008). Association of change in estradiol to lower urinary tract symptoms during the menopausal transition. *Obstetrics and Gynecology, 112*(5), 1045–1052.

Gorter, K. J., Hak, E., Zuithoff, N. P., Hoepelman, A. I., & Rutten, G. E. (2010). Risk of recurrent acute lower urinary tract infections and prescription pattern of antibiotics in women with and without diabetes in primary care. *Family Practice, 27*(4), 379–385. doi:10.1093/fampra/cmg026

Grover, M. L., Bracamonte, J. D., Kanodia, A. K., Edwards, F. D., & Weaver, A. L. (2009). Urinary tract infection in women over the age of 65: Is age alone a marker of complication? *Journal of the American Board of Family Medicine, 22*(3), 266–271. doi:10.3122/jabfm.2009.03.080123

Lakeman, M. M. E., van der Vaart, C. H., Roovers, J. P. (2010). Hysterectomy and lower urinary tract symptoms: A nonrandomized comparison of vaginal and abdominal hysterectomy. *Obstetrical & Gynecological Survey, 65*(8), 498–500. doi:10.1097/OGX.0b013e3181f07ae6

Moore, E. E., Hawes, S. E., Scholes, D., Boyko, E. J., Hughes, J. P., & Fihn, S. D. Sexual intercourse and risk of symptomatic urinary tract infection in post menopausal women. *Journal of General Internal Medicine, 23*(5), 595–599. doi:10.1007/s11606-008-0535-y

VULVAR CONDITIONS

Arnold, L. D., Bachmann, G. A., Rosen, R., & Rhoads, G. G. (2007). Assessment of vulvodynia symptoms in a sample of US women: A prevalence survey with a nested case control study. *American Journal of Obstetrics and Gynecology, 196*(2), 128.e1–e6.

Carrico, D. J., Sheerer, K. L., & Peters, K. M. (2009). The relationship of interstitial cystitis/painful bladder syndome to vulvodynia. *Urology Nursing, 29*(4), 233–238.

Danby, C. S., & Margesson, L. J. (2010). Approach to the diagnosis and treatment of vulvar pain. *Dermatologic Therapy, 23*(5), 485–504. doi:10.1111/j.1529-8019.2010.01352.x

Groysman, V. (2010). Vulvodynia: New concepts and review of the literature. *Dermatologic Clinics, 28*(4), 681–696.

Harlow, B. L., He, W., & Nguyen, R. H. (2009). Allergic reactions and risk of vulvodynia. *Annals of Epidemiology, 19*(11), 771–777.

Harlow, B. L., Vazquez, G., MacLehose, R. F., Erickson, D. J., Oakes, J. M., & Duval, S. J. (2009). Self-reported vulvar pain characteristics and their association with clinically confirmed vestibulodynia. *Journal of Women's Health, 18*(9), 1333–1340.

Kingdon, J. (2009). Vulvodynia: A comprehensive review. *Nursing for Women's Health, 13*(1), 48–57.

Nguyen, R. H., Swanson, D., & Harlow, B. L. (2009). Urogenital infections in relation to the occurrence of vulvodynia. *The Journal of Reproductive Medicine, 54*(6), 385–392.

Petersen, C. D., Kristensen, E., Lundvall, L., & Giraldi, A. (2009). A retrospective study of relevant diagnostic procedures in vulvodynia. *The Journal of Reproductive Medicine, 54*(5), 281–287.

WEIGHT MAINTENANCE

American College of Obstetricians and Gynecologists. (2009). Bariatric surgery and pregnancy. *Obstetrics and Gynecology, 113*(6), 1405–1413.

Annesi, J. J., & Gorjala, S. (2010). Relationship of exercise program participation with weight loss in adults with severe obesity: Assessing psychologically based mediators. *Southern Medical Journal, 103*(11), 1119–1123.

Ayloo, S. M., Addeo, P., Buchs, N. C., Shah, G., & Giulianotti, P. C. (2011). Robot-assisted versus laparoscopic Roux-en-Y gastric bypass: Is there a difference in outcomes? *World Journal of Surgery, 35*(3), 637–642. doi:10.1007/s00268-010-0938-x

Beard, J. H., Bell, R. L., & Duffy, A. J. (2008). Reproductive considerations and pregnancy after bariatric surgery: Current evidence and recommendations. *Obesity Surgery, 18*(8), 1023–1027.

Budd, G. M., & Alpert, P. T. (2011). Impact of nurse practitioner research on the obesity epidemic. *Journal of the American Academy of Nurse Practitioners, 23*(1), 59–116.

Burke, L. E., Wang, J., & Sevick, M. A. (2011). Self-monitoring in weight loss: A systematic review of the literature. *Journal of the American Dietetic Association, 111*(1), 92–102.

Cable, C. T., Colbert, C. Y., Showalter, T., Ahluwalia, R., Song, J., Whitfield, P., & Rodriguez, J. (2011). Prevalence of anemia after Roux-en-Y gastric bypass surgery: What is the right number? *Surgery for Obesity and Related Diseases.* doi:10.1016/j.soard.2010.10.013

Crémieux, P. Y., Ledoux, S., Clerici, C., Cremieux, F., & Buessing, M. (2010). The impact of bariatric surgery on comorbidities and medication use among obese patients. *Obesity Surgery, 20*(7), 861–870.

Field, A. E., Malspeis, S. M., & Willett, W. C. (2009). Weight cycling and mortality among middle-aged or older women. *Archives of Internal Medicine, 169*(9), 881–886.

Grief, S. N., & Miranda, R. L. (2010). Weight loss maintenance. *American Family Physician, 82*(6), 630–634.

Huntington, M. K., & Shewmake, R. A. (2010). Weight-loss supplements: What is the evidence? *South Dakota Medicine, 63*(6), 205–207.

Lapointe, A., Provencher, V., Weisnagel, S. J., Bégin, C., Blanchet, R., Dufour-Bouchard, A. A., . . . Lemieux, S. (2010). Dietary intervention promoting high intakes of fruits and vegetables: Short-term effects on eating behaviors in overweight-obese postmenopausal women. *Eating Behaviors, 11*(4), 305–308. doi:10.1016/j.eatbeh.2010.08.005

Larsen, T. M., Dalskov, S. M., van Baak, M., Jebb, S. A., Papadaki, A., Pfeiffer, A. F., . . . Astrup, A. (2010). Diets with high or low protein content and glycemic index for weight loss maintenance. *New England Journal of Medicine, 363*, 2101–2113.

Lee, M. W., & Fujioka, K. (2011). Dietary prescriptions for the overweight patient: The potential benefits of low-carbohydrate diets in insulin resistance. *Diabetes, Obesity and Metabolism, 13*, 204–206. doi:10.1111/j.1463-1326.2010.01328.x

Ludwig, D. S., & Ebbeling, C. B. (2010). Weight-loss maintenance—mind over matter? *New England Journal of Medicine, 363*, 2159–2161.

Maggard, M. A., Yermilov, I., Li, Z., Maglione, M., Newberry, S., Suttorp, M., . . . Shekelle, P. G. (2008). Pregnancy and fertility following bariatric surgery: A systematic review. *Journal of the American Medical Association, 300*(19), 2286–2296.

Metwally, M., Ong, K. J., Ledger, W. L., & Li, T. C. (2008). Does high body mass index increase the risk of miscarriage after spontaneous and assisted conception? A meta-analysis of the evidence. *Fertility and Sterility, 90*(3), 714–726.

Nejat, E. J., Polotsky, A. J., & Pal, L. (2010). Predictors of chronic disease at midlife and beyond—the health risks of obesity. *Maturitas, 65*(2), 106–111.

Nerfeldt, P., Nilsson, B. Y., Mayor, L., Uddén, J., & Friberg, D. (2010). A two-year weight reduction program in obese sleep apnea patients. *Journal of Clinical Sleep Medicine, 6*(5), 479–486.

Rahman, M., & Berenson, A. B. (2010). Self-perception of weight and its association with weight-related behaviors in young, reproductive-aged women. *Obstetrics and Gynecology, 116*(6), 1274–1280.

Razquin, C., Marti, A., & Martinez, J. A. (2011). Evidences on three relevant obesogenes: MC4R, FTO and PPARγ—Approaches for personalized nutrition. *Molecular Nutrition & Food Research, 55*(1), 136–149.

Rowberg, M. J. (2010). Weight management issues and strategies for success. *Journal for Nurse Practitioners, 6*(7), 540–545.

Shepherd, A. (2010). Current management strategies in the treatment of obesity. *Nursing Standards, 25*(14), 49–56.

Stroh, C., Hohmann, U., Schramm, H., Meyer, F., & Manger, T. (2011). Fourteen-year long-term results after gastric banding. *Journal of Obesity.* 2011:128451. Epub 2010 Dec 22.

Taylor, P. W., Arnet, I., Fischer, A., & Simpson, I. N. (2010). Pharmaceutical quality of nine generic orlistat products compared with Xenical®. *Obesity Facts, 3*(4), 231–237.

Timlin, M. T., Pereira, M. A., Story, M., & Neumark-Sztainer, D. (2008). Breakfast eating and weight change in a 5-year prospective analysis of adolescents: Project EAT (Eating Among Teens). *Pediatrics, 121*(3), e638–e645. doi:10.1542/peds.2007-1035

Zac-Varghese, S., Tan, T., & Bloom, S. R. (2010). Hormonal interactions between gut and brain. *Discovery Medicine, 10*(55), 543–552.

Zitsman, J. L., Fennoy, I., Witt, M. A., Schauben, J., Devlin, M., & Bessler, M. (2011). Laparoscopic adjustable gastric banding in adolescents: Short-term results. *Journal of Pediatric Surgery, 46*(1), 157–162.

WEIGHT MANAGEMENT

American Dietetic Association. Eat Right America Program. Retrieved from http://www.eatright.org

American Obesity Association. Retrieved from http://www.obesity.org

Cyberdiet. Retrieved from http://www.cyberdiet.com

National Heart, Lung, and Blood Institute. Retrieved from http://www.nhlbi.nih.gov/; http://www.nhlbi.nih.gov/guidelines/obesity/ob_home.htm

National Institute of Diabetes and Digestive and Kidney Diseases. Retrieved from http://www2.niddk.nih.gov/

North American Association for the Study of Obesity. Retrieved from http://www.naaso.org

U.S. Department of Agriculture. (2011). Dietary guidelines for Americans. Retrieved from http://www.cnpp.usda.gov/dietaryguidelines.htm

U.S. Department of Agriculture, Nutrient Data Laboratory. Retrieved from http://www.nalusda.gov/fnic/foodcomp

U.S. Department of Commerce. Program specific audit guidelines for Advanced Technology Program (ATP) cooperative agreements with single company. Retrieved from http://www.atp.nist.gov/atp/psag-co.htm

WOMEN AND HEART DISEASE

Aggarwal, B., & Mosca, L. (2009). Heart disease risk for female cardiac caregivers. *The Female Patient, 34*(2), 42–45.

Allen-Peebles, D. (2008, November). A new model for CVD prevention. *The Clinical Advisor,* 119.

American Heart Association. (2011). *The American Heart Association complete guide to women's heart health.* New York, NY: Clarkson Potter Publishers.

Anderson, J. L., May, H. T., Horne, B. D., Bair, T. L., Hall, N. L., Carlquist, J. F., . . . Muhlestein, J. B. (2010). Intermountain Heart Collaborative (IHC) Study Group. Relation of vitamin D deficiency to cardiovascular risk factors, disease status, and incident events in a general healthcare population. *The American Journal of Cardiology, 106*(7), 963–968.

Ashen, D. (2010). Cost-effective prevention of coronary heart disease. *Journal for Nurse Practitioners, 6*(10), 754–764.

Dutkiewicz, M. C. (2008, February). Lifting a fork to heart health. Whole foods as a treatment intervention. *Advance for Nurse Practitioners, 16*(2), 57–60.

Eapen, D. J., Kalra, G. L., Rifai, L., Eapen, C. A., Merchant, N., & Khan, B. V. (2010). Raising HDL cholesterol in women. *International Journal of Women's Health, 1,* 181–191.

Gao, R., & Li, X. (2010). Risk assessment and aspirin use in Asian and Western populations. *Vascular Health and Risk Management, 6,* 943–956.

Harrington, C., Horne, A., Jr., Hasan, R. K., & Blumenthal, R. S. (2010). Statin therapy in primary prevention: New insights regarding women and the elderly. *The American Journal of Cardiology, 106*(9), 1357–1359.

Jneid, H. (2010). Aspirin for primary prevention of cardiovascular disease in women. *Methodist Debakey Cardiovascular Journal, 6*(4), 37–42.

Kerr, C., Murray, E., Noble, L., Morris, R., Bottomley, C., Stevenson, F., . . . Nazareth, I. (2010). The potential of Web-based interventions for heart disease self-management: A mixed methods investigation. *Journal of Medical Internet Research, 12*(4), e56.

Kusnoor, A. V., Ferguson, A. D., & Falik, R. (2011). Ischemic heart disease in women: A review for primary care physicians. *Southern Medical Journal, 104*(3), 200–204.

Levit, R. D., Reynolds, H. R., & Hochman, J. S. (2011). Cardiovascular disease in young women: A population at risk. *Cardiology in Review, 19*(2), 60–65.

McCoy, P. R., & Froelicher, E. S. (2008). Techniques for coronary heart disease risk stratification, *7*(8), 31–43.

McNeal, C. J., & Birchem, J. (2009). Cardiovascular disease in women: The therapeutic spectrum. *The Female Patient, 34,* 44–48.

Monson, E. (2010). An integrative medicine approach to cardiac risk factor modification. *Journal for Nurse Practitioners, 6*(10), 775–782.

Piña, I. L. (2011). Cardiovascular disease in women: Challenge of the middle years. *Cardiology in Review, 19*(2), 71–75.

Sherman, C. (2008). Reducing the risk of heart disease in women. *The Clinical Advisor,* 49–53.

Shirato, S., & Swan, B. A. (2010). Women and cardiovascular disease: An evidentiary review. *Medsurg Nursing, 19*(5), 282–286, 306.

Vassar, K. A. (2009). Promoting cardiovascular health in women. *Women's Health Care: A Practical Journal for Nurse Practitioners, 8*(12), 28–33.

Wolff, T., Miller, T., & Ko, S. (2009). *Aspirin for primary prevention of cardiovascular events: An update of the evidence for the U.S. Preventive Services Task Force.* Retrieved from http://www.uspreventiveservicestaskforce.org/uspstf/uspsasmi.htm

Index